Carolingian Medical Knowledge and Practice, *c.*775–900

Nuncius Series

Studies and Sources in the Material and Visual History of Science Series

VOLUME 14

The titles published in this series are listed at *brill.com/nuns*

Carolingian Medical Knowledge and Practice, *c.*775–900

New Approaches to Recipe Literature

By

Claire Burridge

BRILL

LEIDEN | BOSTON

This book was brought to publication and made available Open Access with the generous assistance of the Wellcome Trust via a Medical Humanities Doctoral Studentship [203431/Z/16/Z].

Cover illustration: St. Gallen, Stiftsbibliothek, Cod. Sang. 751, p. 499. A ninth-century compendium of medical texts (http://www.e-codices.ch/de/csg/0751/499/0). © St. Gallen, Stiftsbibliothek, licensed under CC BY-NC 4.0.

The Library of Congress Cataloging-in-Publication Data is available online at https://catalog.loc.gov
LC record available at https://lccn.loc.gov/2023057889

Typeface for the Latin, Greek, and Cyrillic scripts: “Brill”. See and download: brill.com/brill-typeface.

ISSN 2405-5077
ISBN 978-90-04-46616-6 (hardback)
ISBN 978-90-04-46617-3 (e-book)
DOI 10.1163/9789004466173

This book is printed on acid-free paper and produced in a sustainable manner.

Contents

Conclusion

Appendices

Acknowledgements

With so many people to thank, the only way I can conceive of beginning these acknowledgements is with the biggest and broadest of thank-yous: I wish to express a sincere thank you to everyone involved in the process of producing this book as well as to anyone who gives it a read and builds on this research in the future. And now on to a series of more specific thank-yous:

This book has emerged out of my PhD research at Cambridge. First and foremost, my heartfelt thanks go to Professor Rosamond McKitterick, who supervised my MPhil and PhD and has remained a wonderfully supportive mentor and source of guidance. The wider Cambridge academic community also helped to shape my research, not least by providing me with training in essential skills, from palaeography to palaeopathology. Within the Faculty of History as well as the Departments of Archaeology and ASNC, I should especially like to thank Professor Lesley Abrams, Professor John Arnold, Dr Debby Banham, Dr Jenna Dittmar, Professor Caroline Goodson, Dr Susanne Hakenbeck, Dr Tom Lambert, Dr Piers Mitchell, Professor Tessa Webber, and Dr Neil Wright as well as the early medievalist students with whom I overlapped, including Dr Emma Brownlee, Dr Caitlin Ellis, Revd Dr Robert Evans, Dr Sam Leggett, Dr Eleni Leontidou, Dr Fraser McNair, Dr Sam Ottewill-Soulsby, and Dr Arthur Westwell. I owe an immense debt of gratitude to the Wellcome Trust for making this research possible via a Medical Humanities Doctoral Studentship [203431/Z/16/Z].

I feel incredibly fortunate to have received support and guidance from a host of colleagues and friends in the years since my PhD as I have continued to develop and refine my research. I am extraordinarily grateful to the British School at Rome for two years of postdoctoral fellowships during the first years of the Covid pandemic (as well as to Sidney Sussex College for providing an emergency refuge when I was temporarily repatriated to the UK in March 2020). The BSR community, including Dr Tom Brown, Professors Leslie Brubaker, Stephen Milner, John Osborne, and Chris Wickham, has strongly influenced my work. The Leverhulme Trust has since provided incredible support via an Early Career Fellowship at the University of Sheffield, and I have benefitted from sharing work with my medievalist colleagues, and especially my mentor Professor Charles West, as well as thinking across broader chronologies and geographies with the wide-ranging members of the Department of History, including Dr Caroline Dodds Pennock, Professor Siobhan Lambert-Hurley, Dr Chris Millard, and Professor Phil Withington. The final stages of this book were completed after joining Professor Ildar Garipzanov's MINiTEXTS project at the University of Oslo, and I am very thankful for the warm welcome and support I have received from my new colleagues.

Beyond my own research homes, I am extremely grateful for my network of colleagues and academic friends around the world. In particular, Dr Jeffrey Doolittle, Dr Anna Dorofeeva, Professor Arsenio Ferraces Rodríguez, Professor Klaus-Dietrich Fischer, Professor Peregrine Horden, Dr Meg Leja, Dr Zubin Mistry, Professor James Palmer, Dr Raphaël Panhuysen, and Dr Carine van Rhijn each deserve a heartfelt thank you for their support, suggestions, and critiques. The ensuing book has benefitted immeasurably from their feedback, whether via discussions at conferences, over Zoom, or by email, and, of course, from their own extensive, path-breaking bodies of work. Likewise, I owe my thanks to the wider 'MEDMED' community for sharing their resources and expertise spanning all areas of medieval medicine. In terms of conferences and workshops, I am grateful to have been able to share and discuss elements of the research underpinning the following chapters at Books and Bones (Cambridge), Categorising the Church II (Poitiers), Collecting Knowledge, Creating Knowledge (Cambridge), the Graduate Early Medieval Seminar (Cambridge), the International Congress on Medieval Studies (Kalamazoo), the International Medieval Congress (Leeds), the Medieval Archaeology Group (Cambridge), the Medieval History Research Seminar (Cambridge), and Wissen im Frühen Mittelalter (Göttingen). My thanks to all those involved, organisers and attendees, alike. I must also express an enormous debt of gratitude to the anonymous reviewers selected by Brill for their insightful comments and constructive feedback. All remaining errors are my own.

Numerous other institutions have been instrumental in making this research possible, and foremost among them are the libraries which today hold the manuscripts analysed throughout the following chapters. My thanks to the staff at the Biblioteca Apostolica Vaticana, Bibliothèque nationale de France, and Stiftsbibliothek St. Gallen for enabling me to work with their collections, and especially to the entire team at the Stiftsbibliothek for facilitating my several research stays and allowing me to reproduce images from multiple St. Galler manuscripts. Likewise, I should like to thank Claus Kropp and Dr Hermann Schefers for meeting with me in Lorsch (and later at the Books and Bones workshop in Cambridge) to discuss the excavations at Lorsch and their osteological collections as well as to permit me to use images of skeletal remains from their collections. My sincere thanks, too, to Dr Erik Goosmann of Mappa Mundi Cartography for creating the map seen in the opening pages. Finally, I must also extend an enormous thank you to the team at Brill, including the Nuncius Series' editors, Professors Marco Beretta and Sven Dupré, as well as

Brill editors Rosanna Woensdregt, Simona Casadio, Alessandra Giliberto, and Anita Opdam, for providing such a wonderful home for this book.

My last round of thanks goes to my friends and family, without whom none of this would have been possible. I cannot begin to put my gratitude into words. As a small token of my thanks, this book is dedicated to my biggest supporters and greatest role models: my parents.

Illustrations

Figures

Tables

Maps

Abbreviations

AMTL	Ante-mortem tooth loss
BAV	Biblioteca Apostolica Vaticana
BL	British Library
BnF	Bibliothèque nationale de France
BTML	*Bibliographie des textes médicaux latins: Antiquité et haut Moyen Âge*
Sabbah, Corsetti, and Fischer, *BTML*	Guy Sabbah, Pierre-Paul Corsetti, and Klaus-Dietrich Fischer, *Bibliographie des textes médicaux latins: Antiquité et haut Moyen Âge* (Saint-Étienne: Publications de l'Université de St. Étienne, 1987)
Fischer, *BTML 1*	Klaus-Dietrich Fischer, *Bibliographie des textes médicaux latins: Antiquité et haut Moyen Âge: premier supplement* (Saint-Étienne: Publications de l'Université de St. Étienne, 2000)
Fischer, *BTML 2*	Klaus-Dietrich Fischer, *Bibliographie des textes médicaux latins: Antiquité et haut Moyen Âge: second supplement* (Saint-Étienne: Bibliothèque Interuniversitaire de Médecine, 2000), https://www.biusante.parisdescartes.fr/histoire/medicina/documents/fischer.php
Fischer, *BTML 3*	Klaus-Dietrich Fischer, *Bibliographie des textes médicaux latins: Antiquité et haut Moyen Âge: addendum 2002* (Saint-Étienne: Bibliothèque Interuniversitaire de Médecine, 2002), https://www.biusante.parisdescartes.fr/histoire/medicina/documents/fischer2002.php
CLA	*Codices Latini antiquiores: a palaeographical guide to Latin manuscripts prior to the ninth century*
CEMLM	Corpus of Early Medieval Latin Medicine
Cod. sang.	Codex sangallensis
CMG	*Corpus Medicorum Graecorum*
CML	*Corpus Medicorum Latinorum*
DEH	Dental enamel hypoplasia
ESF	European Science Foundation
HSp	Highly specific

MGH	*Monumenta Germaniae Historica*
Capit.	*Capitularia regum Francorum*
Epp. kar. aevi	*Epistolae Karolini aevi*
Formulae	*Formulae Merowingici et Karolini aevi*
LL	*Leges (in folio)*
Poet.	*Poetae Latini aevi Carolini*
SS	*Scriptores (in folio)*
SS rer. Germ.	*Scriptores rerum Germanicarum in usum scholarum separatim editi*
SS rer. Germ. N. S.	*Scriptores rerum Germanicarum, Nova series*
OA	Osteoarthritis
ÖNB	Österreichische Nationalbibliothek
NSp	Non-specific
PG	*Patrologia Graeca*
PL	*Patrologia Latina*
PMTL	Post-mortem tooth loss
RA	Rheumatoid arthritis
Settimane	Settimane di Studio del Centro italiano di studi sull'alto medioevo
SSp	Semi-specific
UL	University Library

Note on Transcription and Translation

The following transcriptions and translations are my own unless otherwise stated. When recipes are quoted in the text, I provide an edited version of the relevant section of my transcription directly in the text or in the accompanying footnote. Transcriptions of all the individual recipes to which I refer in the text can be found in Appendix 2. For these transcriptions, I use the following conventions:

- Script/colour changes: I have indicated script and/or colour changes (such as titles) with bold text.
- Abbreviations: where I have supplied letters due to an abbreviation in the manuscript, I have indicated this by underlining the letters I have added.
- Corrections/insertions: I have used a back-slash and forward-slash to indicate the corrected/inserted material (i.e., \x/).
- Deletions: I have used brackets to indicate material that has been deleted (i.e., [x]).
- Accidental loss/damage: I have used angle-brackets to indicate the lost/damaged material (i.e., <...>), transcribing partially visible letters where possible.

Note on Weights, Measures, and Their Symbols

When recipes include information on weights and measures, I generally follow the form given in the manuscript, whether that is recorded as a full word, abbreviation, or symbol. Abbreviated forms are italicised in the transcriptions. While there are many standard abbreviations and symbols (outlined below), some can be challenging to interpret; where symbols are unclear or ambiguous, I have recorded them as '(.)'. The symbols listed below are approximations based on current Unicode characters. Finally, it must be remembered that there is some degree of uncertainty and flexibility with respect to the precise volumes and weights described by these metrological terms; while this is perhaps obvious for certain measurements (e.g., one person's *manipulus*, 'handful', could be quite different from someone else's), it should also be kept in mind for the more technical vocabulary in use.

The abbreviations and symbols for weights and measures that appear in the transcriptions are as follows:

Latin term	Approximate English translation	Common abbreviations and symbols
calix	cup	cal
coclearium / coclear	spoon, spoonful	cocl, coclr, etc.
denarius	*denarius* (coin)	denr, dir, dnr, dr, đ[a]
drachma / dragma	*drachma*, dram	drag, drg, z, ∠, ʒ
dimidium	half	dim
fasciculus	bundle, bunch	fascl, fasc, etc.
libra	pound	lib, lb, £
manipulus	handful	man, manp, manip, etc.; rarely m
pondus	pound (or 'weight' more generally)	pond, p
scripulus / scrupulus	scruple	scrip, scrp, sc, ŏ,[b] ∋
semis and/or semuncia	half and/or half ounce	sem.un, s, ʃ, ş[c]
sextarius	*sextarius* (a liquid measure, roughly half a litre)	s, ses, sex, SS, ﬀ, ʃt, ȝ
solidus	*solidus* (coin)	sol
staupus	cup	stau
uncia	ounce	un, unc, ro,[d] ∻, ~, –

Notes:

a There is a potentially some ambiguity and/or overlap for the abbreviations and symbols used to signify *denarius* and *drachma*.

b This is my approximation for one of the symbols that can represent a scruple; an image of this symbol is also reproduced in Henry E. Sigerist, 'Maße und Gewichte in den medizinischen Texten des frühen Mittelalters', *Kyklos* 3 (1930): 439–44; see the table on pp. 442–3.

c This is my approximation for a symbol that resembles an 's' with an additional curved loop; an image of this symbol is also reproduced in Sigerist, 'Maße und Gewichte in den medizinischen Texten des frühen Mittelalters', 442–3.

d This is my approximation for a symbol that looks like a minuscule 'r' or 's' and 'o' joined together; the symbol does not appear frequently, but is seen Appendix 2, entry 6.4.5; an image of this symbol is also reproduced in Sigerist, 'Maße und Gewichte in den medizinischen Texten des frühen Mittelalters', 442–3.

Map

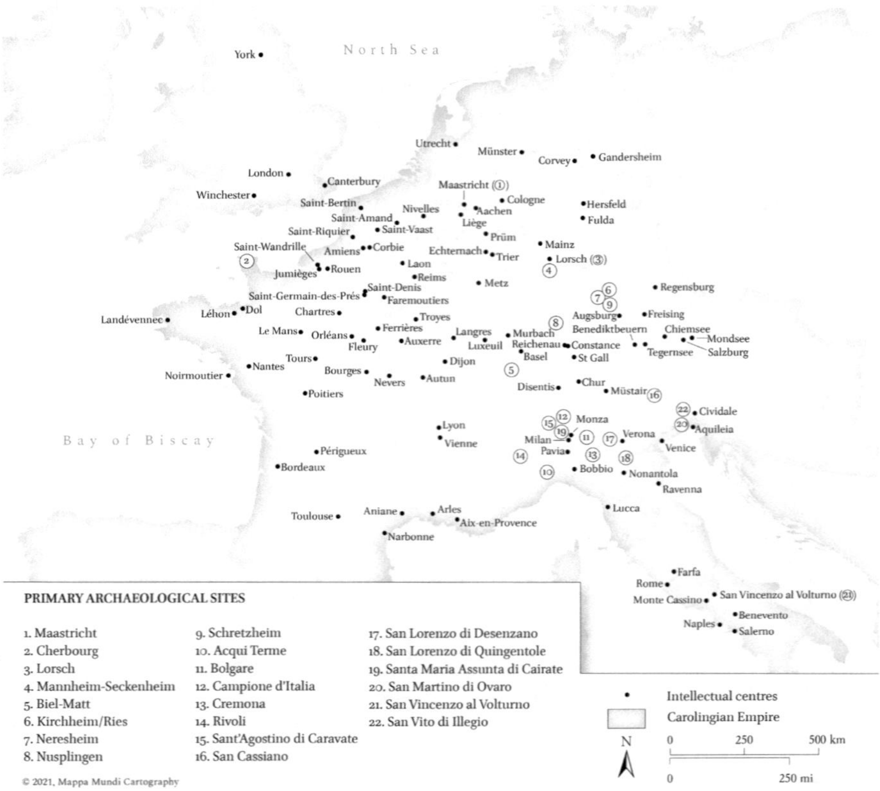

MAP 1 This map highlights important intellectual centres in the Carolingian period and shows the primary archaeological sites that feature in Part 2

© MAPPA MUNDI CARTOGRAPHY

Introduction

CHAPTER 1

Practicality and Applicability

A Dual Approach to Carolingian Medical Knowledge and Practice

1 Introduction: The Case of Terenti(an)us

> A potion for gout, which is called *calapodia*,
> which I, Terentianus, received…[1]

So begins an entry within a collection of medical recipes found in an early ninth-century medical manuscript located in the Stiftsbibliothek St. Gallen, cod. sang. 759 (see Figure 1).[2] This collection, covering roughly the second half of the manuscript (pp. 58–94), includes a vast range of material, from recipes for scented ointments to treatments for blindness, skin conditions, and kidney problems; the recipe in question presents a potion intended to alleviate the agonising pains associated with gout. These opening lines appear to bring a personal dimension to early medieval health and medicine. Terentianus' autobiographical note illustrates the relationship between medical knowledge and practice during this period: his written record not only plays a critical role in the transmission of medical knowledge but testifies to his application of this knowledge in the context of therapy.

An examination of a sample of eighth- and ninth-century manuscripts, however, complicates this neat picture. Another early ninth-century manuscript also located in St Gall, cod. sang. 751, contains a nearly identical phrase at the start of an antidote for gout: *Antidotum podagricum quod dicitur calipodium quod ego Terentius Eoticianus accepi* (see Figure 2).[3] There are intriguing parallels between these two entries: both claim to treat gout, are from early

1 Stiftsbibliothek St. Gallen, cod. sang. 759, p. 60: *Potio ad podagra que dicitur calapodia quem ego Terentianus accipi…* Note: manuscripts held in St Gall are paginated not foliated. For a transcription of the entire recipe, see Appendix 2, entry 11.8; on the textual evidence examined in this book, see Chapter 2. Although *calopodium*, καλοπόδιον, can mean 'clog', the word recorded in the treatment, *calapodium*, is likely from κατάποτον, 'pill', and has undergone some orthographic changes through the process of transmission.

2 On the identification of 'medical manuscripts' as a distinct genre, see Chapter 2; see also Meg Leja, *Embodying the Soul: Medicine and Religion in Carolingian Europe* (Philadelphia: University of Pennsylvania Press, 2022), 12–13.

3 Cod. sang. 751, pp. 489–90. For a transcription of the entire recipe, see Appendix 2, entry 9.38.

© CLAIRE BURRIDGE, 2024 | DOI:10.1163/9789004466173_002

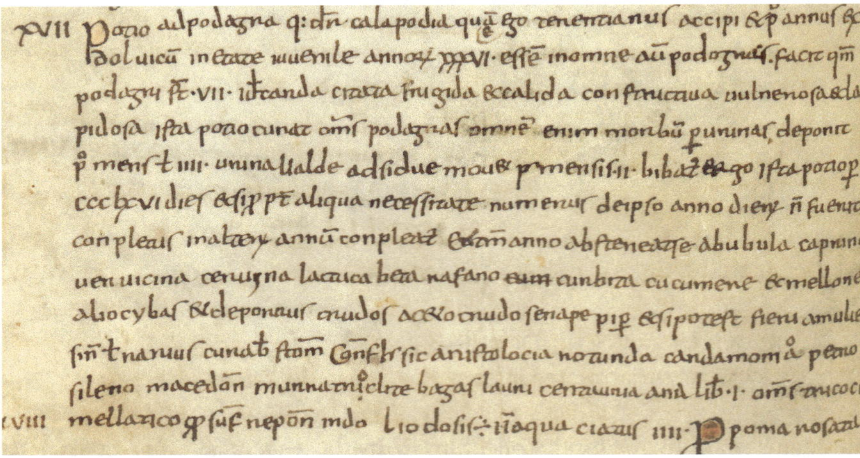

FIGURE 1 *Potio ad podagra* in St. Gallen, Stiftsbibliothek, cod. sang. 759 (p. 60), a ninth-century manuscript with a collection of medical texts (https://www.e-codices.unifr.ch/de/csg/0759/60)

ninth-century medical manuscripts housed in St Gall, and were allegedly used by someone with the name Terenti(an)us. These features demand a closer look. Do the codicological contexts and histories of the two manuscripts indicate that they were written by the same St Gall scribe, a certain Terenti(an)us? Or is there evidence to suggest that these codices have different origins?

Palaeographical analysis supports the latter possibility: an investigation into codd. sang. 751 and 759 indicates that the recipes in question were not written by a single individual. First, it is unlikely that either manuscript originated in St Gall, let alone in the same writing centre. According to Bernhard Bischoff, cod. sang. 751 was probably written at a northern Italian site, whereas cod. sang. 759

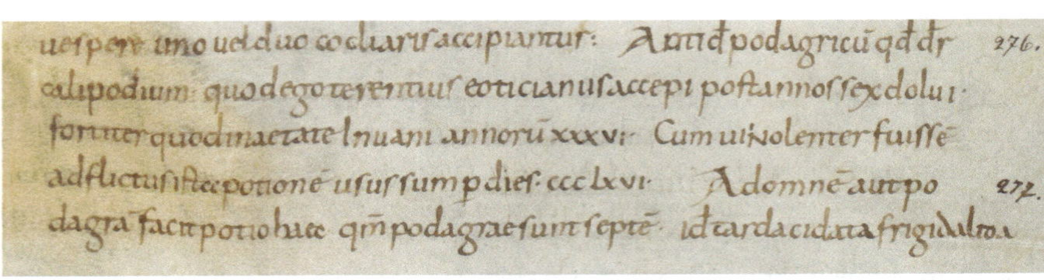

FIGURE 2 *Antidotum podagricum* in St. Gallen, Stiftsbibliothek, cod. sang. 751 (p. 489), a large compendium of medical texts produced in the ninth century (https://www.e-codices.unifr.ch/de/csg/0751/489)

was copied in Brittany (see the map for possible sites of manuscript production in these regions).[4] While the well-documented movement of manuscripts and individuals during this period does not rule out that a scribe such as the hypothetical Terenti(an)us could have moved between multiple intellectual centres, the scripts employed in the two codices are entirely unlike one another, indicating that different scribes were responsible for these compositions.[5] As seen in Figures 1 and 2, the *Potio ad podagra* of cod. sang. 759 is written in a pre-Caroline script with Insular influences, whereas the antidote in cod. sang. 751 is written in a regular, early Caroline hand. These features suggest that codd. sang. 751 and 759 were composed in two different writing centres and by two distinct scribes who copied similar, related recipes.

Indeed, the differences between the contexts in which these treatments are situated—two unique collections of recipes—indicate that they are not based on a single shared exemplar. The collection in cod. sang. 759 is immediately preceded by a contents list on pp. 53–8. While the list contains 446 entries, many pages have been lost from the manuscript, such that only 199 of these entries are extant. The *Potio ad podagra*, located on p. 60, is the seventeenth entry. In contrast, the collection in cod. sang. 751 covers pp. 430–96 and, according to a list of recipe titles on pp. 424–8, contains 319 entries. The *Antidotum podagricum*, found on pp. 489–90, corresponds to entry 277. Although certain individual entries in these collections share overlapping information, it is clear that they represent distinct compilations of medical material.[6]

This example highlights some of the many challenges arising from an investigation into the practice of medicine and its relationship to recorded medical

4 Bernhard Bischoff, *Katalog der festländischen Handschriften des neunten Jahrhunderts (mit Ausnahme der wisigotischen)*, 3 vols. (Wiesbaden: Harrassowitz, 1998–2014), vol. 3, nos. 5844 and 5846.

5 Rosamond McKitterick, *The Carolingians and the Written Word* (Cambridge: Cambridge University Press, 1989). On the movement of early medieval manuscripts with medical texts specifically, see Florence Eliza Glaze, 'The Perforated Wall: The Ownership and Circulation of Medical Books in Medieval Europe, ca. 800–1200' (PhD diss., Duke University, 1999), 73–5, 92–8.

6 At least one additional example of a Terenti(an)us recipe survives: Ernest Wickersheimer recorded another version of the recipe, in this case listed as *Potio ad podagram quae dicitur calapodia quem ego Terrentianus accepi*, in Paris, Bibliothèque nationale de France (hereafter BnF) lat. 11219. While a selection of recipes in this manuscript are also analysed in the present book, its version of the Terenti(an)us recipe is located within a section of the manuscript that does not form part of the textual sample under consideration; see Chapter 2 for further details. Ernest Wickersheimer, *Les manuscrits latins de médecine du haut Moyen Âge dans les bibliothèques de France* (Paris: Éditions du Centre national de la Recherche scientifique, 1966), no. 77.

knowledge in the early Middle Ages. At first glance, Terenti(an)us' seemingly personalised note might have appeared to provide a window into the use of medical texts circulating during the Carolingian period, offering direct evidence for the application of the medical knowledge contained within these writings. Yet, as this case demonstrates, an analysis of individual examples in isolation can easily lead to false conclusions. Since it remains unclear who Terenti(an)us was and when he was writing (or even if he existed), his commentary does not necessarily provide evidence of medical practice during the Carolingian period.

So, what do these recipes tell us? While they can shed light on certain aspects of the medical knowledge circulating in ninth-century Francia, they also indicate a) the dangers of drawing conclusions based on a limited textual sample and reading texts in isolation, and b) the challenge of trying to understand the relationship between medical knowledge and practice in this period. The present book seeks to address both issues. First, this study is grounded in a large and diverse sample of written material: over 5000 newly transcribed and analysed recipes.[7] These recipes are found outside of more established textual traditions (i.e., pharmaceutical writings known from (late) Antiquity)

7 Note: three recipe collections included in this study, all located in cod. sang. 44, were transcribed and published in the early twentieth century (see *Studien und Texte zur frühmittelalterlichen Rezeptliteratur*, ed. Henry E. Sigerist (Leipzig: Johann Ambrosius Barth, 1923), 78–99; *Frühmittelalterliche Rezeptarien*, ed. Julius Jörimann (Zurich: Orell Füssli, 1925), 37–61), while Peter Köpp has published a transcription and translation of a recipe collection I have included from cod. sang. 217 (*Vademecum eines frühmittelalterlichen Arztes: Die gefaltete lateinische Handschrift medizinischen Inhalts im Codex 217 und der Fragmentensammlung 1396 der Stiftsbibliothek in St. Gallen*, ed. and trans. Peter Köpp (Aarau: Sauerländer, 1980)). I have produced new, revised transcriptions in all cases. More recently, material on one folio (p. 392) within a recipe collection in cod. sang. 751 included in this study was published by Rocío Martínez Prieto (Rocío Martínez Prieto, 'A Short Approach to the Analysis of the Textual Tradition of an Extract about Phytotherapy from the Codex Sangallensis 751', in *II Jornadas Predoctorales en Estudios de la Antigüedad y de la Edad Media. Κτῆμα ἐς αἰεὶ: el texto como herramienta común para estudiar el pasado: Proceedings of the Second Postgraduate Conference in Studies of Antiquity and Middle Ages, Universitat Autònoma de Barcelona, 19–21st November 2014*, ed. Núria Olaya Montero, Manuel Montoza Coca, Alba Aguilera Felipe, and Roser Gómez Guiu (Oxford: BAR, 2015), 115–19) and an entire collection in BAV pal. lat. 1088 was published by Arsenio Ferraces Rodríguez after I completed my transcription and analysis of this material (see Arsenio Ferraces Rodríguez, 'Un recetario médico altomedieval (Città del Vaticano, BAV, Pal. lat. 1088, ff. 50r-66r): ensayo de edición crítica', in '*Cui tali cura vel remedio subvenitur*': *De animales y enfermedades en la Edad Media europea*, ed. Gerardo Pérez Barcala (Avellino: Edizioni Sinestesie, 2019), 41–80), so these recipes are still included in the present study. In sum, all analyses of the textual selection delineated in Chapter 2 are based on my own transcriptions; see Appendix 2 for specific examples of recipes cited in the text.

and, consequently, have often been described as 'miscellaneous' collections of recipes or as compilations of brief extracts, assorted recipes, and additional material.[8] That is, while some individual recipes or short sections of text found in these collections are associated with specific sources, the collections as a whole are not derived from a single earlier tradition. Given that past scholarship has tended to focus on the reception and dissemination of classical medical writings (as discussed below), the recipes analysed in this book were often overlooked by earlier generations of philologists and historians. Secondly, by combining investigations into the practicality *and* applicability of this recipe literature, drawing on both textual and osteological evidence, this book casts fresh light on the relationship between medical knowledge and practice. The integration of multiple bodies of evidence in concert with the focus on understudied recipe literature offers new perspectives on medicine in the early Middle Ages, situating the study of early medieval medical texts within the world in which they were produced and read.

Building on the Terenti(an)us example, this opening chapter reviews the existing scholarship on early medieval medicine, explaining the rationale for analysing both the practicality and applicability of the treatments recorded in eighth- and ninth-century manuscripts as well as the significance of setting this work within the long ninth century.

2 Definitions

At the outset, it is essential to define the two key concepts of practicality and applicability that underpin this book. The 'practicality' of recipes considers whether the medical knowledge they present was practical with respect to both intention *and* use in the context of therapy. To evaluate a recipe's intention or design, we can ask: does the text contain user-friendly features suggesting that it was *intended* to be consulted for therapeutic purposes? It might be possible to identify, for example, changes in terminology reflecting adaptations made to accommodate individuals from different linguistic backgrounds. To assess a recipe's potential useability in the context of treatment, it is important to consider whether recipes rely on ingredients that could have been *obtained* in

8 For catalogue descriptions of 'miscellaneous' medical material, see Augusto Beccaria, *I codici di medicina del periodo presalernitano (secoli IX, X e XI)* (Rome: Edizioni di Storia e Letteratura, 1956) and Wickersheimer, *Les manuscrits*. See Chapter 2 for a more detailed discussion of recipe literature and the specific recipes under consideration in this book.

the Carolingian world. That is, would it have been possible to put the recorded knowledge into practice?

The question of applicability, on the other hand, relates to the health needs of individuals during this period. Are the conditions and symptoms described by the texts reflected in the osteological evidence? In other words, did people in early medieval Europe suffer from any of the ailments which the recipes claim to treat? While limitations of both textual and skeletal evidence—as well as the challenges posed by bringing together these two bodies of evidence—complicate this question, it remains possible to investigate the applicability of recipes. By taking account of these limitations and challenges from the start, pursuing carefully selected case studies, and adopting a cautious approach to data analysis and interpretation, we can productively reassess the written record within the framework established by the osteological evidence.

3 Foundations

To explain the significance of this book's aims and evidence base, it is necessary to situate its focus on the questions of practicality and applicability in relation to previous scholarship. Philological approaches to medical texts have long formed the backbone of the study of early medieval medicine and remain vitally important to the field. In addition to reflecting the continuing influence of philological studies, the dual approach pursued over the following chapters builds on and responds to a) the ways in which perceptions of and investigations into early medieval medicine dramatically shifted over the course of the twentieth century, and b) more recent research directions and methodologies in the histories of health and medicine.

3.1 *A Philological Underpinning*

Across many areas of study relating to the ancient and medieval past, philologists have been the pathbreakers: they have been the first scholars to identify and investigate the relevant texts, explore their relationships, and make their content more accessible through the publication of critical editions and commentaries.[9] This is certainly the case for late antique and early medieval medicine, though its current relationship with philological studies differs from many subfields of premodern history. Broadly speaking, the nineteenth and

9 On the development of textual criticism, see Sebastiano Timpanaro, *The Genesis of Lachmann's Method*, trans. Glenn W. Most (Chicago: University of Chicago Press, 2005).

early twentieth centuries can be seen as a heyday of philologically-centred research; consider, for example, major undertakings such as the *Monumenta Germaniae Historica*, the Rolls Series, or the *Patrologia Latina* and *Patrologia Graeca* that have provided the essential foundations on which modern historical research continues to build.[10] While medieval medical writings were studied and published during this period, they received comparatively less attention than the written record of other subfields of medieval history, such as legal texts, patristics, history writing, literature, hagiography, and so on.[11] As a result, the work of transcribing, editing, and translating medical texts remains fundamental to the study of early medieval medicine, and disentangling the relationships between classical, late antique, and early medieval traditions continues to hold a central place. Recent decades have witnessed an efflorescence of research in this area, with scholars such as Arsenio Ferraces Rodríguez, Klaus-Dietrich Fischer, David R. Langslow, Brigitte Maire, María Teresa Santamaría Hernández, and Manuel Enrique Vázquez Buján, among others, producing many much-needed critical editions and commentaries while simultaneously exploring the transmission of (late) ancient texts in the early Middle Ages through rigorous philological studies.[12]

10 Justin Lake, 'Current Approaches to Medieval Historiography', *History Compass* 13, no. 3 (2015): 89–109, https://doi.org/10.1111/hic3.12222, see especially pp. 89–90. On the MGH, see David Knowles, *Great Historical Enterprises. Problems in Monastic History* (London: Nelson, 1963), 66–97; on the Rolls Series, or *Chronicles and Memorials of Great Britain and Ireland during the Middle Ages*, see M. D. Knowles, 'Presidential Address: Great Historical Enterprises IV. The Rolls Series'. *Transactions of the Royal Historical Society* 11 (1961): 137–59 (note: this is reprinted in Knowles, *Great Historical Enterprises*, 99–134); and on Jacques Paul Migne and his *Patrologiae cursus completus*, see R. Howard Bloch, *God's Plagiarist: Being an Account of the Fabulous Industry and Irregular Commerce of the Abbé Migne* (Chicago, University of Chicago Press, 1994).

11 Modern editorial and translation projects continue to play an important role in these areas (e.g., the *Corpus Christianorum* is working to replace the less reliable editions of the *Patrologia Latina*, and the MGH remains highly active), but they are less prominent than in past generations of scholarship. In contrast, as Vivian Nutton highlights, some of the early editorial enterprises that focused on medical writings, such as Karl Gottlob Kühn's monumental twenty-volume edition of Galenic works, were *medical* in purpose rather than philological; see Vivian Nutton, *Galen: A Thinking Doctor in Imperial Rome* (Abingdon: Routledge, 2020) and Galen, *Claudii Galeni Opera Omnia*, ed. K. G. Kühn, 20 vols. (Leipzig: Carl Cnobloch, 1821–33). However, other projects, including the still active *Corpus Medicorum Graecorum* and *Corpus Medicorum Latinorum* series, have always focused on philological research.

12 While it is impossible to do justice to these scholars' extensive outputs in a single footnote, significant contributions in recent years include *Ars medicinalis de animalibus: Estudio introductorio, edición crítica y traducción*, ed. and trans. Arsenio Ferraces Rodríguez (Santiago de Compostela: Andavira Editora, 2016); Arsenio Ferraces Rodríguez,

Yet, paradoxically, as Faith Wallis has noted, the emphasis on producing editions of texts appears to have slowed the development of a broader early medieval medical history due to the ways in which creating editions can generate

ed., *Tradición griega y textos médicos latinos en el período presalernitano: actas del VIII Coloquio Internacional "Textos Médicos Latinos Antiguos" (A Coruña, 2–4 septiembre 2004)* (La Coruña: Servizio de Publicacións, Universidade da Coruña, 2007), including chapters from Arsenio Ferraces Rodríguez, Klaus-Dietrich Fischer, María Teresa Santamaría Hernández, and Manuel Enrique Vázquez Buján; Klaus-Dietrich Fischer, 'A Most Sovereign Herb: Pseudo-Antonius Musa on Betony', *Cuadernos de Filología Clásica. Estudios griegos e indoeuropeos* 30 (2020): 131–48, https://doi.org/10.5209/cfcg.68480; Klaus-Dietrich Fischer, 'Die vorsalernitanischen lateinischen Galenübersetzungen', *Medicina nei secoli* 25, no. 3 (2013); 673–714; Klaus-Dietrich Fischer, 'Unbekannter und seltener Wortschatz in den Pseudosoranischen *Quaestiones medicinales*', *Voces* 23–24 (2012–13): 29–74; Alexander of Tralles, *Alexandri Tralliani Latini Liber tertius: De febribus singulis. Introduction, Edition, Translation, Notes, Indices*, ed. and trans. David R. Langslow (Santiago de Compostela: Andavira Editora, 2020); David Langslow and Brigitte Maire, eds., *Body, Disease and Treatment in a Changing World: Latin Texts and Contexts in Ancient and Medieval Medicine. Proceedings of the Ninth International Conference "Ancient Latin Medical Texts", Hulme Hall, University of Manchester, 5–8 September 2007* (Lausanne: Éditions BHMS, 2010), including chapters from Arsenio Ferraces Rodríguez, Klaus-Dietrich Fischer, Brigitte Maire, and Manuel Enrique Vázquez Buján; Caelius Aurelianus, *Caelii Aureliani operum omnium quae exstant Concordantiae*, ed. Brigitte Maire and Olivier Bianchi, 4 vols. (Hildesheim: Olms-Weidmann, 2003); Cassius Felix, *Cassii Felicis libri de medicina Concordantiae: Accedunt numeri, voces Graecae Graecis Latinisque litteris scriptae, index nominum notabiliorum, index frequentiae decrescentis formarum*, ed. Brigitte Maire and Anne Fraisse (Hildesheim: Olms-Weidmann, 2003); María Teresa Santamaría Hernández, *Estudios sobre Galeno Latino y sus fuentes* (Cuenca: Ediciones de la Universidad de Castilla-La Mancha, 2021); and Manuel Enrique Vázquez Buján, ed., *Tradición e Innovación de la Medicina Latina de la Antigüedad y de la Alta Edad Media: Actas del IV Coloquio Internacional sobre los "textos médicos latinos antiguos"* (Santiago de Compostela: Servicio de Publicacións e Intercambio Científico da Universidade de Santiago de Compostela, 1994), including chapters from Arsenio Ferraces Rodríguez, Klaus-Dietrich Fischer, David R. Langslow, Brigitte Maire, and María Teresa Santamaría Hernández. For lists of editions, translations, commentaries, and lexicographical studies Guy Sabbah, Pierre-Paul Corsetti, and Klaus-Dietrich Fischer, *Bibliographie des textes médicaux latins: Antiquité et haut Moyen Âge* (Saint-Étienne: Publications de l'Université de St. Étienne, 1987); Klaus-Dietrich Fischer, *Bibliographie des textes médicaux latins. Antiquité et haut Moyen Âge: premier supplement* (Saint-Étienne: Publications de l'Université de St. Étienne, 2000); Klaus-Dietrich Fischer, *Bibliographie des textes médicaux latins: Antiquité et haut Moyen Âge: second supplement* (Saint-Étienne: Bibliothèque Interuniversitaire de Médecine, 2000), https://www.biusante.parisdescartes.fr/histoire/medicina/documents/fischer.php; and Klaus-Dietrich Fischer, *Bibliographie des textes médicaux latins. Antiquité et haut Moyen Âge: addendum 2002* (Saint-Étienne: Bibliothèque Interuniversitaire de Médecine, 2002), https://www.biusante.parisdescartes.fr/histoire/medicina/documents/fischer2002.php.

and reinforce assumptions about the texts themselves.[13] The idea that texts are stable constructs that maintain 'a specific and definitive form from manuscript to manuscript', for example, or that 'there is a single author whose intentions the editor can intuit' are problematic suppositions given the complexity, diversity, and dynamism of early medieval medical literature.[14] Moreover, editions tend to focus on tracing a single source or family of texts, isolating the selected material from its wider context, such as the other writings with which it was transmitted.[15] While editorial projects are crucial for understanding individual texts, their relationships, and their linguistic evolution, it is important to build on these studies by a) pursuing complementary types of research that take into account the issues raised by Wallis, and b) expanding the research framework to engage with broader questions of intellectual, social, and cultural history.[16] By reading a text in isolation and without a full consideration of its manuscript context, intended audience(s) and purpose(s), and use over time, we can lose sight of how scribes and readers engaged with a manuscript and its contents and the ways in which the knowledge it transmits was perceived.[17] Ultimately, as Anna Grotans, Julian Hendrix, and Bernice Kaczynski highlight, while editions remain invaluable tools, they are not 'amenable' to all types of research

13 Faith Wallis, 'The Experience of the Book: Manuscripts, Texts, and the Role of Epistemology in Early Medieval Medicine', in *Knowledge and the Scholarly Medical Traditions*, ed. Don G. Bates (Cambridge: Cambridge University Press, 1995), 101–26, at p. 102.

14 Wallis, 'The Experience of the Book', 102.

15 Eric Knibbs, 'How to Use Modern Critical Editions of Medieval Latin Texts'. *History Compass* 5, no. 5 (2007): 1521–49, https://doi.org/10.1111/j.1478-0542.2007.00452.x. See also Sabbah, Corsetti, and Fischer, *BTML*; Fischer, *BTML 1*; Fischer, *BTML 2*; and Fischer, *BTML 3*.

16 Wallis, 'The Experience of the Book', 102; Monica H. Green, 'Moving from Philology to Social History: The Circulation and Uses of Albucasis's Latin *Surgery* in the Middle Ages', in *Between Text and Patient: The Medical Enterprise in Medieval and Early Modern Europe*, ed. Florence Eliza Glaze and Brian K. Nance (Florence: SISMEL Edizioni del Galluzzo, 2011), 331–72.

17 Indeed, a drive to centre manuscripts—which has surely been augmented by the increasing number of libraries and archives that are digitising and making their manuscript collections freely available online—can be felt across many subfields within early medieval history. See, for example, Carine van Rhijn, *Leading the Way to Heaven: Pastoral Care and Salvation in the Carolingian Period* (London: Routledge, 2022); Monique Goullet, Martin Heinzelmann, and Christiane Veyrard-Cosme, eds., *L'hagiographie mérovingienne à travers ses réécritures* (Ostfildern: Thorbecke, 2010); Alice Rio, *Legal Practice and the Written Word in the Early Middle Ages: Frankish Formulae, 500–1000* (Cambridge: Cambridge University Press, 2009); and Rosamond McKitterick, *History and Memory in the Carolingian World* (Cambridge: Cambridge University Press, 2004). On the impact of digitisation projects, see, for example, Benjamin Albritton, Georgia Henley, and Elaine Treharne, eds., *Medieval Manuscripts in the Digital Age* (London: Routledge, 2021).

questions, including those regarding the presentation of material on the page or the interpretation of the signs of how a manuscript was used or a text was read and/or adapted over time.[18]

Related to the emphasis on philological research within the traditional approach to the study of early medieval medicine, there has been an understandable prioritisation of those writings that can be linked to a known classical or late antique tradition.[19] Consequently, medical writings with clearer (late) ancient pedigrees have typically received more focus than the many so-called 'miscellaneous' medical writings and compendia that draw on combinations of sources, though there are a number of important early exceptions, such as the early medieval recipe collections published by Henry Sigerist and Julius Jörimann in the 1920s.[20] The field's interests, however, have shifted and expanded over time, such that many studies in recent decades are now focusing on precisely the type of material that was overlooked in the past. Much of the recent work by scholars such as Arsenio Ferraces Rodríguez and Klaus-Dietrich Fischer has recalibrated and enriched our understanding of the composition of early medieval compilations, tracing the links between recipe collections, extracts, or even individual recipes that appear across a range of manuscripts. Their research emphasises the degree to which (late) ancient medical knowledge underpinned the so-called 'miscellaneous' and previously

18 Anna Grotans, Julian Hendrix, and Bernice Kaczynski. 'Understanding Medieval Manuscripts: St. Gall's Virtual Library'. *History Compass* 7, no. 3 (2009): 955–80, https://doi.org/10.1111/j.1478-0542.2009.00603.x, at p. 955–6.

19 For editions and the categorisation of texts, see Sabbah, Corsetti, and Fischer, *BTML*; Fischer, *BTML 1*; Fischer, *BTML 2*; and Fischer, *BTML 3* as well as Beccaria, *I codici* and Wickersheimer, *Les manuscrits*.

20 On the emphasis on classical and late antique medical writings in earlier research, see, for example, the publications of the *CML*, including Celsus, *A. Cornelii Celsii quae supersunt*, ed. Friedrich Marx, *CML* 1 (Leipzig: Teubner, 1915); Quintus Serenus, *Liber medicinalis*, ed. F. Vollmer, *CML* 2 (Leipzig: Teubner, 1916); *Plinii Secundi Iunioris qui feruntur De medicina libri tres*, ed. Alf Önnerfors, *CML* 3 (Berlin: Akademie-Verlag, 1964); *Antonii Musae De herba vettonica liber. Pseudoapulei Herbarius. Anonymi De taxone liber. Sextii Placiti Liber medicinae ex animalibus etc.*, ed. Ernst Howald and Henry E. Sigerist, *CML* 4 (Leipzig; Teubner, 1927); Marcellus, *De medicamentis liber*, ed. Eduard Liechtenhan and Maximilian Niedermann, trans. Jutta Kollesch and Diethard Nickel, *CML* 5, 2 vols. (Berlin: Akademie-Verlag, 1968); Caelius Aurelianus, *Celerum Passionum Libri III. Tardarum Passionum Libri V*, ed. Gerhard Bendz, trans. Ingeborg Pape, *CML* 6, 2 vols. (Berlin: Akademie-Verlag, 1990–93); and Anthimus, *De observatione ciborum ad Theodoricum regem Francorum epistula*, ed. and trans. Eduard Liechtenhan, *CML* 8 (Berlin: Akademie-Verlag, 1963). On early exceptions, see *Studien und Texte*, ed. Sigerist; *Frühmittelalterliche Rezeptarien*, ed. Jörimann.

unidentified material.[21] At the same time, more work has turned to individual manuscripts: Ulrich Stoll, for example, published an edition and translation of the *Lorscher Arzneibuch*, while Peter Köpp and Monica Niederer have each produced studies of distinct recipe collections in cod. sang. 217 (with the former including related fragments in cod. sang. 1396).[22]

By concentrating on material found outside the established corpus, such as recipes in anonymous collections that appear to have been compiled in the early Middle Ages as well as individual recipes added to manuscripts during this period, this book builds on and contributes to these studies, continuing to broaden the current discourse on early medieval recipe literature. These recipes and their contexts will be discussed in Chapter 2 (and see Appendix 1 for a more detailed review of the specific manuscripts involved in this study).

3.2 *Histories of Early Medieval Medicine: From Negative Stereotypes to Revisionist Approaches*

Scholars of the early Middle Ages have been relatively slow to turn to the history of medicine: Loren MacKinney's *Early Medieval Medicine, With Special Reference to France and Chartres*, now over eighty years old, remains the only general monograph on the topic, and discussions of health and medicine have rarely featured in more general studies of the period.[23] As Meg Leja has

---

21 Arsenio Ferraces Rodríguez, 'Reutilización de fuentes en recetarios médicos de la antigüedad tardía: Teodoro Prisciano-*Teraupetica-Tereoperica*', *Acta Classica: Proceedings of the Classical Association of South Africa* 64, no. 1 (2021): 212–36; Arsenio Ferraces Rodríguez, 'El recetario *Ut pili evulsi non recrescant* (Paris, BNF, Lat. 13955, ff. 146r-147v)', *Galenos* 5 (2011): 71–90; Klaus-Dietrich Fischer, 'Two Latin Pre-Salernitan medical manuals, the *Liber passionalis* and the *Tereoperica* (Ps. Petroncellus)', in *Medical Books in the Byzantine World*, ed. Barbara Zipser (Bologna: Università di Bologna, 2013), 35–56; and Klaus-Dietrich Fischer, '*Antidotum cui nomen est acharistum*', in *Between Text and Patient: The Medical Enterprise in Medieval and Early Modern Europe*, ed. Florence Eliza Glaze and Brian K. Nance (Florence: SISMEL Edizioni del Galluzzo, 2011), 173–99.

22 *Das 'Lorscher Arzneibuch': Ein medizinisches Kompendium des 8. Jahrhunderts (Codex Bambergensis medicinalis 1): Text, Übersetzung und Fachglossar*, ed. and trans. Ulrich Stoll (Stuttgart: Franz Steiner, 1992); *Vademecum eines frühmittelalterlichen Arztes*, ed. and trans. Köpp; and *Der St. Galler* Botanicus*: Ein frühmittelalterliches Herbar: Kritische Edition, Übersetzung und Kommentar*, ed. and trans. Monica Niederer (Bern: Peter Lang, 2005).

23 Loren C. MacKinney, *Early Medieval Medicine, With Special Reference to France and Chartres* (Baltimore: Johns Hopkins Press, 1937). For overviews of Carolingian history and culture, and the conspicuous absence of health and medicine from these works, see, for example, Marios Costambeys, Matthew Innes, and Simon MacLean, *The Carolingian World* (Cambridge: Cambridge University Press, 2011); Rosamond McKitterick, ed., *The New Cambridge Medieval History* II, *c. 700-c. 900* (Cambridge: Cambridge University Press, 1995); Rosamond McKitterick, *The Frankish Kingdoms under the Carolingians,*

suggested, perhaps Einhard's claim that Charlemagne did not listen to his physicians has coloured modern historians' approach to this area: 'scholars have followed Einhard's lead—unconsciously or not—in discounting medicine as an important aspect of the Carolingian renaissance'.[24] Regardless of Einhard's influence, however, the realm of medicine has traditionally been seen as a field comparatively unaffected by the Carolingian focus on learning and writing. Although the copying of classical and late antique medical texts during this period may seem to fit with the more general Carolingian interest in studying writings from Antiquity, it has been shown that few of these medical texts were actually rediscovered at this time.[25] The surviving written record has thus been interpreted as continuing late antique trends rather than marking a new phase in relation to Carolingian cultural and intellectual developments. As a result, the primary medical achievement of this period has often been characterised as an increase in the production of manuscripts containing medical content rather than as an increase in the production of *new* medical material.[26]

If early medievalists have, by and large, begun to engage with medical history only in relatively recent years (as discussed below), earlier generations of historians of medicine often dismissed the early Middle Ages entirely. The now outdated, though still influential, teleological approach to medical history understood medicine to be on a path of inevitable progress from Antiquity to the present day, excepting a period of stagnation coinciding with the 'Dark Ages'.[27] These centuries—the millennium or so between the heights of classical learning and the reintroduction of Greek medical knowledge in the central

---

751–987 (London: Longman, 1983); and Joanna Story, ed., *Charlemagne: Empire and Society* (Manchester: Manchester University Press, 2005). Michael McCormick's contribution to *The Long Morning of Medieval Europe: New Directions in Early Medieval Studies* is a notable exception: Michael McCormick, 'Molecular Middle Ages: Early Medieval Economic History in the Twenty-First Century', in *The Long Morning of Medieval Europe: New Directions in Early Medieval Studies*, ed. Jennifer R. Davis and Michael McCormick (Aldershot: Ashgate, 2008), 83–97.

24 Meg Leja, 'The Sacred Art: Medicine in the Carolingian Renaissance', *Viator* 47, no. 2 (2016): 1–34, https://doi.org/10.1484/J.VIATOR.5.111224; see especially pp. 1–2.

25 Vivian Nutton, 'Early Medieval Medicine and Natural Science', in *The Cambridge History of Science 2: Medieval Science*, ed. David C. Lindberg and Michael H. Shank (Cambridge: Cambridge University Press, 2013), 323–40, at p. 336.

26 MacKinney, *Early Medieval Medicine*, 99; Peregrine Horden, 'What's Wrong with Early Medieval Medicine?' *Social History of Medicine* 24, no. 1 (2011): 5–25, https://doi.org/10.1093/shm/hkp052, at p. 17. For a reassessment of medicine's place in the Carolingian world, see Leja, *Embodying the Soul*.

27 See, for example, the general assessments of late antique medicine in Vivian Nutton, 'From Galen to Alexander, Aspects of Medicine and Medical Practice in Late Antiquity', *Dumbarton Oaks Papers* 38 (1984): 1–14, https://doi.org/10.2307/1291489, and for a more

and later Middle Ages thanks to the translation of Arabic texts—have been described as a 'refrigerator, in which the medical knowledge of antiquity [was] merely preserved'.[28] Early medieval medicine, therefore, was largely ignored (or even ridiculed) by numerous earlier scholars.[29] Accordingly, it remains less well established than many other comparable subfields in both Carolingian history *and* medical history.[30]

Already in the early twentieth century, however, a handful of researchers, including Henry Sigerist and Loren MacKinney, bucked the general trends and took seriously the study of early medieval medicine.[31] Although their landmark

recent assessment, Vivian Nutton, *Ancient Medicine*, 2nd ed. (Abingdon: Routledge, 2013), 299–317.

28 Peter van Minnen, 'Medical care in late antiquity', in *Ancient Medicine in Its Socio-Cultural Context, Volume 1: Papers Read at the Congress Held at Leiden University, 13–15 April 1992*, ed. H. F. J. Horstmanshoff, Philip J. van der Eijk, and P. H. Schrijvers (Amsterdam: Rodopi, 1995), 153–169, at p. 153.

29 While many earlier historians may have viewed medieval medical writings simply as witnesses to the blind copying of older sources, others went further, comparing early medieval pharmacy to the potion produced by the witches in Macbeth and even labelling some material as 'absurd and childish'; Charles Singer, 'A Review of the Medical Literature of the Dark Ages, with a New Text of about 1110', *Proceedings of the Royal Society of Medicine* 10 (1917): 107–60, see especially pp. 158–60. Similar views are espoused in J. H. G. Grattan and Charles Singer, *Anglo-Saxon Magic and Medicine: Illustrated Specially from the Semi-Pagan Text* Lacnunga (Oxford: Oxford University Press, 1952). On the development of these perceptions, see *Medieval Herbal Remedies: The* Old English Herbarium *and Anglo-Saxon Medicine*, trans. Anne Van Arsdall (New York: Routledge, 2002), 35–100.

30 On general Carolingian histories, see n. 23 above. For an overview of western medical history, and the relatively limited space given to early medieval medicine, see Lawrence I. Conrad, Michael Neve, Vivian Nutton, Roy Porter, and Andrew Wear, *The Western Medical Tradition: 800 BC to AD 1800* (Cambridge: Cambridge University Press, 1995). For medicine in the ancient world, see especially Nutton, *Ancient Medicine*; and for later medieval medicine, see, for example, Nancy G. Siraisi, *Medieval and Early Renaissance Medicine: An Introduction to Knowledge and Practice* (Chicago, University of Chicago Press, 1990); Monica H. Green, 'Bodies, Gender, Health, Disease: Recent Work on Medieval Women's Medicine', *Studies in Medieval and Renaissance History* 3 (2005): 1–46; Michael R. McVaugh, *Medicine before the Plague: Practitioners and their Patients in the Crown of Aragon, 1285–1345* (Cambridge: Cambridge University Press, 1993); Michael McVaugh, *The Rational Surgery of the Middle Ages* (Florence: SISMEL Edizioni del Galluzzo, 2006); and Piers D. Mitchell, *Medicine in the Crusades: Warfare, Wounds and the Medieval Surgeon* (Cambridge: Cambridge University Press, 2004). These titles offer only a fraction of the available scholarship on these topics.

31 See, for example, MacKinney, *Early Medieval Medicine*; *Studien und Texte*, ed. Sigerist; Henry E. Sigerist, 'A Summer of Research in European Libraries', *Bulletin of the Institute of the History of Medicine* 2, no. 10 (1934): 559–610; Henry E. Sigerist, 'The Latin Medical Literature of the Early Middle Ages', *Journal of the History of Medicine and Allied Sciences* 13, no. 2 (1958): 127–45.

studies remain valuable today, they still perpetuated many of the prevailing ideas about medical knowledge and practice during this period, such as its perceived backwardness and superstitious nature. Consider how, on the one hand, Sigerist's opening remarks in *Studien und Texte zur frühmittelalterlichen Rezeptliteratur* assumed medicine's stagnation in the 'Dark Ages' while, on the other hand, his concluding analyses recognized the production of new, original compilations that reflected the needs and conditions of the communities in which they were produced.[32] Negative stereotypes of medieval medicine may persist in popular culture but, thanks to these pioneering scholars, more researchers began to question these assumptions.[33]

Expanding from this foundation, the study of early medieval medicine experienced a significant swing of the historiographical pendulum in the second half of the twentieth century. Led by historians such as John M. Riddle, Jerry Stannard, and Linda Ehrsam Voigts, a wave of revisionist scholarship radically altered the field, and especially with respect to topics concerning the relationship between medical knowledge and practice.[34] Although Riddle and Stannard concentrated on continental material, much of the research into the practicality of medical texts has been rooted in the study of Old English recipe literature.[35] Voigts's 1979 article, 'Anglo-Saxon Plant Remedies and the Anglo-Saxons', for example, provided one of the first in-depth reassessments of early English herbal medicine and contends that texts such as the *Old English*

---

32 *Studien und Texte*, ed. Sigerist, iii-v and 182–95.

33 On medieval medicine and popular culture, see Lucy Barnhouse and Winston Black, eds., *Beyond Cadfael: Medieval Medicine and Medical Medievalism* (Budapest: Trivent Publishing, 2023).

34 See, for example, John M. Riddle, 'The Introduction and Use of Eastern Drugs in the Early Middle Ages', *Sudhoffs Archiv für Geschichte der Medizin und der Naturwissenschaften* 49, no. 2 (1965): 185–98; John M. Riddle, 'Theory and Practice in Medieval Medicine'. *Viator* 5 (1974): 157–84, https://doi.org/10.1484/J.VIATOR.2.301620; John M. Riddle, 'Pseudo-Dioscorides' *Ex herbis femininis* and Early Medieval Medical Botany', *Journal of the History of Biology* 14, no. 1 (1981): 43–81; Jerry Stannard, 'The Herbal as a Medical Document', *Bulletin of the History of Medicine*' 43, no. 3 (1969): 212–20; Jerry Stannard, 'Marcellus of Bordeaux and the Beginnings of Medieval *Materia Medica*', *Pharmacy in History* 15, no. 2 (1973): 47–53; Linda Ehrsam Voigts, 'The Significance of the Name Apuleius to the *Herbarium Apulei*', *Bulletin of the History of Medicine* 52, no. 2 (1978): 214–27; and Linda E. Voigts, 'Anglo-Saxon Plant Remedies and the Anglo-Saxons', *Isis* 70, no. 2 (1979): 250–68. For collections of Riddle's and Stannard's groundbreaking articles, see John M. Riddle, *Quid pro quo: Studies in the History of Drugs* (Aldershot: Variorum, 1992); Jerry Stannard, *Pristina Medicamenta: Ancient and Medieval Medical Botany* (Aldershot: Ashgate, 1999); and Jerry Stannard, *Herbs and Herbalism in the Middle Ages and Renaissance* (Aldershot: Ashgate, 1999).

35 Horden, 'What's Wrong with Early Medieval Medicine?', 6.

Herbarium could have been used in practice.[36] While arguments for the practicality of early medieval recipes will be reviewed in more detail below, Voigts's analysis, alongside Riddle's work on the evolving relationship between medical theory and practice, has proved pivotal. In particular, Malcolm L. Cameron, Anne Van Arsdall, Maria Amalia D'Aronco, and Audrey Meaney, among others, have built on Voigts's arguments by exploring the transmission of medical information, the processes involved in translating knowledge into practice, the allegedly 'magical' or 'superstitious' elements within recipes, as well as their potential efficacy.[37]

Although this significant body of scholarship has provided great insights into early medieval medicine whilst simultaneously overturning the traditional,

36 Voigts, 'Anglo-Saxon Plant Remedies'. On medieval herbals more generally, see Minta Collins, *Medieval Herbals: The Illustrative Traditions* (London: British Library, 2000) and on the Old English *Herbarium*, see Maria Amalia D'Aronco and Malcolm L. Cameron, *The Old English Illustrated Pharmacopoeia* (Copenhagen: Rosenkilde and Bagger, 1998) and *Medieval Herbal Remedies*, trans. Van Arsdall.

37 M. L. Cameron, *Anglo-Saxon Medicine* (Cambridge: Cambridge University Press, 1993); M. L. Cameron, 'Anglo-Saxon Medicine and Magic', *Anglo-Saxon England* 17 (1988): 191–215; Anne Van Arsdall, 'Challenging the "Eye of Newt" Image of Medieval Medicine', in *The Medieval Hospital and Medical Practice*, ed. Barbara Bowers (Aldershot: Ashgate, 2007), 195–205; Anne Van Arsdall, 'The Transmission of Knowledge in Early Medieval Medical Texts: An Exploration', in *Between Text and Patient: The Medical Enterprise in Medieval and Early Modern Europe*, ed. Florence Eliza Glaze and Brian K. Nance (Florence: SISMEL Edizioni del Galluzzo, 2011), 201–15; Maria Amalia D'Aronco, 'Anglo-Saxon Plant Pharmacy and the Latin Medical Tradition', in *From Earth to Art: The Many Aspects of the Plant-World in Anglo-Saxon England. Proceedings of the First ASPNS Symposium, University of Glasgow, 5–7 April 2000*, ed. C. P. Biggam (Amsterdam: Rodopi: 2003), 133–51; Maria Amalia D'Aronco, 'The Transmission of Medical Knowledge in Anglo-Saxon England: The Voices of Manuscripts', in *Form and Content of Instruction in Anglo-Saxon England in the Light of Contemporary Manuscript Evidence: Papers Presented at the International Conference, Udine, 6–8 April 2006*, ed. Patrizia Lendinara, Loredana Lazzari, and Maria Amalia D'Aronco (Turnhout: Brepols, 2007), 35–58; *Medieval Herbal Remedies*, trans. Van Arsdall; Audrey Meaney, 'The Practice of Medicine in England about the Year 1000', *Social History of Medicine* 13, no. 2 (2000): 221–37, https://doi.org/10.1093/shm/13.2.221; and Audrey L. Meaney, 'Extra-Medical Elements in Anglo-Saxon Medicine', *Social History of Medicine* 24, no. 1 (2011): 41–56, https://doi.org/10.1093/shm/hkq105. For more recent work on efficacy since Cameron's research, see Barbara Brennessel, Michael D. C. Drout, and Robyn Gravel, 'A Reassessment of the Efficacy of Anglo-Saxon Medicine', *Anglo-Saxon England* 34 (2005): 183–95; Freya Harrison, Aled E. L. Roberts, Rebecca Gabrilska, Kendra P. Rumbaugh, Christina Lee, and Stephen P. Diggle, 'A 1,000-Year-Old Antimicrobial Remedy with Antistaphylococcal Activity', *mBio* 6, no. 4 (2015), https://doi.org/10.1128/mBio.01129-15; and Rebecca Brackmann, '"It Will Help Him Wonderfully": Placebo and Meaning Responses in Early Medieval English Medicine', *Speculum* 97, no. 4 (2022): 1012–39, https://doi.org/10.1086/721680.

disparaging stereotypes regarding the topic, there are certain limitations with its scope as well as potential pitfalls in its approach. On the one hand, the extensive focus on Insular material has yet to be replicated for continental sources, though claims for the practicality of the latter are sometimes based on extrapolating from analyses of the Old English texts. On the other hand, much of the work investigating the relationship between medical knowledge and practice has started with assumption that the texts were, by their very nature, intended to be used in practice, creating a circular argument. The present book aims to offer an intervention that addresses both points.

While the heightened focus on Insular recipe literature may stem largely from the interest it has generated as medical knowledge recorded in the vernacular, it has also been facilitated by its size. As Peregrine Horden explains, scholars of Old English medicine 'have to work with a substantial corpus of around 500 folios but embodying only five major works, three of which survive in unique manuscripts. Many difficulties remain, but the focus is at least clear'.[38] By comparison, the Latin continental material, with over one hundred extant early medieval manuscripts containing medical texts, presents a rather different picture than the handful of codices with Old English medical writings.[39] Yet, despite the challenges raised by this considerably larger volume of recipe literature, it deserves to be studied in its own right as well as in comparison with the Old English corpus, (late) ancient texts, and later medieval writings.

Although earlier scholars' emphasis on the distinctiveness of the Insular medical texts has been revised and the significance of pan-European medical traditions recognised, it is still dangerous to base claims for continental recipe literature's practicality primarily on the analyses of the Old English

38 Horden, 'What's Wrong with Early Medieval Medicine?', 6. The major surviving recipe collections in Old English include three *Leechbooks* (*Bald's Leechbook I* and *II* as well as *Leechbook III*), the *Lacnunga*, and translations/adaptations of several late antique Latin recipe collections.

39 On the numbers of surviving manuscripts, see Beccaria, *I codici* and Wickersheimer, *Les manuscrits*; the former includes 158 manuscripts produced between the ninth and eleventh centuries while the latter, which only focuses on manuscripts held in French collections, gives 119 manuscripts for the same period. Both catalogues, however, are in need of revision and the Corpus of Early Medieval Latin Medicine (CEMLM, formerly the Beyond Beccaria Project (2020–23)), a British Academy-funded cataloging project (https://cemlm.wp.st-andrews.ac.uk/), is working to produce a new, expanded catalogue of early medieval manuscripts containing medical texts that includes manuscripts missed by Beccaria and Wickersheimer. A preliminary handlist is in preparation that covers these additional manuscripts (approximately 200 in number).

corpus.[40] In contrast to the evidence for practicality identified by Voigts and others, Florence Eliza Glaze, in a critical study of Latin continental medical manuscripts, challenges the idea that the texts in these codices were inherently useable, writing, 'after examining numerous manuscripts studded with Greek anatomical terminology, much of it hopelessly corrupt, it has become clear that in many cases, neither scribes nor readers had the critical linguistic skills to grasp appreciably the meaning of the material in hand, to unlock the obscurity of the Greek, and parse the texts before them'.[41] Faith Wallis, too, has questioned the utility of certain medieval medical writings, in her case treatises on urine and pulse analysis, having identified corrupted passages that would have changed their meaning.[42] Wallis suggests that such treatises would have had limited practical use in the context of therapy. These examples serve as helpful cautions, reminders of not only the possible differences between the Latin and Old English traditions but also the potential dangers of overemphasising signs of practicality in medical texts. Consequently, arguments regarding recipe practicality that are built on extrapolations from Insular evidence or that rely on the handful of early published Latin collections, such as the works of Sigerist and Jörimann, are in need of reassessment and must take into account a larger sample of the surviving recipe literature. This book, though not comprehensive in its analysis of early medieval Latin recipes, examines a much more extensive body of the extant recipes and thus begins the process of re-evaluating earlier scholarship while offering new insights.

The second issue raised above, namely, that much recent research on the practicality of recipes begins with the assumption that pharmaceutical writings were naturally intended to be used in therapy, reflects how far the field has moved: this idea stands in stark contrast to the traditional view of *Mönchsmedizin*, monastic medicine, in which medical writings were understood to be the result of the blind copying of earlier texts. The number of surviving early medieval manuscripts containing medical texts, for example, has

40 On pan-European traditions, see Gundolf Keil and Paul Schnitzer, eds., *Das Lorscher Arzneibuch und die frühmittelalterliche Medizin: Verhandlungen des medizinhistorischen Symposiums im September 1989 in Lorsch* (Lorsch: Laurissa, 1991); *Medieval Herbal Remedies*, trans. Van Arsdall, 68–100; Riddle, 'Theory and Practice'. On the Latin sources of Old English medical writings, see Conan T. Doyle, *The Reception of Latin Medicine in Anglo-Saxon England: Evidence from Old English Medical Texts* (York: York Medieval Press, forthcoming).

41 Glaze, 'The Perforated Wall', 5–6.

42 Faith Wallis, 'Signs and Senses: Diagnosis and Prognosis in Early Medieval Pulse and Urine Texts', *Social History of Medicine* 13, no. 2 (2000): 265–78, https://doi.org/10.1093/shm/13.2.265, at p. 273.

been interpreted as evidence for their practical value.[43] Yet the sheer number of extant manuscripts containing a certain genre of texts does not indicate *how* these texts were used. Furthermore, these manuscripts actually comprise a relatively small percentage of the total number of codices that survive from this period. According to Vivian Nutton, 'out of roughly 9,000 codices surviving from the ninth century, barely 100 can be classed as medical'.[44] While the full story of the manuscript evidence is more complicated—not least because hundreds of recipes have also been identified as additions to fly-leaves, margins, and other blank spaces in early medieval manuscripts otherwise unrelated to medicine—Nutton's point still stands: medical writings make up but a small percentage of the surviving textual record. The simple existence of medical literature should not be read as evidence of its use in medical practice.

A variety of other features, including signs of wear and tear, the presence of glosses, the lack of theoretical writings, and the size and shape of manuscripts, have also been employed as indications of the use of these texts in medical practice.[45] The dimensions and folds of several manuscripts containing recipes considered in this study, such as Paris, BnF lat. 11218 and cod. sang. 217, have been interpreted as evidence of their use by medical practitioners. In the case of BnF lat. 11218, this small, rectangular manuscript dated to the late eighth or early ninth centuries contains a diverse collection of medical and pharmaceutical texts.[46] Based on its proportions (23.2 cm x 13.3 cm) and lack of writings on medical theory, it has been described as having 'the appearance of a manual [intended] for practical use'.[47] While the portability of a manuscript does indicate that it could have travelled with ease—and thus could have accompanied a Carolingian *medicus*—its size cannot be conclusively linked to its deployment in medical contexts. Small volumes may have been made for many reasons entirely unrelated to their use in therapy, such as the constraints of available parchment and other resources. The jump from portability to practicality, moreover, assumes much about how medicine was practised and imagines that a physician-figure would have needed a portable medical guide

43 Van Arsdall, 'The Transmission of Knowledge', 210.

44 Nutton, 'Early Medieval Medicine and Natural Science', 336.

45 Voigts, 'Anglo-Saxon Plant Remedies'; Riddle, 'Theory and Practice'; Bernhard Bischoff, 'Über gefaltete Handschriften, vornehmlich hagiographischen Inhalts', in *Mittelalterliche Studien. Ausgewählte Aufsätze zur Schriftkunde und Literaturgeschichte*, ed. Bernhard Bischoff, vol. 1 (Stuttgart: Hiersemann, 1966), 93–100, at p. 99; Horden, 'What's Wrong with Early Medieval Medicine?', 10 and 16.

46 See Chapter 2 for more information about this manuscript and the others under analysis.

47 Beccaria, *I codici*, no. 34: 'Il volume, che nelle proporzioni ha l'aspetto di un manuale per l'uso practico' (p. 161).

to assist in his or her practice.[48] And what does this say about medical manuscripts with larger folia? Would the use of wider or longer pieces of parchment, as seen in many of the manuscripts considered in this book, suggest that such compendia were impractical with respect to medical practice?

Regarding glosses, consider, for example, those in cod. sang. 878, Walahfrid Strabo's *vademecum*, another manuscript analysed in this study. On p. 333, a number of recipes have been glossed in Old High German, translating many of the ingredients into the vernacular.[49] In mixed linguistic communities, this would have been a very practical addition for an individual who was less familiar with Latin. Such glosses, however, could also reflect the manuscript's role in teaching vocabulary. Regardless, in this case, they date to the eleventh century and therefore cannot be used to comment on the Carolingian use of these texts. London, BL Harley MS 585, a manuscript containing the *Lacnunga*, a copy of the *Old English Herbarium*, and other medical texts, provides a parallel from the Insular world. It has been described as 'a complete manual for a physician's use', which 'has the aspect of a manuscript intended for use, study, and/or reference'.[50] While its texts do include many recipes and other writings related to therapy, as Katharine Park highlights, the degree to which they were intended for use in the practice of medicine remains unknown, even in manuscripts that that appear 'decidedly practical in orientation' to a modern reader.[51] This final point is crucial: while it is tempting to assume that medical texts that *look* practical were intended for medical practice—and then to read all evidence of practical features as supporting this conclusion—it is a circular argument and ignores the possibility that such texts may have been used in other ways.[52] While the evidence mobilised in these arguments does confirm the *use* of these manuscripts, rarely does it pinpoint the specific contexts in which they were read, handled, annotated, and otherwise used. In fact, with respect to the glosses in London, BL Harley MS 585, the comments that most

48 All surviving records of a term for a professional medical practitioner are masculine (*medicus*), though the possibility of female healers with access to medical texts should not be automatically discounted. See also Leja, *Embodying the Soul*, 137.

49 Emil Elias von Steinmeyer and Eduard Sievers, *Die althochdeutschen Glossen*. 5 vols. (Berlin: Weidmann, 1879–1922), vol. 4, 455.

50 D'Aronco, 'The Transmission of Medical Knowledge', 50.

51 Katharine Park, 'Medicine and Society in Medieval Europe, 500–1500', in *Medicine in Society: Historical Essays*, ed. Andrew Wear (Cambridge: Cambridge University Press, 1992), 59–90, at p. 66.

52 Peregrine Horden, 'Prefatory Note: The Uses of Medical Manuscripts', in *Medical Books in the Byzantine World*, ed. Barbara Zipser (Bologna: Università di Bologna, 2013), 1–6.

clearly connect the texts to the practice of medicine have been dated to the fourteenth century, reinforcing the need for caution.[53]

Studies of cod. sang. 217 paint a similar picture. Based on its 'very practical orientation and simple decoration', it has been argued that the manuscript served as the *vademecum* of an early medieval physician.[54] A number of elements, including its a) shape, size, and folds, b) exclusive focus on recipes and bloodletting treatises, c) lack of writings on medical theory, d) simplicity of decoration, and e) signs of wear and tear, support this as a possibility. That is, the evidence suggests that it *could* have been used in the context of therapy and *could* have accompanied a practising early medieval *medicus*. Yet to understand these features as proof of the manuscript's use in medical practice assumes that it was designed with this single purpose in mind: the argument presupposes that *any* signs of use are indicative of its use by a medical practitioner in the context of therapy.[55]

Instead, as Peregrine Horden emphasises, it is essential to recognise the variety of ways in which medical texts could have been used.[56] Although the 'simple preservation of a text for its own sake … should be automatically suspect', we should not entirely rule out the possible influence of antiquarian impulses in the drive to copy certain texts.[57] Alternatively, some surviving medical manuscripts, such as the richly decorated Vienna Dioscorides, may have been intended as markers of prestige and involved in elite gift exchange.[58]

53 D'Aronco, 'The Transmission of Medical Knowledge', 52.

54 Clare Pilsworth, *Healthcare in Early Medieval Northern Italy: More to Life than Leeches?* (Turnhout: Brepols, 2014), 81. On the interpretation of the manuscript's use, see the studies by Monica Niederer and Peter Köpp: *Der St. Galler* Botanicus, ed. and trans. Niederer (see especially pp. 9–23, 51–61); *Vademecum eines frühmittelalterlichen Arztes*, ed. and trans. Köpp (see especially pp. 12–13). The manuscript itself is discussed further in Chapter 2.

55 Despite reiterating many of the standard views regarding the use of cod. sang. 217, Clare Pilsworth also cautions against assuming that medical texts were intended exclusively for use in therapy and extends the discussion of manuscripts' potential to be used in multiple ways based on her analysis of Modena, Archivio Capitolare, O.I.11: Pilsworth, *Healthcare in Early Medieval Northern Italy*, 81–93.

56 Horden, 'Prefatory Note', 1–6. See also Horden, 'What's Wrong with Early Medieval Medicine?', 5–25.

57 Horden, 'Prefatory Note', 4.

58 Vienna, Österreichische Nationalbibliothek, Med. gr. 1. On this manuscript, see, for example, Leslie Brubaker, 'The Vienna Dioskorides and Anicia Juliana', in *Byzantine Garden Culture*, ed. Antony Robert Littlewood, Henry Maguire, and Joachim Wolschke-Bulmahn (Washington, D.C.: Dumbarton Oaks, 2002), 189–214 and Ernst Gamillscheg, 'Das Geschenk für Juliana Anicia: Überlegungen zur Struktur und Entstehung des Wiener Dioskurides', in *Byzantina Mediterranea. Festschrift für Johannes Koder zum 65. Geburtstag*, ed. Klaus Belke, Ewald Kislinger, Andreas Külzer, and Maria A. Stassinopoulou (Vienna: Böhlau, 2007), 187–95. On illustrated herbals, see Collins, *Medieval Herbals*. See also Monica

Medical texts also seemed to have a played an important role in scholarly pursuits more broadly, ranging from literary models to works of scientific information, thereby offering additional non-therapeutic uses of medical writings.[59] The presence of medical texts alongside works on the liberal arts and technical subjects, such as computus, in a number of manuscripts involved in this book, certainly supports the possibility that they were used in teaching, whether they were intended to provide guidance for specific medical matters or form part of the broader curriculum—or both.[60] Indeed, these varied purposes should not be seen as mutually exclusive: a single medical text may have been copied, read, and consulted for multiple reasons and its use(s) may have evolved over time.

Overall, in the process of reclaiming the study of early medieval medicine, historians have, at times, been overly positive in reading the evidence, falling into circular arguments and reaching premature conclusions. Claims regarding the relationship between knowledge and practice that have been built on the idea that a text's practical adaptations present proof of its consultation *in* medical practice and, relatedly, that any signs of a manuscript's use indicate its use *in* medical practice, must be reassessed. Although medical texts *could* have been used in the practice of medicine, it is inappropriate to jump to such a finding without additional evidence. The relationship between knowledge and practice must be interrogated more critically, and that investigation lies at the heart of this book. At the same time, given the past focus on Old English medical texts, further assessment of Carolingian material is particularly needed. As this book demonstrates, a more thorough contextualisation of the manuscript evidence and the analysis of a larger volume of data have significant implications for the question of practicality. The examination of an extensive sample of understudied recipes and recipe collections enables a re-evaluation of the conclusions of earlier research. This investigation begins without presuming that medical texts were exclusively intended for use in medical practice. Rather, *that* is the question: do recipes provide evidence that can shed light on not only whether they were used but also how they were used? Part 1 tackles

---

Green's compelling argument regarding the advertising purposes of deluxe, illustrated surgical treatises in Green, 'Moving from Philology to Social History'.

59 Horden, 'Prefatory Note', 4; Glaze, 'The Perforated Wall', 103.

60 Horden, 'Prefatory Note', 1–6. Faith Wallis also links the arrangement of manuscripts to the context of education, connecting 'the transmission of texts through florilegia' to medical training; Wallis, 'The Experience of the Book', 106. On medicine's place within a general education, see James T. Palmer, 'Merovingian Medicine between Practical Art and Philosophy', *Traditio* (forthcoming).

these questions through the lens of practicality. In doing so, it takes the topic in a new direction by distinguishing between general evidence for the use of these texts and more specific signs suggesting that they were intended to be used in medical practice.

3.3 *New Directions in Early Medieval Medical Research*

In recent decades, there has been a significant increase in the number of scholars studying early medieval Europe who either specialise in the history of health and medicine or integrate this field into their work on other areas of early medieval history. As a result, early medieval medical history is now being productively connected to a wide range of different subfields, intersecting with and contributing to research in social, cultural, intellectual, political, religious, legal, and environmental history and beyond.[61] Among the most important developments have been the diversification of the types of evidence employed in analyses and the drive to explore health as part of medical history.[62] The history of medicine, moreover, has traditionally taken a top-down approach that has primarily concentrated on practitioners—and, more specifically, the subset of practitioners who left a written record of their practice (or at least appear in the surviving written record), thereby privileging an elite, western, and male perspective. By concentrating on this limited group of individuals, not only have other types of practitioners been largely ignored, but so, too, have patients. In earlier generations of scholarship, the lack of attention given to patients, their experiences, and the wider cultures of healing in which they

61 For connections between medicine and other subfields of Carolingian history, see, for example, Leja, *Embodying the Soul*; Zubin Mistry, *Abortion in the Early Middle Ages, c. 500–900* (Woodbridge: Boydell & Brewer, 2015); Palmer, 'Merovingian Medicine'; and Faith Wallis, 'Medicine in Medieval Calendar Manuscripts', in *Manuscript Sources of Medieval Medicine*, ed. Margaret R. Schleissner (London: Garland, 1995), 105–43. For more focused assessments of health and disease, medicine, and medical practitioners in early medieval Europe, see, for example, Timothy P. Newfield, 'Malaria and Malaria-like Disease in the Early Middle Ages', *Early Medieval Europe* 25, no. 3 (2017): 251–300, https://doi.org/10.1111/emed.12212; Pilsworth, *Healthcare in Early Medieval Northern Italy*; and Patricia Skinner, *Health and Medicine in Early Medieval Southern Italy* (Leiden: Brill, 1997); and on the integration of medicine into the study of medieval history, see Monica H. Green, 'Integrative Medicine: Incorporating Medicine and Health into the Canon of Medieval European History', *History Compass* 7, no. 4 (2009): 1218–45, https://doi.org/10.1111/j.1478-0542.2009.00618.x.

62 On the increasing range of evidence and methodologies available to historians, see McCormick, 'Molecular Middle Ages'. On the history of health vs. the history of medicine, see, for example, Monica H. Green, ''History of Medicine' or 'History of Health'?', *Past and Future: The Magazine of the Institute of Historical Research* 9 (2011): 7–9.

lived and died is striking.[63] Indeed, the general dearth of named practitioners and few glimpses of *medici* in the early medieval west may help to explain why this period's medical history has suffered neglect in comparison to earlier and later periods: though *medici* occasionally appear as witnesses in charters and their presence is alluded to in law codes, poems, and other documentary evidence, only two royal *medici*, Wintar and Zedechias, are named in the surviving sources.[64] This book, through its examination of the lived experiences, and especially the experiences of injury and disease, of individuals in early medieval Europe, in concert with the textual record, thus expands on current trends in the field by drawing together different types of evidence to investigate questions of health alongside the transmission of medical knowledge.

Sources outside of the standard textual corpus are of particular interest and relevance to the study of health and disease in past populations. Genetics, for example, now provides previously unimaginable evidence for tracing the histories of pathogens, while the integration of the osteological record can, as Robin Fleming writes, help historians 'to re-animate the historical dead'.[65] Indeed, combinations of multiple lines of written and archaeological evidence

63 Monica H. Green, 'Gendering the History of Women's Healthcare', *Gender & History* 20, no. 3 (2008): 487–518, https://doi.org/10.1111/j.1468-0424.2008.00534.x, at p. 492. On the framework of 'cultures of healing', see Peregrine Horden, *Cultures of Healing: Medieval and After* (Abingdon: Routledge, 2019), ix-xi.

64 On Wintar, see Heiric of Auxerre, *Miracula S. Germani* 86, *PL* 124, cols. 1207–72, at col.1248B and Eigil of Fulda, *Vita Sturmi* 25, in Eigil of Fulda, *Die Vita Sturmi des Eigil von Fulda: Literarkritisch-historische Untersuchung und Edition*, ed. Pius Engelbert (Marburg: N. G. Elwert, 1968), 161. On Zedechias, see the *Annales Bertiniani*, ed. G. Waitz, *MGH SS Rer. Germ.* 5 (Hanover: Hahn, 1883), 136–7 (note: his name recorded as 'Sedechias') and *The Annals of St-Bertin*, trans. Janet L. Nelson (Manchester: Manchester University Press, 1991), 202. For examples of *medici* named in charters, see Pilsworth, *Healthcare in Early Medieval Northern Italy* and Skinner, *Health and Medicine in Early Medieval Southern Italy*. On doctors in early medieval law codes, see Lisi Oliver, *The Body Legal in Barbarian Law* (Toronto: University of Toronto Press, 2011).

65 Maria A. Spyrou, Kirsten I. Bos, Alexander Herbig, and Johannes Krause, 'Ancient pathogen genomics as an emerging tool for infectious disease research', *Nature Reviews Genetics* 20 (2019): 323–40, https://doi.org/10.1038/s41576-019-0119-1; Monica H. Green, 'Genetics as a Historicist Discipline: A New Player in Disease History', *Perspectives on History* 52, no. 9 (1 December 2014), https://www.historians.org/research-and-publications/perspectives-on-history/december-2014/genetics-as-a-historicist-discipline; Monica H. Green, ed., *Pandemic Disease in the Medieval World: Rethinking the Black Death* (Kalamazoo, MI: Arc Humanities Press, 2015); Robin Fleming, 'Bones for Historians: Putting the Body Back into Biography', in *Writing Medieval Biography, 750–1250: Essays in Honour of Frank Barlow*, ed. David Bates, Julia Crick, and Sarah Hamilton (Woodbridge: Boydell & Brewer, 2006), 29–48 (note: quotation is from p. 29); and Robin Fleming, 'Writing Biography at the Edge of History', *The American Historical Review* 114, no. 3 (2009): 606–14.

have been productively incorporated in a growing number of social and cultural histories of early medieval Europe, such as Paolo Squatriti's studies of chestnuts and weeds, Jamie Kreiner's work on pigs, and Caroline Goodson's investigation of urban gardening.[66] Human osteological material, however, has not often been studied in these types of histories that effectively draw on multidisciplinary evidence bases (though notable exceptions, such as Piers Mitchell's discipline-bridging research, will be addressed below). Overall, as Michael McCormick stresses, 'the mortal remains of people are among the most abundant yet least scrutinized archaeological remains to have survived from the Middle Ages,' despite their potential to enrich our understanding of past population's lived experiences.[67]

Osteological evidence can provide information about individuals' diets, living and working conditions, and experiences of injury and disease. Crucially, this source material is not limited to those whose lives are recorded in the texts. The possibility of investigating the health of people who lived in early medieval Europe therefore adds another angle to studying the practice of medicine in this period, and especially the relationship between medical knowledge and practice. Part 2 of this book surveys osteological evidence to gain insights into the health of individuals who lived in the early Middle Ages and then reconsiders the recipe literature from this new perpsective. As Jennifer Davis and Michael McCormick underline, 'in the light of archaeological results, the texts must be reanalyzed, and our conventional wisdom, rewritten'.[68] It is necessary to ask whether skeletal remains preserve evidence of the conditions recorded in the texts. To put it another way, were the treatments listed in eighth- and ninth-century manuscripts applicable to individuals in this period?

It may seem surprising that this book questions the applicability of recipes to the medical needs of individuals in early medieval Europe: a remedy

66 Paolo Squatriti, *Landscape and Change in Early Medieval Italy: Chestnuts, Economy, and Culture* (Cambridge: Cambridge University Press, 2013); Paolo Squatriti, *Weeds and the Carolingians: Empire, Culture, and Nature in Frankish Europe, AD 750–900* (Cambridge: Cambridge University Press, 2022); Jamie Kreiner, *Legions of Pigs in the Early Medieval West* (New Haven: Yale University Press, 2020); and Caroline Goodson, *Cultivating the City in Early Medieval Italy* (Cambridge: Cambridge University Press, 2021).

67 McCormick, 'Molecular Middle Ages', 90. See also Raphaël G. A. M Panhuysen, 'Demography and Health in Early Medieval Maastricht: Prosopographical Observations on Two Cemeteries' (Diss., Universiteit Maastricht, 2005), 10–12.

68 Jennifer R. Davis and Michael McCormick, 'The Early Middle Ages: Europe's Long Morning', in *The Long Morning of Medieval Europe: New Directions in Early Medieval Studies*, ed. Jennifer R. Davis and Michael McCormick (Aldershot: Ashgate, 2008), 1–10, at p. 5.

for, say, gout must have been preserved because people suffered from gout. Much scholarship has made this assumption, but there is little direct evidence to indicate that the recording of recipes represented a response to the medical concerns of individuals in early medieval Europe.[69] There are no case notes accompanying these texts and, as the opening example of Terenti(an)us demonstrated, even seemingly personal comments should not be automatically interpreted as a reflection of the scribe's experience with a treatment. Just as with the question of practicality (where it is tempting to assume that medical texts were, by definition, used in medical practice), the existence of medical writings does not *prove* their applicability. Many of the recipes analysed in this study, though they are not directly attributable to classical and late antique writings, are related to this body of knowledge. As Peregrine Horden succinctly puts it, 'early medieval medicine is ancient medicine'.[70] Although there are important developments in the recorded medical knowledge of the early Middle Ages (on which, see Chapters 3–5), the content is largely derived from (late) ancient texts. The overarching influence of classical medical traditions demands that we question the texts' assumed applicability because the climate, living conditions, and lifestyles of the Mediterranean world of Antiquity and of ninth-century western Europe were different in many ways. These fundamental differences may have resulted in vastly altered experiences of disease, injury, and overall health between the original authors of these medical writings and the scribes responsible for the manuscripts discussed in this book. The question of a text's relevance to contemporary individuals is therefore essential for understanding the relationship between medical knowledge and practice, and recent research trends have laid the groundwork for such an investigation.

Although there has traditionally been a 'non-relationship between historians and researchers in more scientific disciplines', historical studies integrating evidence from the archaeological sciences have greatly increased in recent years.[71] Scholarship relating to past experiences of and responses to health and

---

69 Take, for example, Vivian Nutton's comment on the content of early medieval medical manuscripts: 'most medical manuscripts before 1100 are largely recipe lists, often well organized and well suited to the needs of the community'; Nutton, 'Early Medieval Medicine and Natural Science', 335.

70 Horden, 'What's Wrong with Early Medieval Medicine?', 19.

71 Fleming, 'Writing Biography', 614. For an overview, see McCormick, 'Molecular Middle Ages', and for a sample of the current diversity of research areas uniting evidence from archaeological sciences with traditional historical sources, see, for example, A. Radini, M. Tromp, A. Beach, E. Tong, C. Speller, M. McCormick, J. V. Dudgeon, et al., 'Medieval women's early involvement in manuscript production suggested by lapis lazuli

disease has been particularly enriched by a number of historians' multidisciplinary approaches incorporating various palaeo- and archaeological sciences, such as Monica Green's pioneering work on plague genetics and Timothy Newfield's analyses of palaeoclimate data in relation to disease outbreaks.[72] Turning to osteological evidence, as Piers Mitchell has demonstrated, the skeletal record can be effectively studied alongside the written record.[73] Mitchell's work, however, concentrates on the central and later Middle Ages, and few of the studies involving early medieval skeletal remains have assessed the osteological record in concert with medical writings.[74] Yet, some scholars, such

identification in dental calculus', *Science Advances* 5, no. 1 (2019), https://doi.org/10.1126/sciadv.aau7126; Sam Leggett, 'A Hierarchical Meta-Analytical Approach to Western European Dietary Transitions in the First Millennium AD', *European Journal of Archaeology* 25, no. 4 (2022): 523–43, https://doi.org/10.1017/eaa.2022.23; Tianyi Wang, Craig Cessford, Jenna M. Dittmar, Sarah Inskip, Peter M. Jones, and Piers D. Mitchell, 'Intestinal parasite infection in the Augustinian friars and general population of medieval Cambridge, UK', *International Journal of Paleopathology* 39 (2022): 115–21, https://doi.org/10.1016/j.ijpp.2022.06.001; and Sarah Fiddyment, Natalie J. Goodison, Elma Brenner, Stefania Signorello, Kierri Price, and Matthew J. Collins, 'Girding the loins? Direct evidence of the use of a medieval English parchment birthing girdle from biomolecular analysis', *Royal Society Open Science* 8, no. 3 (2021), https://doi.org/10.1098/rsos.202055.

72 Monica H. Green, 'A New Definition of the Black Death: Genetic Findings and Historical Interpretations', *De Medio Aevo* 11, no. 2 (2022): 139–55, https://doi.org/10.5209/dmae.83788; Robert Hymes and Monica H. Green, *New Evidence for the Dating and Impact of the Black Death in Asia*, ed. Carol Symes (Leeds: Arc Humanities Press, 2022); Monica H. Green, 'The Four Black Deaths', *American Historical Review* 125, no. 5 (2020): 1601–31, https://doi.org/10.1093/ahr/rhaa511; Joris Roosen and Monica H. Green, 'The Mother of All Pandemics: The State of Black Death Research in the Era of COVID-19—Bibliography,' last modified 26 February 2024, last accessed 3 March 2024, https://drive.google.com/file/d/1xoD_dwyAwp9xi9sMCW5UvpGfEVH5J2ZA/view?usp=sharing; Timothy P. Newfield, 'Mysterious and Mortiferous Clouds: The Climate Cooling and Disease Burden of Late Antiquity', in *Environment and Society in the Long Late Antiquity*, ed. Adam Izdebski and Michael Mulryan (Leiden: Brill, 2019), 271–97; Newfield, 'Malaria and Malaria-like Disease'; and Timothy P. Newfield, 'Domesticates, Disease and Climate in Early Post-Classical Europe: The Cattle Plague of c.940 and its Environmental Context', *Postclassical Archaeologies* 5 (2015): 95–126.

73 Piers D. Mitchell, 'Palaeopathology of the Crusades', in *Crusader Landscapes in the Medieval Levant: The Archaeology and History of the Latin East*, ed. Micaela Sinibaldi, Kevin J. Lewis, Balázs Major, and Jennifer A. Thompson (Cardiff: University of Wales Press, 2016), 349–59; Piers D. Mitchell, 'Improving the Use of Historical Written Sources in Paleopathology', *International Journal of Paleopathology* 19 (2017): 88–95, https://doi.org/10.1016/j.ijpp.2016.02.005; and Mitchell, *Medicine in the Crusades*.

74 E.g., Simon Mays, 'A Biomechanical Study of Activity Patterns in a Medieval Human Skeletal Assemblage', *International Journal of Osteoarchaeology* 9, no. 1 (1999): 68–73, https://doi.org/10.1002/(SICI)1099-1212(199901/02)9:1%3C68::AID-OA468%3E3.0.CO;2-M; Joanna R. Sofaer Derevenski, 'Sex Differences in Activity-related Osseous Change

as Clare Pilsworth, have made initial moves in this direction, and these brief investigations have served to emphasise that further research is desperately needed to reassess recipes in the light of skeletal evidence.[75] Part 2 responds to this need, using osteological evidence to reinform our understanding of the recipe literature and its potential applicability to early medieval individuals.

3.4 *Summary*

As the example of Terenti(an)us revealed, the relationship between medical knowledge and practice in the Carolingian world is far from straightforward and, as the preceding pages have demonstrated, requires further study and critical re-examination. This book's dual investigation of the possible practicality and applicability of the medical knowledge recorded in recipes bridge the knowledge-practice divide and provide new perspectives on early medieval medicine. This study, therefore, explores, first, the potential practicality of the recorded knowledge, questioning its useability in the context of therapy rather than presuming an intended use in therapy. That is, do recipes recommend ingredients that could have been sourced in Carolingian Europe? Do recipe collections contain user-friendly features suggestive of their application in medical practice? And secondly, this book investigates whether there is a correlation, a connection, or any overlap between the medical issues recorded in the texts and those seen on skeletons dated to the same period. In other words, is there evidence to suggest that individuals in the early medieval west suffered from the conditions and symptoms described in the texts? These guiding questions consider whether it was possible that those individuals in possession of the recorded medical knowledge could have used the texts in an attempt to treat people during this period. The twin concepts of practicality and applicability thus provide the analytical framework for the book and delineate its use of evidence, with Part 1 a study of practicality and Part 2 an examination of applicability. This dual approach, in conjunction with the examination of a large sample of understudied material, breaks new ground in the field of Carolingian medicine.

---

in the Spine and the Gendered Division of Labor at Ensay and Wharram Percy, UK', *American Journal of Biological Anthropology* 111, no. 3 (2000): 333–54, https://doi.org/10.1002/(sici)1096-8644(200003)111:3%3C333::aid-ajpa4%3E3.0.co;2-k; Fleming, 'Bones for Historians'; and Fleming, 'Writing Biography'.

75 Clare Pilsworth's chapter on diet and health within her study of healthcare in early medieval northern Italy offers one such exception: Pilsworth, *Healthcare in Early Medieval Northern Italy*, 47–72, see especially pp. 68–71 for the section on joint diseases and fractures, 'Joint Conditions and Fractures in the Osteo-Archaeological Evidence'.

4 The Carolingian Context

Before outlining the following chapters, it is essential to address the book's chronological positioning. The date range, *c.* 775–900, covers the 'long ninth century', from the late eighth century to the cusp of the tenth century. This period has been selected on the basis of the manuscript evidence. While this context is discussed in more detail in the following chapter (and the codices themselves are reviewed in Appendix 1), there are several key features to note with respect to the selection of this timeframe. First, based on the surviving evidence, a burst of manuscript production followed the reforming legislation promulgated by Charlemagne's court in the late eighth and early ninth centuries; this increase in the written record can be seen across many genres, and, as noted above, medicine is no exception.[76] While this intensification of manuscript production has meant that a significantly larger number of codices containing medical writings have survived from this period than the preceding centuries, the selected dates are underpinned by more than the sheer number of extant manuscripts.

Although the concept of a Carolingian 'renaissance' has been revised in recent years, the intellectual culture that developed in the wake of the reforms stemming from Charlemagne's court provides the framework within which the written sources must be understood.[77] Despite the fact that, as noted above,

76 On the extant medical manuscripts see Beccaria, *I codici* and Wickersheimer, *Les manuscrits*. On medical texts listed in Carolingian library catalogues, see Glaze, 'The Perforated Wall', 268–71. On writing and manuscript production in the Carolingian period, see McKitterick, *The Carolingians and the Written Word* and Rosamond McKitterick, 'Eighth-Century Foundations', in *The New Cambridge Medieval History* II, *c. 700-c. 900*, ed. Rosamond McKitterick (Cambridge: Cambridge University Press, 1995), 681–94. James Palmer, however, highlights the need for caution when comparing numbers of surviving manuscripts, especially with respect to medicine; see Palmer, 'Merovingian Medicine' and, on the shift from papyrus to parchment, see Dario Internullo, 'Du papyrus au parchemin. Les origines médiévales de la mémoire archivistique en Europe occidentale', *Annales. Histoire, Sciences Sociales* 74, nos. 3–4 (2019): 523–57, https://doi.org/10.1017/ahss.2020.52.

77 Much has been written about the related topics of reform, manuscript production, and literacy in the Carolingian world; for a sample of the range of assessments of the Carolingian 'renaissance' in recent decades, see Giles Brown, 'Introduction: The Carolingian Renaissance', in *Carolingian Culture: Emulation and Innovation*, ed. Rosamond McKitterick (Cambridge: Cambridge University Press, 1994), 1–51; Rosamond McKitterick, 'The Carolingian Renaissance of Culture and Learning', in *Charlemagne: Empire and Society*, ed. Joanna Story (Manchester: Manchester University Press, 2005), 151–66; van Rhijn, *Leading the Way to Heaven*; Carine van Rhijn, 'Manuscripts for local priests and the Carolingian Reforms', in *Men in the Middle: Local Priests in Early Medieval Europe*, ed. Steffen Patzold and Carine van Rhijn (Berlin: De Gruyter, 2016), 177–98; Carine van Rhijn,

early medieval historians have not tended to see medical writing as affected by or contributing to this evolving intellectual culture, Meg Leja has convincingly argued for medicine's direct engagement with these developments.[78] Many of the same impulses seen in other genres of writing, such as legal, liturgical, exegetical, grammatical, and computistical texts, are likewise apparent in the medical literature produced in this period. Recipe collections, for example, bear witness to an interest in compiling and reordering knowledge from earlier sources, a strong focus on the presentation and structure of texts, intersections with other fields of learning, and engagement with contemporary theological discourses.[79] It is therefore essential to study the medical texts written at this time within the particular intellectual and cultural climate in which they were produced in order to grasp more fully their significance.

By beginning this study in *c.* 775, it captures the start of the major increase in manuscript production.[80] This upswing not only provides the sources of this book but also documents the evolving intellectual and cultural environment of the Carolingian world, an environment inherently linked to the ecclesiastical and elite networks of the period. The movement of manuscripts and dissemination of knowledge, themes that emerge in Part 1, were dependent on the intellectual, socio-cultural, ecclesiastical, and political dynamics of this period. In the decades after *c.* 900, changes in these dynamics, including in the intellectual culture of medicine, begin to emerge. Building on the increasing number of medical texts in circulation, scribes and scholars started moving in new directions. A growth in cathedral schools can be seen in France, with centres such as Laon, Chartres, and Reims recorded as places of medical teaching

---

'Charlemagne's *correctio*: A Local Perspective', in *Charlemagne: les temps, les espaces, les hommes. Construction et déconstruction d'un règne*, ed. Rolf Grosse and Michel Sot (Turnhout: Brepols, 2018), 43–59; Janet L. Nelson, 'Revisiting the Carolingian Renaissance', in *Motions of Late Antiquity: Essays on Religion, Politics, and Society in Honour of Peter Brown*, ed. Jamie Kreiner and Helmut Reimitz (Turnhout: Brepols, 2016), 331–46; Rutger Kramer, 'Monasticism, Reform, and Authority in the Carolingian Era', in *The Cambridge History of Medieval Monasticism in the Latin West*, ed. Alison I. Beach and Isabelle Cochelin, vol. 1 (Cambridge: Cambridge University Press, 2020), 432–49; and Rutger Kramer, *Rethinking Authority in the Carolingian Empire: Ideals and Expectations during the Reign of Louis the Pious (813–828)* (Amsterdam: Amsterdam University Press, 2019).

78 Leja, *Embodying the Soul*; Leja, 'The Sacred Art'.

79 Leja, *Embodying the Soul*; Wallis, 'Medicine in Medieval Calendar Manuscripts'; and Claire Burridge, 'Healing Body and Soul in Early Medieval Europe: Medical Remedies with Christian Elements', *Studies in Church History* 58 (2022): 46–67, https://doi.org/10.1017/stc.2022.3.

80 See n. 76 above.

in the tenth century.[81] Around the same period, sites in southern Italy, including Montecassino and Salerno, appear to have begun to reintroduce more theoretical elements into their medical writings.[82] While the growth of a tenth-century 'School of Salerno' continues to be debated, recent work on Cassinese and early Salernitan manuscripts has suggested that new impulses can be seen in the medical literature produced in this period.[83] Simultaneously, the introduction of a basic vocabulary that differentiated between various kinds of medical specialists (i.e., terminology that named physicians, surgeons, herbalists, and bleeders as distinct types of practitioners), reflects further changes in the medical culture of the Latin west around the turn of the millennium.[84]

Determining *c.* 775 to *c.* 900 as the book's chronological focus thus centres the manuscript sample around the shared cultural and intellectual framework of the Carolingian world while avoiding overlap with new developments in the study and recording of medical knowledge that emerged in the wake of the long ninth century. It must be remembered, however, that the selected dates are guidelines rather than strict boundaries, and manuscripts whose dating has been debated or that contain hands dated beyond this timeframe are discussed further in Appendix 1. The dating of archaeological sites, and the osteological remains found within them, must likewise be approached with some degree of flexibility given that a) many sites were used over a longer period of time than the years considered in this book, and b) much dating is relative rather than exact. The specific challenges presented by this material are considered in Chapter 6.

81 Loren C. MacKinney, 'Tenth-Century Medicine as Seen in the *Historia* of Richer of Rheims', *Bulletin of the Institute of the History of Medicine* 2, no. 6 (1934): 347–75; Park, 'Medicine and Society', 66–7; Nutton, 'Early Medieval Medicine and Natural Science', 337; Florence Eliza Glaze, 'Master-Student Medical Dialogues: The Evidence of London, British Library, Sloane 2839', in *Form and Content of Instruction in Anglo-Saxon England in the Light of Contemporary Manuscript Evidence: Papers Presented at the International Conference, Udine, 6–8 April 2006*, ed. Patrizia Lendinara, Loredana Lazzari, and Maria Amalia D'Aronco (Turnhout: Brepols, 2007), 467–94.

82 Wallis, 'The Experience of the Book', 119.

83 Florence Eliza Glaze, 'Gariopontus and the Salernitans: Textual Traditions in the Eleventh and Twelfth Centuries', in *La* Collectio Salernitana *di Salvatore De Renzi. Convegno internazionale, Università degli Studi di Salerno, 18–19 giugno 2007*, ed. Danielle Jacquart and Agostino Paravicini Bagliani (Florence: SISMEL Edizioni del Galluzzo, 2008), 149–90; regarding developments in Cassinese manuscripts, I have also benefitted from hearing Glaze's papers at several conferences, including 'The Confluence of Latin, Byzantine, and Arabic Pharmacy: Southern Italy c. 1050–1150 CE', a paper delivered at 'Drugs in the Medieval World (ca. 1050-ca. 1400)' (King's College London, 7 December 2018).

84 Park, 'Medicine and Society', 70.

5 Structuring the Dual Approach

As noted above, this book is divided into two parts, aligning with its dual approach. Part 1 focuses on the textual evidence for practicality. Chapter 2 introduces the investigation into the question of the recipes' practicality by reviewing the relationship between medical knowledge and practice as documented by the written record and outlining the recipe literature under analysis. Chapters 3–5 each explore a different aspect of the recipe literature's practicality, shedding light on these treatments' potential useability in the context of therapy from multiple directions. Chapter 3 traces the introduction (or, in some cases, reintroduction) of *materia medica* from the east, following the appearance of ingredients such as camphor, musk, and ambergris. Recipes that include these types of exotic products highlight the dynamic nature of this body of knowledge in the Carolingian world and may reflect the practicality of these treatments—if only for a very restricted and elite clientele. Chapter 4 then looks at the other end of the spectrum, turning to the appearance of beer and mead (specifically as *medus*) in medical contexts. The assimilation of these non-classical beverages in medical texts points to the active adaptation of the written record to meet local conditions. While Chapters 3 and 4 concentrate on case studies of ingredients, Chapter 5 examines other features within recipes: units of measurement and the inclusion of instructions for substituting ingredients. By considering how knowledge is presented in recipes, these two aspects explore the practicality of their design, complementing the preceding chapters' focus on the possibility of their use via the availability of ingredients. The combination of case studies thus addresses the potential practicality of the recipe sample from a variety of perspectives to reconsider whether this material was intended to be used in medical practice.

Part 2 unites the textual and skeletal evidence to investigate the potential applicability of this body of knowledge. Chapter 6 introduces the process of reconsidering the recipe literature in view of the evidence provided by the osteological record, addressing key conceptual challenges, such as retrospective diagnosis, and outlining the analytical approach to the following case studies. Chapters 7–9 each concentrate on different types of pathologies that have the potential to be recorded in skeletal remains, using palaeopathological reports from excavations of early medieval burials to re-evaluate the texts. More specifically, Chapter 7 examines dental disease, Chapter 8 considers joint diseases, and Chapter 9 focuses on surgery and trauma.

Bringing together the two approaches, Chapter 10 assesses the findings from both Parts 1 and 2. This chapter concludes with a final reflection on the practicality and applicability of the medical knowledge circulating during the

Carolingian period, the relationship between medical knowledge and practice, and the question of whether these texts may have been used in the practice of medicine. Ultimately, this book's joint investigation of practicality and applicability—underpinned by analyses of traditionally understudied textual sources in concert with osteological evidence—results in the emergence of a more nuanced picture of early medieval health and medicine.

PART 1

Practicality

CHAPTER 2

Setting the Scene

The Texts, Their Contexts, and the Need for a Re-examination of Practicality

1 Introduction: a Mixed Picture of (Im)practicality

Linda Ehrsam Voigts's pathbreaking article, 'Anglo-Saxon Plant Remedies and the Anglo-Saxons', focuses, as its title suggests, on recipe literature in early medieval England.[1] Latin, continental material, however, is never far from view. When detailing the ways in which the Old English translations of Pseudo-Apuleius' *Herbarius* adapted the Latin text and its structure, Voigts makes a direct comparison to a herbal in cod. sang. 217, a ninth-century manuscript produced on the continent and today held in the Stiftsbibliothek St. Gallen.[2] Building on Erhard Landgraf's study of this recipe collection, the *St. Galler Botanicus*, she notes that, of the sixty-two plants it lists, just over half of the entries 'derive from the *Herbarium Apulei*, but twenty-six have no known source, and a number of those seem to be the addition of alpine plants. One finds as well entries which vary from the *Herbarium Apulei* in the addition of such details as *nascitur in excelsis montis juxta aquas*', i.e., a note explaining that the plant in question grows in high mountains.[3] These features have been used to argue that the herbal was composed in a centre of manuscript production within an alpine environment, such as St Gall or a northern Italian site, and by someone familiar with the added plants. Such an interpretation speaks to the practical nature of the herbal and its recipes.[4]

At first glance, this might appear to strengthen the argument that the *St. Galler Botanicus*, and other recipe collections like it, were intended to be used for therapeutic purposes. A closer examination, however, reveals that the evidence cannot provide a concrete foundation for such claims. As Monica

1 Voigts, 'Anglo-Saxon Plant Remedies'. See Chapter 1 for further discussion of this piece and its influence on the field.

2 Voigts, 'Anglo-Saxon Plant Remedies', 256. For an edition of Pseudo-Apuleius' *Herbarius*, see Pseudo-Apuleius. *Herbarius*, in *Antonii Musae De herba vettonica liber. Pseudoapulei Herbarius. Anonymi De taxone liber. Sexti Placiti Liber medicinae ex animalibus etc.*, ed. Ernst Howald and Henry E. Sigerist. CML 4 (Leipzig: Teubner, 1927), 15–225.

3 Voigts, 'Anglo-Saxon Plant Remedies', 256; Erhard Landgraf, 'Ein frühmittelalterlicher Botanicus', *Kyklos* 1 (1928): 114–46.

4 Ibid.

 | DOI:10.1163/9789004466173_003

Niederer, who has more recently published a critical edition, translation, and commentary of the *St. Galler Botanicus*, points out, it is dangerous to jump to conclusions regarding the manuscript's context of production and intended use(s) based on this evidence alone since such textual adaptations could have occurred for a host of reasons:

> The only certainty is that some exotic, oriental plants are actually left out of the work and that some of the newly added [plants] are said to grow in the mountains. As the only argument, however, this is not enough for localisation: exotic drugs were difficult to obtain and very expensive throughout the Latin west and therefore could easily have been deleted from the recipe texts. And 'mountains' as a way to localise the origin of the text is far too imprecise: even if one assumes that the Alps are meant, that is still a very large area.[5]

Niederer's perceptive analysis offers an important counterbalance to many of the arguments regarding the practicality of recipe literature—and the assumption, constructed partly on these arguments, that such writings were, by definition, intended to be used in practice (see Chapter 1). Likewise, as Florence Eliza Glaze and Faith Wallis have highlighted, some medical texts, including recipes, appear to have been so altered by the process of copying and re-copying (resulting in, for example, changed meanings, Greek to Latin translation errors, and other corruptions), that they would not have been useable in the context of therapy.[6] Peregrine Horden's emphasis on the multiple ways in which medical manuscripts could have been read is also essential to bear in mind: although a recipe collection may have been recorded with the intention to use the recipes in practice, this remains but one possibility.[7]

Overall, while many scholars have put forward compelling arguments for the practical features exhibited by recipe collections and documented evidence for the use of the manuscripts in which they are located, the cautionary

5 *Der St. Galler* Botanicus, ed. and trans. Niederer, 29: 'Sicher ist nur, dass tatsächlich manche exotischen, orientalischen Pflanzen aus der Vorlage weggelassen sind, und dass von manchen der neu hinzugefügten gesagt wird, sie wüchsen im Gebirge. Als einziges Argument reicht das jedoch nicht aus zur Lokalisierung: Exotische Drogen waren im ganzen lateinischen Abendland schwer zu beschaffen und sehr teuer und hätten daher leicht aus den Rezepttexten gestrichen werden können. Und 'Gebirge' als Lokalisierungshilfe für die Entstehung des Textes ist viel zu ungenau: Selbst wenn man annimmt, dass damit die Alpen gemeint sind, ist das immer noch ein sehr grosses Gebiet'.

6 Glaze, 'The Perforated Wall', 5–6; Wallis, 'Signs and Senses', 273.

7 Horden, 'Prefatory Note'.

remarks of Niederer, Glaze, Wallis, and Horden underscore the need for more critical analyses that approach the texts without assuming that they were necessarily intended to be used in the practice of medicine. This chapter, therefore, provides an introduction to Part 1 by opening with the bigger picture: I survey textual sources beyond the recipe literature to consider a wider range of evidence for the potential practicality (or impracticality) of recipes and examine whether there are external signs that these texts were consulted for therapeutic purposes. I then turn to the recipes under analysis and their manuscript contexts, reviewing the textual evidence that underpins this book.

2 Contextualising Medicine's Place in Early Medieval Europe and the Question of Practicality

Chapter 1 showcased how research into the corpus of surviving Old English recipes has moved the study of the relationship between medical knowledge and practice in new directions, often positing that these texts were not only *intended* to be used in the context of therapy but that they were, in fact, *useable* texts. Such arguments have offered direct challenges to the traditional view that the presumed non-local nature of many of the ingredients named in recipes would have rendered them useless in practice.[8] Voigts's aforementioned landmark article challenges this assumption, among others; she contends that a wider range of plants could have been growing in England than might have been expected due to a combination of 'auspicious climatic conditions' and careful cultivation. Voigts also suggests that other, non-local *materia medica* could have been acquired through trade.[9] Regarding the latter possibility, however, a letter from the Insular world exchanged between Cynehard (d. *c.* 778), bishop of Winchester, and Lull (d. 786), archbishop of Mainz (though originally from Wessex), presents a different scenario: it documents instead the challenge posed by procuring particular ingredients and underlines that, for all their practical features, recipes could still present impracticalities.

In his letter, Cynehard complains to Lull that many exotic ingredients listed in medical texts 'are unknown to us and difficult to come by', asking his continental colleague to send supplies.[10] Despite coming from beyond the

8 E.g., Grattan and Singer, *Anglo-Saxon Magic and Medicine*, 28.

9 Voigts, 'Anglo-Saxon Plant Remedies', 266.

10 Faith Wallis, *Medieval Medicine: A Reader* (Toronto: University of Toronto Press, 2010), 110–11; 'Epistula 114', in *Die Briefe des heiligen Bonifatius und Lullus*, ed. Michael Tangl, *MGH Epistulae selectae* 1 (Berlin: Weidmann, 1916), 247 (see n. 13 below for the Latin text).

Carolingian world, this epistle has three significant implications for the present study. First, Cynehard's complaint indicates that some communities in eighth-century England were encountering challenges in sourcing all the ingredients listed in recipes, raising the possibility that people in Carolingian Francia may have experienced similar problems. This lack of access would have made certain recipes impractical since, at least in their recorded state, they would have been unusable. Although Cynehard's attempts to obtain the specified ingredients exhibit no signs of attempted substitutions, it remains possible that recipes could have been adapted *in situ* by replacing unavailable *materia medica* with local products.[11] Two chapters in Part 1 address these topics specifically, with Chapter 3 investigating the potential practicality of recipes in relation to their inclusion of non-local *materia medica* and Chapter 5 considering the presence of instructions for the substitution of ingredients.

On the other hand, Cynehard's letter reflects that Lull, situated in the middle of the Frankish Empire, may have had better access to foreign products, or at least that Cynehard expected (or hoped) this was the case. Indeed, Lull, along with two other missionaries, Denehard and Burchard, is recorded as having sent a gift of frankincense, pepper, and cinnamon to the English abbess Cuneburg earlier in the eighth century—did Cynehard know of this gift?[12] Was he, in effect, asking for a similar package to be sent in his direction? As will be explored in Chapter 3, a number of records of elite gift exchange on the continent feature non-local products that could have served as *materia medica*—was Cynehard trying to insert himself into this gift economy?

Finally, the letter indicates that Cynehard was, in fact, consulting the medical remedies listed in his codices with the intention of preparing them. In the same letter, he also writes, 'if you should come into the possession of any books of secular learning unknown to us, for example, concerning medicines—of which we have a goodly quantity here ... you might consider sharing them [with us]'.[13] Cynehard's comments thus provide direct evidence for the desire

11 Voigts, 'Anglo-Saxon Plant Remedies', 250–68.

12 'Epistula 49', in *Die Briefe des heiligen Bonifatius und Lullus*, ed. Tangl, 78–80. The gifts are described on p. 80: *Parva quoque munusculorum transmisio scedulam istam comitatur, quae sunt tria, id est turis et piperis et cinnamomi permodi*[*c*]*a* [*x*]*enia, sed omni mentis affectione destinata.*

13 Wallis, *Medieval Medicine*, 110–11; 'Epistula 114', in *Die Briefe des heiligen Bonifatius und Lullus*, ed. Tangl, 246–7: *Et hoc petimus, si qua apud vos solamina nobis necessaria vel ignota, spiritalis quidem scientiae sive in libris antiquis, qui a nobis habentur, sive in aliis ecclesiasticis administrationibus, ut nobis libenter participare non negetis. Nec non et, si quos saecularis scientiae libros nobis ignotos adepturi sitis, ut sunt de medicinalibus, quorum copia est aliqua apud nos, sed tamen* [*p*]*igmenta ultramarina, quae in eis scripta conperimus, ignota nobis sunt et difficilia adipiscendum, vel si qua in aliis quibuslibet negotiis*

to apply the medical knowledge recorded in the texts in practice. Crucially, this letter highlights that an intention to follow a recipe does not necessarily reflect its practicality with respect to use: Cynehard was unable to put his recorded medical knowledge *into* practice because he lacked certain ingredients. The following sections review additional evidence from non-medical texts that speak to the potential (im)practicality of recipes. As Cynehard's experience demonstrates, it is essential to consider practicality at two levels: intention (i.e., were recipes understood as being intended for therapeutic purposes?) and use (i.e., if they were intended to be used, could they be followed?). Cynehard's unequivocal statement regarding his attempt to prepare treatments based on his recipe collections provides a notable window onto the relationship between medical knowledge and practice, especially because, as will become apparent over the following pages, such clear evidence testifying to the use of recipes in the context of therapy, whether intended or actualised, is exceedingly rare in the Carolingian world.

Before reviewing non-medical textual evidence for the perception and practice of medicine in Carolingian Francia, it is important to acknowledge some of the major ways in which the general healthscape of the Latin west evolved over the preceding centuries. The interrelated social, cultural, intellectual, political, economic, and religious shifts of late Antiquity altered not only the medical marketplace and approaches to healing, but also the study and transmission of medical knowledge.[14] Such changes likewise had major implications for the survival of evidence relating to medicine, from the ways in which it was studied, practised, and perceived to the types of medical texts recorded, excerpted, compiled, and (re)copied. Much has been written about these topics in recent years and what follows presents a brief overview in relation to evidence that

---

vel speciebus nobis necessariis providetis, communicare dignemini, ut fecistis villosam mittendo.

14 For broader overviews of late Antiquity and the transition to the early Middle Ages, see, for example, Peter Brown, *The Making of Late Antiquity* (Cambridge, MA: Harvard University Press, 1978); Averil Cameron, *The Mediterranean World of Late Antiquity, 395–700 AD*, 2nd ed. Abingdon: Routledge, 2012); G. W. Bowersock, Peter Brown, and Oleg Grabar, eds., *Late Antiquity: A Guide to the Postclassical World* (Cambridge, MA: Belknap Press, 1999); and the volumes stemming from the ESF project 'Transformation of the Roman World' (1992–97), e.g., Inge Lyse Hansen and Chris Wickham, eds., *The Long Eighth Century. Production, Distribution and Demand* (Leiden: Brill, 2000); Richard Corradini, Max Diesenberger, and Helmut Reimitz, eds., *The Construction of Communities in the Early Middle Ages. Texts, Resources and Artefacts* (Leiden: Brill, 2003); and Frans Theuws and Janet L. Nelson, eds., *Rituals of Power: From Late Antiquity to the Early Middle Ages* (Leiden: Brill, 2000).

helps to elucidate how, why, and where medical texts, and especially those concerning pharmacy, were read and written in the Latin west.[15]

Given medicine's complex relationship with the Church, the spread of Christianity, and its concomitant restructuring of communities and power dynamics, is among the most significant developments to highlight during this period. Notably, this evolving relationship is documented by a wealth of non-medical sources, ranging from hagiographies and histories to the writings of the Church Fathers.[16] Some texts paint doctors and classical medical traditions—a 'religion of Hippocrates' as described by Owsei Temkin—in a negative light by recording the ineffectiveness of medicine in comparison with divine healing or raising concerns with its pre-Christian roots.[17] A number of Church authorities, including Gregory the Great (d. 604), even questioned the appropriateness of human intervention in matters of health and disease, life and death.[18] Yet, as Peregrine Horden cautions, the apparent 'tensions between religion and medicine should not be overstressed'.[19] Not only do diatribes against doctors and medical practice *underline* their presence and perceived efficacy among the general populace, but, more significantly, 'secular' medicine was often viewed positively and as a divinely provided complement to spiritual healing.[20] Indeed, the Christian emphasis on charity made caring for the sick a virtuous act and fostered the rise of hospitals, while theologians turned to

15 For more detailed accounts of the state of medicine in late Antiquity and the transition to the early Middle Ages in relation to wider social, cultural, intellectual, political, economic, and religious shifts, see, for example, Nutton, *Ancient Medicine*, 299–317; Horden, 'What's Wrong with Early Medieval Medicine?'; Peregrine Horden, 'Sickness and Healing', in *The Cambridge History of Christianity 3: Early Medieval Christianities, c. 600–1100*, ed. Thomas F. X. Noble and Julia M. H. Smith (Cambridge: Cambridge University Press, 2008), 416–32; Palmer, 'Merovingian Medicine'.

16 Jonathan L. Zecher, *Spiritual Direction as a Medical Art in Early Christian Monasticism* (Oxford: Oxford University Press, 2022); Andrew Crislip, *Thorns in the Flesh: Illness and Sanctity in Late Ancient Christianity* (Philadelphia: University of Pennsylvania Press, 2013); Gary B. Ferngren, *Medicine and Health Care in Early Christianity* (Baltimore: Johns Hopkins University Press, 2009).

17 Owsei Temkin, *Hippocrates in a World of Pagans and Christians* (Baltimore: Johns Hopkins University Press, 1995), 181. Healing miracles make frequent appearances in hagiographical writings; on Caesarius of Arles' concerns about pagan influences, see Caesarius of Arles, *Sermons*, trans. Mary Magdeleine Mueller, 3 vols. (Washington, D.C.: Catholic University of America Press, 1956), vol. 1, Sermons 52 and 53, at pp. 259–65.

18 Gregory the Great wrote that the 'gift' of sickness should be endured (though he does not appear to have always heeded his own advice): Gregory the Great, *The Book of Pastoral Rule*, trans. James Barmby (Buffalo: Christian Literature Publishing Co., 1895), 35.

19 Horden, 'Sickness and Healing', 101.

20 Nutton, *Ancient Medicine*, 312–17; Horden, 'Sickness and Healing', 100–3.

medical imagery, such as the *Christus medicus* metaphor, and engaged with a 'Galenic logic of practice' to convey their interpretations of doctrine and provide guidance to their communities.[21] The accommodation or appropriation of classical and late antique medical knowledge had profound effects, marking this body of scholarship as (largely) acceptable within a Christian intellectual culture, if used with the acknowledgement that successful healing ultimately depended on God.

With theologians in the Greek east presenting more (and more diverse) examples of sustained engagement with medical writings in their works, the relatively few Latin authorities, such as Cassiodorus (d. *c.* 585) and Isidore (d. 636), who offered explicit statements on the practice and study of medicine became particularly impactful in shaping perspectives in the early medieval west. Cassiodorus, a scholar and Roman civil servant of the Ostrogothic regime, founded a monastery in southern Italy, Vivarium, and composed a text, the *Institutiones*, to guide this community in their pursuit of both divine and secular learning.[22] Medical matters feature within his guidance: in line with the positive attitude towards healing evinced by many intellectuals of the period, he admonished the monks to help those afflicted by illness and disease with medicines and with hope in God, 'emphasizing the eternal rewards granted to

21 Ferngren, *Medicine and Health Care*. On hospitals, see Andrew T. Crislip, *From Monastery to Hospital: Christian Monasticism & the Transformation of Health Care in Late Antiquity* (Ann Arbor: University of Michigan Press, 2005); and especially the work of Peregrine Horden, including, Peregrine Horden, 'Alms and the Man: Hospital Founders in Byzantium', in *The Impact of Hospitals, 300–2000*, ed. John Henderson, Peregrine Horden, and Alessandro Pastore (Oxford: Peter Lang, 2007), 59–76; Peregrine Horden, 'Poverty, Charity, and the Invention of the Hospital', in *The Oxford Handbook of Late Antiquity*, ed. Scott Fitzgerald Johnson (Oxford: Oxford University Press, 2012), 715–43; and Peregrine Horden, 'Cities Within Cities: Early Hospital Foundations and Urban Space', in *Stiftungen zwischen Politik und Wirtshaft. Ein Dialog zwischen Geschichte und Gegenwart*, ed. Sitta von Reden (Berlin: De Gruyter, 2015), 157–75. On the use of medical imagery and ideas in theological writings, see, for example, Marie-Anne Vannier, 'L'image du Christ médecin chez les pères', in *Les Pères de l'Église face à la science médicale de leur temps*, ed. Véronique Boudon-Millot and Bernard Pouderon (Paris: Beauchesne, 2005), 525–34; Michael Dörnemann, 'Einer ist Arzt, Christus: Medizinales Verständnis von Erlösung in der Theologie der griechischen Kirchenväter des zweiten bis vierten Jahrhunderts', *Zeitschrift für antikes Christentum/Journal of Ancient Christianity* 17 (2013): 102–24, https://doi.org/10.1515/zac-2013-0006; and, on the 'Galenic logic of practice', Zecher, *Spiritual Direction*, 23–196, and especially at pp. 32–3.

22 Cassiodorus, *Cassiodori Senatoris Institutiones*, ed. R. A. B. Mynors (Oxford: Clarendon Press, 1937); for an English translation, see Cassiodorus, *Institutions of Divine and Secular Learning*, in *Cassiodorus,* Institutions of Divine and Secular Learning *and* On the Soul, trans. James W. Halporn (Liverpool: Liverpool University Press, 2004).

those who charitably heal the sick'.[23] Carolingian theologians would build on Cassiodorus' instructions, framing the practice of medicine as a 'sacred art'.[24]

In addition to articulating a general conception of medicine's place in a Christian community, Cassiodorus also provided very specific details for the monks of Vivarium, recommending a selection of Greek medical writings in Latin translations.[25] This list reveals a group of treatises that were accessible to a primarily Latin-speaking community and that he considered acceptable for a Christian audience. Cassiodorus included a herbal of Dioscorides, Latin translations of Hippocrates and Galen, 'a certain anonymous work that has been collected from various authors', Caelius Aurelius' *Medicine*, and 'various other works ... I have left to you'.[26] Although Cassiodorus' ambiguous phrasing and nonstandard names of authors and their works have puzzled modern historians (e.g., should 'Caelius Aurelius' be interpreted as 'Caelius Aurelianus'?), surviving Carolingian copies of the texts it is thought that he suggested, in concert with evidence from extant ninth-century library catalogues, illustrate that these writings circulated in Carolingian Europe.[27] Such findings not only bear witness to his long-term impact on the perception of medicine but also reflect his influence on the transmission of medical knowledge itself.

Moreover, Cassiodorus' practical approach to medicine aligns with comments on medical care recorded in monastic rules, such as the *Rule of St Benedict*. Chapter 36 of this rule, for example, instructs monastic communities to care for their sick brothers, stipulating that there should be a designated

---

23 Cassiodorus, *Cassiodori Senatoris Institutiones*, 78; Leja, *Embodying the Soul*, 106.

24 Leja, *Embodying the Soul*; Leja, 'The Sacred Art'.

25 Cassiodorus, *Cassiodori Senatoris Institutiones*, 78–9.

26 Cassiodorus, *Cassiodori Senatoris Institutiones*, 78–9: *Quod si vobis non fuerit Graecarum litterarum nota facundia, in primis habetis* Herbarium *Dioscoridis, qui herbas agrorum mirabili proprietate disseruit atque depinxit; post haec legite Hippocratem atque Galienum Latina lingua conversos, id est* Tharapeutica *Galieni ad philosophum Glauconem destinata, et anonymum quendam, qui ex diversis auctoribus probatur esse collectus. Deinde Caeli Aureli* de Medicina *et Hippocratis* de Herbis et Curis *diversosque alios medendi arte compositos, quos vobis in bibliothecae nostrae sinibus reconditos Deo auxiliante dereliqui.* Translation from: Cassiodorus, *Institutions of Divine and Secular Learning*, trans. Halporn, 166.

27 On the question of identifying the texts, see Pierre Courcelle, *Late Latin Writers and Their Greek Sources*, trans. Harry E. Wedeck (Cambridge, MA: Harvard University Press, 1969), 403. For mentions of medical texts in surviving early medieval library catalogues, see Glaze, 'The Perforated Wall', 268–91. On early medieval catalogues (with a focus on those from Lorsch), see Angelika Häse, *Mittelalterliche Bücherverzeichnisse aus Kloster Lorsch. Einleitung, Edition und Kommentar* (Wiesbaden: Harrassowitz, 2002).

room, complete with a 'God-fearing' attendant, for the ill and infirm.[28] Certain regulations, such as the prohibition on meat consumption (or at least the meat of four-footed animals), were also relaxed for the sick.[29] While recent scholarship has challenged the 'misleadingly tidy picture' presented by Benedict of Aniane regarding the evolution of monastic rules as well as the immediate impact of the series of councils at Aachen in the early ninth century that established the *Rule of St Benedict* as the standard rule guiding monastic communities, the prescriptive perspective of such a text can illuminate common ideals and underlying attitudes.[30] In this case, it suggests that caring for a community's infirm and elderly members was an expected feature of monastic life.

However, just as with hospitals in this period, 'care' should not be conflated with 'cure'. Furthermore, acts of both caring and curing could concern the health of the soul rather than or alongside the body.[31] In other words, although the *Rule of St Benedict* supports caring for the sick, its instructions do not refer to medical interventions as part of this care (aside from the possible therapeutic benefits resulting from relaxed bathing and dietary rules). On this point, the so-called *Plan of St Gall*, cod. sang. 1092, offers further insights.[32] While this manuscript, sent by the monks of Reichenau to Abbot Gozbert of St Gall (816–37), may look like an architectural blueprint, the diagram is now

---

28 *RB 1980: The Rule of St. Benedict in Latin and English with Notes*, ed. and trans. Timothy Fry (Collegeville, MN: Liturgical Press, 1981), Chapter 36.

29 *RB 1980*, ed. and trans. Fry, Chapters 36–7, 39.

30 Felice Lifshitz, 'The Historiography of Central Medieval Western Monasticism', in *The Cambridge History of Medieval Monasticism in the Latin West*, ed. Alison I. Beach and Isabelle Cochelin, vol. 1 (Cambridge: Cambridge University Press, 2020), 365–81. For recent approaches, see especially Albrecht Diem, 'Inventing the Holy Rule: Some Observations on the History of Monastic Normative Observance in the Early Medieval West', in *Western Monasticism* ante litteram*: The Spaces of Monastic Observance in Late Antiquity and the Early Middle Ages*, ed. Hendrik Dey and Elizabeth Fentress (Turnhout: Brepols, 2011), 53–84; Albrecht Diem and Claudia Rapp, 'The Monastic Laboratory: Perspectives of Research in Late Antique and Early Medieval Monasticism', in *The Cambridge History of Medieval Monasticism in the Latin West*, ed. Alison I. Beach and Isabelle Cochelin, vol. 1 (Cambridge: Cambridge University Press, 2020), 19–39; Albrecht Diem and Philip Rousseau, 'Monastic Rules (Fourth to Ninth Century)', in *The Cambridge History of Medieval Monasticism in the Latin West*, ed. Alison I. Beach and Isabelle Cochelin, vol. 1 (Cambridge: Cambridge University Press, 2020), 162–94 (quotation at p. 163); and Kramer, 'Monasticism, Reform, and Authority in the Carolingian Era'.

31 Horden, 'Sickness and Healing'; Nutton, *Ancient Medicine*, 315.

32 Cod. sang. 1092. On the *Plan*, see Barbara Schedl, *Der Plan von St. Gallen: Ein Modell europäischer Klosterkultur* (Vienna: Böhlau, 2014) and Walter Horn and Ernest Born, *The Plan of St. Gall: A Study of the Architecture and Economy of, and Life in a Paradigmatic Carolingian Monastery*, 3 vols. (Berkeley, CA: University of California Press, 1979).

thought to represent an idealised vision of a monastic centre. The detailed drawing provides a wealth of information, specifying even the plants growing in the diagram's three gardens. Within the *Plan*, a substantial amount of space is dedicated not simply to caring for the sick but also to therapeutic practices: in addition to separate quarters for the sick, as required by the *Rule of St Benedict*, the *Plan* includes a bloodletting room, physician's quarters, and even a storeroom for the drugs involved in treatment (*armarium pigmentorum*). Complementing these therapeutic spaces, one of the *Plan*'s gardens, appropriately located next to the infirmary, is designed to grow medicinal plants; named herbs include costmary, mint, pennyroyal, rue, and sage—all products that feature as ingredients in medical recipes.[33]

Like the preceding examples, however, it is important recognise the normative nature of this remarkable source: it reflects an ideal rather than direct evidence for medical practices on the ground. Yet, it remains noteworthy that this diagram affords medical care so much space *and* depicts it in such detail. Even though such a plan was never actualised in St Gall, it reveals a positive attitude towards healing and healthcare. Nevertheless, despite the detailed nature of the *Plan*, the manuscript does not shed light on the relationship between medical knowledge and practice. Was there a space for books in the infirmary or would the medical manuscripts of St Gall have been located in the monastery's main library? Given Cassiodorus' general advice and list of works intended to be used in the context of therapy, it seems likely that the community's medical and pharmaceutical writings—some of which have survived and are central to the following chapters' analyses—were expected to be consulted for therapeutic purposes. The works of Isidore of Seville, however, offer a cogent reminder that such a purpose was but one of many possible options and that, especially within the Christian environments in which such material was copied and read, texts could have multiple, layered functions.

Isidore's *Etymologiae*, a twenty-book encyclopaedia addressing all areas of knowledge, represents one of the most influential works of the period: the latest survey of early medieval manuscripts containing the text (including fragments) has identified over 400 manuscript witnesses from before the year 1000.[34] Significantly, medicine is allocated an entire book, *De medicina*, and

33 In cod. sang. 1092, these are listed as *costo*, *menta*, *pulegio*, *ruta*, and *saluia*; Horn and Born, *The Plan of St. Gall*, 181–3. See Chapter 4 for further discussion of gardens and local *materia medica*.

34 Evina Steinová, 'The Oldest Manuscript Tradition of the *Etymologiae* (Eighty Years after A. E. Anspach)', *Visigothic Symposium* 4 (2020–21): 100–43, https://doi.org/10.17613/ehr8-5c39. For the text, see Isidore of Seville, *Etymologiarum sive originum, libri xx*, ed. W. M. Lindsay, 2 vols. (Oxford: Oxford University Press, 1911); and for an English translation, see

appears immediately after the three opening books on the liberal arts, though topics related to health and medicine can also be found throughout the entire encyclopaedia.[35] Book 11, 'The human being and portents' (*De homine et portentis*), Book 17, 'Rural matters' (*De rebus rusticis*), and Book 20, 'Provisions and various implements' (untitled in early manuscripts), for example, each contain content with direct relevance to medical knowledge, such as a description of the human body as well as information regarding substances that could have been used as *materia medica*. Within *De medicina*, Isidore reviews a wide range of medical matters, including the history of medicine, the concept of the four humours, acute and chronic diseases, types of remedies and medications, varieties of medical books, physicians' instruments, and scents and ointments, ending with a section on the 'foundations of medicine' (*De initiis medicinae*), which outlines the basic educational requirements of this 'Second Philosophy'.[36]

While Isidore's overview of medicine covers much ground, it is fairly superficial and would have provided little in the way of practical guidance. Rather, it demonstrates how medical knowledge could be redeployed for Christian learning: the medical information he recorded was 'intended to be studied as words'.[37] And, as Meg Leja points out, by focusing attention on the art of medicine and its various components, Isidore 'implicitly classified it as something essential for future Christian societies'; that is, medical knowledge, including material derived from non-Christian classical and late antique writers, had a place within the pastoral and pedagogical project of the early medieval west.[38] Moreover, as Jacques Fontaine has argued, the Carolingian reception of the *Etymologiae* introduced new layers of allegorical interpretation.[39] Hrabanus Maurus (d. 856), archbishop of Mainz, for example, produced an encyclopaedia, *De rerum naturis* (also known as *De universo*) that reordered and adapted

Isidore of Seville, *The Etymologies of Isidore of Seville*, trans. Stephen A. Barney, W. J. Lewis, J. A. Beach, and Oliver Berghof (Cambridge: Cambridge University Press, 2006). On the general reception of the *Etymologiae*, see Andrew T. Fear and Jamie Wood, eds., *Isidore of Seville and His Reception in the Early Middle Ages: Transmitting and Transforming Knowledge* (Amsterdam: Amsterdam University Press, 2016).

35 See Isidore, *Etymologiae*, Book 4. On Isidore and medicine, see especially Arsenio Ferraces Rodríguez, ed., *"Isidorus medicus": Isidoro de Sevilla y los textos de medicina* (A Coruña: Servizio de Publicacións, Universidade da Coruña, 2005).

36 On *De initiis medicinae*, see Isidore, *Etymologiae*, 4.13.

37 Nutton, *Ancient Medicine*, 301.

38 Leja, *Embodying the Soul*, 105.

39 Jacques Fontaine, 'Isidore de Séville et la mutation de l'encyclopédisme antique', *Cahiers d'Histoire Mondiale* 9, no. 1 (1966): 519–38.

the *Etymologiae*, creating a new composition that was designed to be used as 'a reference tool for the practice of biblical interpretation'.[40] While Hrabanus included comments on medicine within his work, he excerpted only a fraction of the content covered by Isidore's *De medicina* and, according to Frederick Paxton, placed this material 'in the least prominent position possible, at the end of book eighteen, after a series of chapters on weights, measures, numbers, and music and its parts'.[41] Hrabanus' other writings that touch on medicine, such as his commentary on *Ecclesiasticus*, underscore his position on the subject. Although Hrabanus concurred with this biblical book's praise for doctors—praise rooted in the argument that earthly medicine was, after all, created by God and thus inherently good—he immediately reinterpreted the passage, taking it as commentary on spiritual physicians: 'Ben Sira's praise for doctors and medicine is read as praise for clerics and the methods they use to cure sick souls'.[42]

While Hrabanus' positive references to medicine have long been seen as his support not only for medical practice but also medicine's inclusion in the standard curriculum, Paxton's close readings of his metaphorical uses and allegorical interpretations of the medical art suggest otherwise.[43] Yet, even if Hrabanus' medical metaphors cannot be used as strong evidence for the subject's integration within a general educational programme in the Carolingian period, the frameworks provided by the writings of Cassiodorus and Isidore still suggest that this was a possibility. In fact, until at least the seventh century, there appears to have been a specialised medical school in Ravenna that followed a curriculum based on the Galenic canon established at Alexandria.[44]

40 Frederick S. Paxton, 'Curing Bodies—Curing Souls: Hrabanus Maurus, Medical Education, and the Clergy in Ninth-Century Francia', *Journal of the History of Medicine and Allied Sciences* 50, no. 2 (1995): 230–52, at p. 241.

41 Paxton, 'Curing Bodies—Curing Souls', 247; Hrabanus Maurus, *De universo* 18.5, *PL* 111, cols. 500–4.

42 Paxton, 'Curing Bodies—Curing Souls', 243.

43 Paxton, 'Curing Bodies—Curing Souls'. Cf. MacKinney, *Early Medieval Medicine*, 94–5; Loren C. MacKinney, 'Medical Education in the Middle Ages', *Cahiers d'histoire mondiale* 2, no. 4 (1955): 835–61, at p. 846; Richard Kieckhefer, *Magic in the Middle Ages* (Cambridge: Cambridge University Press, 1990), 58.

44 On Ravenna's medical school, see Nicoletta Palmieri, 'Il galenismo alessandrino in Italia tra antichità tarda e alto medioevo', in *La conoscenza scientifica nell'alto medioevo: Spoleto, 25 aprile-1 maggio 2019*, Settimane 67, vol. 1 (Spoleto: Fondazione Centro italiano di studi sull'alto medioevo, 2020), 237–70; Nicoletta Palmieri, 'Nouvelles remarques sur les commentaires à Galien de l'école médicale de Ravenne', in *«Docente natura». Mélanges de médecine ancienne et médiévale offerts à Guy Sabbah*, ed. Armelle Debru and Nicoletta Palmieri (Saint-Étienne: Publications de l'Université de Saint-Étienne, 2001), 209–46; and, for a summary of current scholarship, Judith Herrin, *Ravenna: Capital of Empire, Crucible*

However, while some scholars, such as Loren MacKinney and John Contreni, have identified a handful of intellectual centres, such as Laon and Chartres, as possible hubs of medical learning in the early medieval west, it would be inappropriate to see these cathedral schools as continuations of the classical and late antique medical schools.[45] On the other hand, additional indirect evidence, including the writings of individual Carolingian intellectuals, such as Walahfrid Strabo (d. 849), Lupus of Ferrières (d. *c.* 862), and Pardulus of Laon (d. *c.* 865), reveal that their authors acquired some level of medical knowledge, supporting the idea that medicine did, in fact, feature within the general curriculum in many communities.[46]

In a letter sent by Pardulus to Hincmar of Reims (d. 882), for example, Pardulus shares dietary advice with his unwell superior, aiming to rebalance his humours and restore his health. As part of his recommendations, he writes, 'when rising from table, one should take a measure of beans that have been thoroughly purged and cooked with very clear fat. Although according to the philosophers this is said to dull the senses, it is nonetheless believed to evacuate and dry out phlegm'.[47] While this epistle documents ecclesiastical elites engaging with learned medicine in a practical, hands-on way, Pardulus does not comment on where he gained his medical knowledge. His references to philosophers, descriptions of dietetic approaches to finding humoral balance, and use of specific terminology (such as *hygeia*) imply a familiarity with the types of writings circulating during this period. Pardulus' letter is thus highly suggestive that recipes and other medical texts were studied with the intent

of Europe (London: Allen Lane, 2020), 239–44. On the Alexandrian curriculum, see, in addition to Nicoletta Palmieri's works cited above, Ivan Garofalo and Amneris Roselli, eds., *Galenismo e medicina tardoantica. Fonti greche, latine e arabe. Atti del Seminario internazionale di Siena, Certosa di Pontignano, 9 e 10 settembre 2002* (Naples: Istituto Universitario Orientale, 2003).

45 MacKinney, *Early Medieval Medicine*; MacKinney, 'Tenth-Century Medicine'; John J. Contreni, 'Masters and Medicine in Northern France in the Reign of Charles the Bald', in *Charles the Bald: Court and Kingdom. Papers Based on a Colloquium Held in London in April 1979*, edited by Margaret T. Gibson and Janet Nelson, 2nd ed. (Aldershot: Variorum, 1990), 267–82.

46 For examples of Carolingian intellectuals who demonstrate some degree of medical learning in their surviving writings, see especially Contreni, 'Masters and Medicine'. On medicine as part of a general education, see Palmer, 'Merovingian Medicine'.

47 Contreni, 'Masters and Medicine', 282: *In ultimo, antequam surgatur a mensa, faba purgatissima cum purissimo pingui ad mensuram decocta sumatur; quae licet secundum philosophos sensum obtundere dicatur, tamen phlegmata et deponere et exsiccare creditur.* Translation from Wallis, *Medieval Medicine*, 111–12.

of applying this knowledge in therapy, though it does not provide explicit evidence of this practice.

In contrast, in the tenth and eleventh centuries, the period immediately following this study, the use of medical texts, and specifically pharmaceutical prescriptions, for therapeutic purposes is clearly recorded in letters exchanged among the ecclesiastical elite. The writings of Richer of Reims (d. after 998) or Fulbert of Chartres (d. 1028), for instance, indicate that medical texts were studied and consulted to prepare medications.[48] In a letter to Bishop Adalbero of Laon, Fulbert writes that he is sending several medications to help treat Ebalus, Adalbero's secretary, who is suffering from an unnamed illness.[49] Fulbert specifically recommends referring to the *antidotaria* (books of antidotes) in Laon if Adalbero needs guidance on 'what these [medications] are good for and how to take or to administer them'.[50] Yet, given the shifting landscape of medical learning discussed in Chapter 1, the comments of Richer and Fulbert should not be assumed to reflect the ways in which Carolingian scribes, readers, and medical practitioners engaged with their medical texts.

Returning to the ninth century, Walahfrid Strabo's poem *Hortulus* offers a window onto the author's first-hand knowledge of gardening while also showcasing his familiarity with possible medical uses for many of the plants growing in his 'little garden'. Significantly, Walahfrid begins the poem with a comment on how he has learnt about gardening, listing his own experiences in the garden alongside the knowledge he has acquired from books and picked up from oral traditions:

> A quiet life has many rewards: not least of these
> Is the joy that comes to him who devotes himself to the art
> They knew at Paestum, and learns the ancient skill of obscene
> Priapus—the joy that comes of devoting himself to a garden…
> This I have learnt not only from common opinion
> And searching about in old books, but from experience—
> Experience of hard work and sacrifice of many days
> When I might have rested, but chose instead to labor.[51]

48 Richer of Reims, *Histoire de France*, ed. and trans. Robert Latouche, 2 vols. (Paris: H. Champion, 1930), vol. 2, 224–30; Fulbert of Chartres, *The Letters and Poems of Fulbert of Chartres*, ed. and trans. Frederick Behrends (Oxford: Clarendon Press, 1976), see, for example, Letters 24, 47, 48, and 71 (at pp. 45–7, 83–4, 84–5, and 119–20, respectively).

49 Fulbert, *The Letters and Poems of Fulbert of Chartres*, Letter 47 (at pp. 83–4).

50 Ibid, and translation from Wallis, *Medieval Medicine*, 15.

51 Walahfrid Strabo, *De cultura hortorum*, ed. Ernst Dümmler, *MGH Poet.* 2 (Berlin: Weidmann, 1884), 335–49. Latin text and translation from Walahfrid Strabo, *Hortulus*, trans. Raef

While it is noteworthy that Walahfrid mentions book learning, this comment refers only to his knowledge of gardening rather than to the medical information that follows. His recording of remedies in this text and others (see the discussion of cod. sang. 878 in Appendix 1) is, as with the case of Pardulus, particularly suggestive that he was well-versed in the medical texts circulating during this period, even if his autobiographical comments are not as explicit as those found in the letters of Cynehard, Richer, or Fulbert.[52] Ultimately, the testimonies of the literate elite of Carolingian Francia do not provide direct evidence for the application of practical medical texts in the context of therapy though they strongly support this possibility.

Furthermore, although these leading Carolingian scholars appear to have engaged with medical knowledge and practice, they are not described in the surviving textual evidence as *medici*, i.e., professional practitioners. As Horden laments, 'we know more about the medicine of the period, for all its obscurities, than we do about doctors'.[53] Consider a reference to *medici* in a poem composed by Alcuin (d. 804), Charlemagne's famed Northumbrian scholar. Describing the entrance of the *medici* at court, he writes:

> Forthwith flock in the doctors [*medici*], disciples of Hippocrates:
> This one opens veins, this one mixes herbs in a pot,
> That one cooks up a poultice, another offers potions.[54]

Alcuin offers a tantalising glimpse into the practices of these largely invisible professionals, noting what the *medici* do—and these activities fit with those recorded in the medical texts—but he provides no further evidence regarding their identity, training, sources of information, and so on.[55] As noted in Chapter 1, named medical practitioners are few and far between, though *medici*

Payne (Pittsburgh: Hunt Botanical Library, 1966), 24–5: *Plurima tranquillae cum sint insignia vitae, / Non minimum est, si quis Paestanae deditus artis / Noverit obsceni curas tractare Priapi. / … Haec non sola mihi patefecit opinio famae / Vulgaris, quaesita libris nec lectio priscis; / Sed labor et studium, quibus otia longa dierum / Postposui, expertum rebus docuere probatis.*

52 Voigts uses Walahfrid's comments in the *Hortulus* as evidence of his use of medical texts in the practice of medicine. Walahfrid's references to book learning, however, do not explicitly confirm this. See Voigts, 'Anglo-Saxon Plant Remedies', 268.

53 Horden, 'Sickness and Healing', 96.

54 Alcuin, *Carmina*, 26, ed. Ernst Dümmler, MGH *Poet.* 1 (Berlin: Weidmann, 1881), 245: *Accurrunt medici mox, Hippocratica secta: | Hic venas fundit, herbas hic miscet in olla, | Ille coquit pultes, alter sed pocula praefert.* Translation from Wallis, *Medieval Medicine*, 80.

55 For additional comments on *medici* by Alcuin, see Alcuin, *Epistola*, 213, ed. Ernst Dümmler, MGH *Epp. kar. aevi* 2 (Berlin: Weidmann, 1895), 356–7.

can be found in charters and law codes.[56] Their appearance in these contexts, however, offers little sense of their medical practice and no direct evidence regarding their possible use of medical texts as part of this practice. On the other hand, these sources shed light on certain aspects of their lives, such as their position in society and apparent literacy, that are typically lacking in the documentary evidence reviewed above.[57] It seems plausible, therefore, that these literate medical practitioners consulted medical writings during their general education, training in medicine, and possibly in their practice, too.

It must also be remembered that the written record captures only a fraction of the variety of medical practitioners active during this period.[58] While the textual evidence reveals the existence of elite male practitioners, it rarely sheds light on 'informal healthcare delivered by men and women in their communities'.[59] Yet, the general absence of evidence regarding the provision of healthcare beyond elite networks should not be read as evidence of absence; as Patricia Skinner cautions, 'we must remain alive to the possibility that [informal healthcare] existed, and that the picture we build up from the surviving sources may only be a small part of the whole'.[60] When considering the potential diversity of the medical marketplace, it is important to recognise that many of the individuals involved in healing practices, and especially those unrecorded by the texts, may not have had the skills or resources (including access to the manuscripts) to incorporate medical texts in their practice or that they worked within complementary healing systems (e.g., miraculous cures).[61] The literate *medici*, who, given their connections and education, are more likely to have consulted texts as part of their practice, may have represented only a small percentage of the available practitioners during this period. Consequently, their practices and potential engagement with the medical literature in circulation likely reflect just one of the many interwoven threads within the complex web of healing traditions in early medieval Europe.

While acknowledging that the medical writings recorded in manuscripts capture only a partial picture of the wider healthscape, as the other types of documentary evidence surveyed above make clear, these texts remain

56 Skinner, *Health and Medicine in Early Medieval Southern Italy*; Pilsworth, *Healthcare in Early Medieval Northern Italy*, 187–209.

57 Pilsworth, *Healthcare in Early Medieval Northern Italy*, 187.

58 Horden, 'Sickness and Healing', 92–3.

59 Skinner, *Health and Medicine in Early Medieval Southern Italy*, 83.

60 Ibid.

61 Valerie J. Flint, 'The Early Medieval 'Medicus', the Saint—and the Enchanter', *Social History of Medicine* 2, no. 2 (1989): 127–45, https://doi.org/10.1093/shm/2.2.127; Park, 'Medicine and Society'.

fundamentally important for understanding medicine's place in the early medieval Latin west, and it is thus essential to consider the contexts in which medical manuscripts were produced. According to Florence Eliza Glaze, all extant early medieval medical manuscripts are 'likely monastic products'.[62] This monastic setting has helped to give rise to the problematic concept of *Mönchsmedizin*, monastic medicine, i.e., the idea that 'the medieval medical literature ... comes from and belongs in monasteries'.[63] While this conclusion may, at first glance, appear to be justified if all texts were written in monastic contexts, it is an unhelpful and reductive assumption that has accumulated negative connotations. The restriction of early medieval medical knowledge and practice to monastic environments has limited the field's understanding of the texts and contexts in which they could have been used. Although there is strong evidence for the production of these manuscripts in monastic scriptoria and for their continued existence in these communities, there is also evidence of their presence in lay households. The Carolingian counts Eberhard of Friuli (d. 867) and Ekkehard of Mâcon (d. 876) are both recorded as owning one medical manuscript.[64] Therefore, although no surviving eighth- and ninth-century medically-focused codices appear to have been produced outside of monastic centres, it is evident that the manuscripts themselves could have moved beyond these cloistered communities.

That being said, given the large number of manuscripts that remained in monastic contexts, such as the libraries of Lorsch, St Gall, Reichenau, and Corbie, it is also important to reflect on this particular type of environment. Under the influence of *Mönchsmedizin*, the inclusion of certain types of medical writings, such as treatises on or including gynaecology, in these codices was used to argue that ancient texts were blindly copied and had little practical value. Countering this interpretation, Peregrine Horden has shown that texts on such 'problematic' topics could have been used in multiple ways and in multiple settings—even within the cloister.[65] In a monastic environment without

62 Glaze, 'The Perforated Wall', 1.

63 Bernhard Schnell, 'Prolegomena to a History of Medieval German Medical Literature: The Twelfth Century', in *Manuscript Sources of Medieval Medicine: A Book of Essays*, ed. Margaret R. Schleissner (London: Garland, 1995), 3–15, at p. 12. For early studies commenting on the monastic context of early medieval medicine see *Studien und Texte*, ed. Sigerist (especially p. 186) and *Frühmittelalterliche Rezeptarien*, ed. Jörimann (especially p. 1).

64 On the evidence for the circulation of medical manuscripts specifically, see Glaze, 'The Perforated Wall', 69–79; on lay medical book ownership, see Glaze, 'The Perforated Wall', 13–14, n. 6. It is also useful to remember that in the early medieval Greek east, luxury or display copies of medical writings, such as Vienna, ÖNB, Med. gr. 1, appear to have circulated within royal and aristocratic households.

65 Horden, 'What's Wrong with Early Medieval Medicine?', 12–13.

childbearing community members, for example, a gynaecological treatise could have been read as a work on natural history.[66] Alternatively, given the 'comings and goings of elite patronesses; of the mothers, sisters, daughters and former wives of monks; of labourers on the monastery's estates', it is possible that the texts were, in fact, studied in relation to therapy.[67] Ultimately, it must be remembered that, as Horden writes, 'what has often been called monks' medicine was not especially monastic. It simply comes to us from monastic manuscripts'.[68] The monastic context thus presents a setting in which early medieval scribes, readers, and potentially even medical practitioners engaged with medical writings for a number of different, potentially overlapping reasons—but, simultaneously, this was not the *only* possible environment in which these activities could have occurred.

2.1 *Summary*

While past scholarship has uncovered evidence for a number of different ways to practise medicine and pursue healing in the Carolingian world, there are few clear signs that medical texts were consulted as part of this practice. That is not to say that texts were ignored in the context of therapy, but rather to remember that explicit evidence for this type of use, such as Cynehard's letter, is exceedingly rare. Therefore, although it may be tempting to extrapolate from the evidence presented in the writings of Cassiodorus, the medical features depicted in the *Plan of St Gall*, or the comments of later authors, and presume that medical writings were used in medical practice, it would be inappropriate to make such an assumption. Between the repurposing of medical knowledge seen in the works of Isidore and Hrabanus, the 'unintelligibility' exhibited by some medical texts, as well as Cynehard's inability to access ingredients, it becomes clear that medical writings, including seemingly practical recipe collections, could be used in multiple ways or become unusable for therapeutic purposes.[69]

An in-depth reconsideration of recipe practicality, in terms of both intention/design and use, is therefore much needed. Can the evidence for both practicality and impracticality be reconciled? Cynehard's letter documents his experiences across the channel, but what was the situation in Carolingian Francia? Before turning to case studies on the question of practicality

66 Horden, 'What's Wrong with Early Medieval Medicine?', 12; Horden, 'Prefatory Note'.
67 Horden, 'What's Wrong with Early Medieval Medicine?', 13.
68 Ibid.
69 Horden, 'Sickness and Healing', 96: 'other, lesser, texts often degenerate into unintelligibility through repeated copying'.

(Chapters 3–5), it is essential to provide an overview of the recipe literature and sample of recipes involved in this study.

3 Outlining the Recipe Literature

Over 100 codices containing medical texts have survived from the eighth and ninth centuries alone.[70] Most of these can be termed 'medical manuscripts', i.e., their contents focus largely, if not entirely, on texts relating to health and medicine. Given the vocabulary used in manuscript catalogues from the period, this label parallels Carolingian descriptions of these codices.[71] It must be remembered, however, that although this terminology suggests that medical writings were understood to belong to a distinct subject area, such writings could also appear outside of strictly medical manuscripts. Medicine often travelled with calendrical material, for example, due to the significant links between these areas of learning.[72] Medical texts also appear in seemingly unexpected contexts, such as the addition of medical material—sometimes no more than a single recipe—to a blank space in a manuscript otherwise unconnected to health, medicine, and related fields.[73] While these finds are important, especially when considering the spread of medical knowledge, they provide only a fraction of the total number of surviving texts, and the majority of the recipes analysed in this book are located in medical manuscripts. It is therefore worth pausing to highlight the complex, unstable nature of these codices before reviewing the recipe literature contained within them, especially since many

70 On the numbers of surviving manuscripts, see Beccaria, *I codici* and Wickersheimer, *Les manuscrits*; the former includes 158 manuscripts produced between the ninth and eleventh centuries while the latter, which only focuses on manuscripts held in French collections, gives 119 manuscripts for the same period. As noted in Chapter 1, the CEMLM has identified roughly 200 manuscripts missed by Beccaria and Wickersheimer.

71 Leja, *Embodying the Soul*, 12.

72 On the links between medicine and calendars, see Wallis, 'Medicine in Medieval Calendar Manuscripts' and Faith Wallis, 'Counting All the Bones: Measure, Number and Weight in Early Medieval Texts About the Body', in *Was zählt Ordnungsangebote, Gebrauchsformen und Erfahrungsmodalitäten des "numerus" im Mittelalter*, ed. Moritz Wedell (Cologne: Böhlau, 2012), 185–208.

73 For examples of non-medical manuscripts to which recipes have been added, see, for example, Cambridge, Corpus Christi College, MS 223, a ninth-century codex containing a variety of non-medical texts, such as works by Prudentius, with recipes added to its opening flyleaf, or Laon, Bibliothèque Municipale, MS 199, a ninth-century codex covering the Lateran Council of 649 in which a recipe has been added to the final half folio.

of the manuscripts' general characteristics likewise apply to their constituent recipe collections.

While texts relating to pharmacy represent a substantial proportion of the writings preserved within medical manuscripts, this area of medicine was one of many that interested Carolingian compilers. Other popular topics include phlebotomy, diagnosis and prognosis, and dietetics and preventative medicine, to name but a few.[74] Faith Wallis and Peregrine Horden, in particular, have provided important and perceptive syntheses of the manuscript evidence and the challenges it poses to modern researchers given its inconsistencies, variability, and paradoxical 'reverence for authority coincid[ing] with extraordinary indifference to textual authenticity'.[75] As Wallis recognises, 'the more important the text was for the early medieval reader ... the more it was subject to dismemberment, rearrangement, abbreviation, and so forth'.[76] With texts concerning pharmaceutical information comprising one of the most popular areas of medical writing, the surviving recipe literature reflects this dismemberment, rearrangement, and abbreviation.

Since Antiquity, recipes have been gathered to form collections of various sizes, structures, and thematic concentrations, as described below. Copies of classical and late antique collections continued to circulate in the early medieval west, though often in 'decanonised' and adapted versions.[77] Alongside these established (if unstable) texts, new compilations were produced that brought together multiple earlier sources as well as outside influences, combining and recombining pharmaceutical information in novel ways. This book focuses on recipes from these new compositions as well as 'miscellaneous' prescriptions found outside of large collections. As described in Chapter 1, the relative lack of engagement with these types of recipes in past scholarship, combined with the field's changing research trends, provides an ideal opportunity to analyse a large sample of previously overlooked and/or understudied material. These recipes, moreover, are particularly useful for investigating questions of practicality and applicability given that they combine a variety of sources rather than presenting the work of a single author or more established tradition. In

74 For a full breakdown of the genres of medical writing and number of texts associated with each during this period, see Wallis, 'The Experience of the Book', 112, n. 30.

75 For particularly insightful syntheses of early medieval medicine in relation to the manuscript evidence, see Wallis, 'The Experience of the Book' (quotation at p. 107) and Horden, 'What's Wrong with Early Medieval Medicine?', though these themes are also addressed in their other work; see the bibliography for more examples.

76 Wallis, 'The Experience of the Book', 103–4.

77 Wallis, 'The Experience of the Book'.

other words, while the recipes under analysis are intimately related to earlier medical writings (and, in some cases, individual recipes can be traced to a particular classical or late antique source), additional influences from beyond the classical corpus are also apparent (see Chapters 3 and 4).[78] Early medieval recipe collections, each presenting a distinct blend of sources, thus present fertile ground for exploring the evolution of medical knowledge during this period.

Over the following pages, I introduce the recipes under consideration, first reviewing the typical ways in which prescriptions were presented and ordered into collections. This starts with an emphasis on classical and late antique traditions due to their influence on early medieval compilations. Indeed, the shared manuscript contexts in which all these texts are located highlight both the differences between collections as well as their innate entanglements and commonalities. This leads, therefore, to an overview of the specific manuscripts involved in the present study.

3.1 *Recipes and Recipe Collections*

The recipes recorded in early medieval manuscripts—whether in copies of classical and late antique pharmaceutical treatises or in new compositions—appear in a range of formats and with varied levels of detail and complexity. One of the most fundamental distinctions is that between simple and compound medicines.[79] The former, *simplicia*, offer treatments based on a single primary ingredient (the active drug). Although the selected substance was sometimes intended to be used completely alone (e.g., a treatment might simply advise that a herbal product should be ingested), many recipes provide instructions that combine the primary ingredient with at least one additional substance that served as a liquefying agent, binder, etc., and that was not perceived as having a therapeutic effect. In contrast, compound medicines, *compositiones*, involve a mixture of *materia medica* and, rather than targeting a single ailment, were often presented as treatments for multiple conditions.[80] While compound medicines could include just a handful of active ingredients,

78 Horden, 'What's Wrong with Early Medieval Medicine?', 19. For examples of the identification of individual extracts and transmission of earlier sources within early medieval recipe collections, see the work of Arsenio Ferraces Rodríguez and Klaus-Dietrich Fischer highlighted in Chapter 1.

79 Ferraces Rodríguez, 'Un recetario médico altomedieval', 41.

80 Alain Touwaide, 'Pharmaceutic Handbooks', in *Medieval Science, Technology and Medicine: An Encyclopedia*, ed. Thomas Glick, Steven J. Livesey, and Faith Wallis (London: Routledge, 2005), 393–4; Alain Touwaide, 'Pharmacy and *Materia medica*', in *Medieval Science, Technology and Medicine: An Encyclopedia*, ed. Thomas Glick, Steven J. Livesey, and Faith Wallis (London: Routledge, 2005), 397–9.

recipe collections also contain many complicated recipes that feature long lists of exotic ingredients and claim to treat a host of different diseases, from common maladies (headaches, stomach pains, and the like) to more extreme illnesses and injuries (including rabid dog bites, scorpion stings, and epilepsy, to name but a few examples). Such sweeping panaceas often provide treatments for poisons and encounters with venomous animals and appear to be derived from and modelled on ancient compound medicines, such as Mithridates' antidote, reflecting the influence of classical treatises on toxicology.[81]

Simples and compounds were traditionally associated with different types of recipe collections, though these divisions and organising principles were somewhat fluid, especially in early medieval compendia. Texts focused on and ordered by *materia medica*, such as herbals and bestiaries, concentrate on *simplicia*.[82] In these collections, each chapter covers a different ingredient and often provides some information about the substance in question (e.g., synonyms, instructions for collection and/or preparation, etc.) in addition to its medical uses. Dioscorides' (*c.* 40–90) *De materia medica*, an enormous composition with individual chapters dedicated to nearly 800 plants and over 100 animals and minerals, respectively, is the most comprehensive of the ancient works following this general schematic and had a lasting impact.[83] New compositions were created not only by following Dioscorides' model but also by directly excerpting, rearranging, and translating his text and, later, its descendants.

In surviving manuscripts, the widespread circulation of recipe collections ordered by *materia medica* suggests that they were a popular genre within pharmaceutical writing.[84] In particular, a group of late antique herbals and

81 Laurence M. V. Totelin, 'Mithridates' Antidote—A Pharmacological Ghost'. *Early Science and Medicine* 9, no. 1 (2004): 1–19; Philip Wexler, ed., *Toxicology in Antiquity*, 2nd ed. (London: Academic Press, 2019).

82 For more on the genre of herbals, see, for example, the collected essays of Jerry Stannard and John Riddle: Stannard, *Pristina Medicamenta*; Stannard, *Herbs and Herbalism in the Middle Ages and Renaissance*; and Riddle, *Quid pro quo*. On the illustrated traditions specifically, see Collins, *Medieval Herbals*.

83 Dioscorides, *Pedanii Dioscuridis Anazarbei De materia medica libri quinque*, ed. Max Wellmann, 3 vols. (Berlin: Weidmann, 1906–14); for an English translation, see Dioscorides, *De materia medica*, trans. Lily Y. Beck (Hildesheim: Olms-Weidmann, 2005). On Dioscorides' reception, see John M. Riddle, *Dioscorides on Pharmacy and Medicine* (Austin: University of Texas Press, 1985); Riddle, 'Pseudo-Dioscorides' *Ex herbis femininis*', 43–81; Alain Touwaide, 'Dioscorides', in *Medieval Science, Technology and Medicine: An Encyclopedia*, ed. Thomas Glick, Steven J. Livesey, and Faith Wallis (London: Routledge, 2005), 152–4.

84 Beccaria, *I codici*; Wickersheimer, *Les manuscrits*.

bestiaries, labelled the *Herbariencorpus* by Gerhard Baader, are often found transmitted together; these texts include Pseudo-Antonius Musa's *De herba vettonica liber*, Pseudo-Apuleius' *Herbarius* (noted in Chapter 1 in relation to its translation into Old English), Pseudo-Dioscorides' *Ex herbis femininis*, Pseudo-Sextus Placitus' *Liber medicinae ex animalibus, pecoribus et bestiis*, and the anonymous *De taxone liber*.[85] Baader has traced their connection to sixth- or seventh-century Ravenna, a city already noted for its medical importance. In addition to its school of medicine, Ravenna seems to have played an important role in the translation of several Greek medical texts into Latin, cementing its significance in relation to the transmission of medical knowledge during this period.[86] At the same time, the widespread popularity of herbal medicine can also be seen through Isidore's brief comments on different types of medical books, as he included two terms for texts concerning plants in this section of Book 4: *dinamidia*, collections of herbal remedies, and *butanicum*, a botanical treatise.[87]

In contrast to simples, the multipart nature of compound medicines, such as antidotes, is less suited to treatises ordered by individual *materia medica*; instead, *compositiones* tend to be found in separate collections, *antidotaria*. In these texts, prescriptions are typically named after a) a primary or noteworthy ingredient(s), b) their (alleged) creator or a famous user, or c) a principal

85 Gerhard Baader, 'Die Anfänge der medizinischen Ausbildung im Abendland bis 1100', in *La scuola nell'Occidente latino dell'alto medioevo, 15–21 aprile 1971*, Settimane 19, vol. 2 (Spoleto: Fondazione Centro italiano di studi sull'alto medioevo, 1972), 669–772. Voigts, 'The Significance of the Name Apuleius', 215; Riddle, 'Pseudo-Dioscorides' *Ex herbis femininis*', 43–81. Ernst Howald and Henry Sigerist produced a *CML* volume (4) featuring many of these texts: *Antonii Musae De herba vettonica liber. Pseudoapulei Herbarius. Anonymi De taxone liber. Sextii Placiti Liber medicinae ex animalibus etc.*

86 Baader, 'Die Anfange der medizinischen Ausbildung'. On Ravenna's medical school, see n. 44 above. On translation at Ravenna, see also Innocenzo Mazzini, 'Les traductions latines d'Oribase et d'Hippocrate', in *Les écoles médicales à Rome: Actes du 2ème Colloque international sur les textes médicaux latins antiques, Lausanne, septembre 1986*, ed. Philippe Mudry and Jackie Pigeaud (Geneva: Droz, 1991), 286–93.

87 For Isidore's discussion of medical books, see Isidore, *Etymologiae*, 4.10.1–4. On *dynamidia*, see Arsenio Ferraces Rodríguez, 'El Pseudo-Dioscórides *De herbis femininis*, los *Dynamidia* e Isidoro de Sevilla, *Etym*. xvii, 7–11', in *Tradición e Innovación de la Medicina Latina de la Antigüedad y de la Alta Edad Media: Actas del iv Coloquio Internacional sobre los "textos medicos latinos antiguos"*, ed. Manuel Enrique Vázquez Buján (Santiago de Compostela: Servicio de Publicacións e Intercambio Científico da Universidade de Santiago de Compostela, 1994), 183–203; John M. Riddle, 'The Pseudo-Hippocratic *Dynamidia*', *Sudhoffs Archiv für Geschichte der Medizin und der Naturwissenschaften* 27 (1989): 283–311; and Loren C. MacKinney, '"Dynamidia" in Medieval Medical Literature', *Isis* 24, no. 2 (1936): 400–14.

therapeutic property, and follow the precedent set by Galen's (*c.* 129-*c.* 216) *On Antidotes*.[88] The textual boundaries between simple and compound medicines are blurred, however, in collections ordered by diseases (generally following a head-to-toe, *a capite ad calcem*, arrangement) or by style/method of treatment. In the former, each chapter focuses on the treatment of a disease, condition, or cluster of symptoms, presenting at least one prescription, though multiple options are often listed. While *simplicia* comprise the core of these collections, compound medicines also appear. In recipe collections ordered by style/method, following Galen's *On Medicines by Genres*, the prescriptions are arranged into different groups based on their final form, distinguishing between, for example, oils, unguents, plasters, electuaries, pessaries, collyria, and so on.[89] While some of these preparations align with the simple model and centre on a single active drug, many involve more complicated mixtures.

The *a capite ad calcem* arrangement can already be seen in some texts attributed to Galen and became a very popular ordering strategy in late antique adaptations of earlier works. Consider, for example, the Plinian family of pharmaceutical writings. Medical recipes are scattered throughout Pliny the Elder's (23–79) monumental and unwieldy *Natural History*.[90] Anonymous compilers excerpted the medical sections and reordered them from head to toe, producing new texts, the *Medicina Plinii* and *Physica Plinii*, in the fourth and sixth centuries, respectively.[91] Similar processes of reworking, excerpting, condensing, and translating ancient medical writings can be observed in the works of numerous late antique authors, including Oribasius (*c.* 320–400), Caelius

88 Touwaide, 'Pharmaceutic Handbooks', 393–4. For work on specific antidote traditions, see, for example, Fischer, '*Antidotum cui nomen est acharistum*' and Fischer, 'Die Antidotos des Zopyros und andere Fundstücke zu Scribonius Largus', in *Body, Disease and Treatment in a Changing World: Latin Texts and Contexts in Ancient and Medieval Medicine. Proceedings of the Ninth International Conference "Ancient Latin Medical Texts", Hulme Hall, University of Manchester, 5–8 September 2007*, ed. David Langslow and Brigitte Maire (Lausanne: Éditions BHMS, 2010), 147-60.

89 Touwaide, 'Pharmaceutic Handbooks', 393. See also Isidore, *Etymologiae*, 4.9.8–11 for a list of different types of preparations.

90 Pliny the Elder, *Natural History*, trans. Harris Rackham, William Henry Samuel Jones, and D. E. Eichholz. 10 vols. (Cambridge, MA: Harvard University Press, 1938–63).

91 *Plinii Secundi Iunioris qui feruntur De medicina libri tres*, ed. Önnerfors; *The* Medicina Plinii*: Latin Text, Translation, and Commentary*, trans. Yvette Hunt (Abingdon: Routledge, 2020); *Physica Plinii Bambergensis (Cod. Bamb. med. 2, fol. 93^v-232^r)*, ed. Alf Önnerfors (Hildesheim: Olms, 1975); Aude Doody, 'Authority and Authorship in the *Medicina Plinii*', in *Authorial Voices in Greco-Roman Technical Writing*, ed. Liba Taub and Aude Doody (Trier: Wissenschaftlicher Verlag, 2009), 93–105; Aude Doody, *Pliny's Encyclopedia: The Reception of the* Natural History (Cambridge: Cambridge University Press, 2010).

Aurelianus (fl. *c.* 400), Marcellus of Bordeaux (fl. late fourth/early fifth centuries), Alexander of Tralles (*c.* 525–605), and Paul of Aegina (*c.* 625–90).[92] While such efforts were formerly seen as the unsophisticated repackaging and simplification of earlier texts that resulted in the stagnation of medical progress, more recent scholarship has viewed this work as indicative of an environment in which the study of medicine flourished.[93] In the context of the present study, it is important to recognise how the reordering of texts, composition of commentaries on existing works, and translations of Greek writings into Latin suggest that late antique compilers, authors, and translators worked to make this body of knowledge more user-friendly: older texts were revised to create more practical medical guidebooks.[94]

When producing new compilations, late antique authors did not simply work from a single text, reordering or excerpting material in isolation; rather, just like the ancient medical writers before them and the early medieval compilers who would follow, they often brought together multiple sources. In these late antique syntheses, as Nutton highlights, 'extracts from earlier writers are assembled, often verbatim and duly acknowledged, into a coherent mosaic of opinions, ideas and remedies'.[95] In some cases, the authorities cited were near contemporaries: Marcellus, for example, refers to the 'two Plinies', i.e., Pliny the Elder and the anonymous compiler of the *Medicina Plinii*, as sources for his extensive recipe collection, *De medicamentis liber*.[96] The production of new compendia in the early Middle Ages continued these practices of excerpting and reordering earlier sources, if with certain differences. While some trends appear amplified, such as the reduction of theoretical material and emphasis on texts with a seemingly practical orientation, others speak to evolving contexts of production: material unrecorded in the classical corpus, ranging from the inclusion of Christian elements to new *materia medica*, also comes into view.[97] Overall, these developments suggest that broadly similar impulses underpinned the creation of new compendia in both late Antiquity

92 Nutton, *Ancient Medicine*, 299–308.

93 Nutton, *Ancient Medicine*, 300; Stannard, 'Marcellus of Bordeaux', 47–53; Glaze, 'The Perforated Wall', 18–46.

94 Owsei Temkin, *The Double Face of Janus and Other Essays in the History of Medicine* (Baltimore: Johns Hopkins University Press, 1977), 202.

95 Nutton, *Ancient Medicine*, 302.

96 Marcellus, *De medicamentis liber*, ed. Liechtenhan and Niedermann, trans. Kollesch and Nickel; Stannard, 'Marcellus of Bordeaux'; Doody, *Pliny's Encyclopedia*, 138.

97 Horden, 'Sickness and Healing', 94–6; Nutton, *Ancient Medicine*, 303. On Christian elements, see Burridge, 'Healing Body and Soul'; on previously unrecorded ingredients, see Chapters 3 and 4.

and the early Middle Ages, supporting the idea that many of these compilations were intended to be used in the context of therapy—just as Cassiodorus recommended.

Significantly, although, like earlier compilations, many early medieval compendia brought together material from classical and late antique recipe collections that followed multiple organisational principles, in contrast to earlier compilers, early medieval compilers did not necessarily impose a single overarching structure on their new compositions.[98] As a result, many of these early medieval products only loosely follow one of the standard organisational strategies or alternate between several approaches, suggesting that clusters of information were derived from specific sources. For example, entries following the herbal model (i.e., a section of text that names a plant, provides some basic information about it, and lists a series of simples using it) sometimes punctuate a collection in which recipes are more frequently listed under headings reflecting the ailment they aim to treat, though the headings may not be ordered *a capite ad calcem*.[99] Although such varied assemblages might raise questions about their potential usability in practice (how would a practitioner know where to find a particular recipe within this assortment?), many compendia begin with lists of their contents that would have helped readers to navigate these multi-layered collections.[100]

Furthermore, it is important to recognise that these compilations, like the manuscripts in which they are found, often include more than recipes alone. In addition to prescriptions, pharmaceutical collections commonly incorporate supplementary, related material, such as brief tracts on weights and measures, urine analysis, or phlebotomy.[101] Such inclusions reinforce the

98 It must be remembered, however, that in cases where an organisational principle seems to be lacking, it remains possible that the compilers' strategy is simply unclear to modern readers and that it followed a logical system that was recognised within the environment in which the text was produced.

99 On the less uniform grouping of treatments, see, for example, Paris, BnF lat. 11218: although it does not follow the *a capite ad calcem* pattern consistently, many types of similar treatments are located in clusters, such as a notably gynaecological section on ff. 108r–109r that contains thirty-four recipes entirely related to menstruation, conception, childbirth, etc. Several folia later, there is a section that could be described as an *antidotaria* as it contains mostly antidotes and complex, composite prescriptions (ff. 113v–118v).

100 Extensive collections in codd. sang. 44, 751, 759, and Biblioteca Apostolica Vaticana (hereafter BAV) pal. lat. 1088, for instance, are all preceded by contents lists. A list also survives in BnF lat. 6882A, though the collection itself has been lost. With the exception of BAV pal. lat. 1088, where a duplication error in the list has confused the numbering, the contents lists and collections are usually near perfect matches.

101 Beccaria, *I codici*; Wickersheimer, *Les manuscrits*.

impression that they were conceived of as general handbooks for medical care, and, notably, when lists of contents are recorded, they also include these extra-pharmaceutical elements, thereby indicating that they were understood as integral parts of the collection rather than as unplanned addenda. Given the comprehensiveness of these works, this book's use of 'recipe collection' must be clarified. Under this label, I include textual units that a) consist *primarily* of recipes, and b) contain at least three recipes. Collections vary enormously in size and scope: some feature hundreds of numbered entries, each containing one or more recipes, and are accompanied by lists of contents, while others list only a handful of recipes. Though the latter present a significant contrast with the much larger collections, they still appear as a coherent textual unit recording pharmaceutical information. Additionally, some collections involve multiple hands and were corrected and/or added to over time, whereas others appear to have been the work of a single scribe.

Here, it is also necessary to elaborate on the term 'recipe'. Excepting the extra-pharmaceutical extracts mentioned above, most of the entries within recipe collections could be classified as 'remedies'; that is, 'a medicine or treatment that promotes healing or alleviates symptoms'.[102] Some, however, are broader in scope, such as instructions for the preparation of composite ingredients, including oxymel, various oils and unguents, and incense. Recipes for these products can be found alongside remedies.[103] Although such ingredients may not have been intended to treat a disease or alleviate symptoms, they still had a medical purpose, serving as components within remedies. Moreover, some of these composite ingredients may have, in fact, been used both as the constituent parts of a remedy *and* as treatments themselves. The term 'recipe', therefore, more accurately describes the material at hand and, in the analyses that follow, all recorded recipes have been considered, rather than exclusively focusing those entries that can be clearly shown to be remedies, given the potential ambiguities and overlap between categories.

Related to defining what constitutes a recipe within the context of this study is the question of how to count recipes. In line with classical and late antique pharmaceutical writings, titled entries within recipe collections often represent discrete chapters, within which multiple recipes may be listed. Contents lists record these titles, meaning that their numbering is based on chapters rather than individual recipes. In the following analyses, all recipes

102 For a definition of the word, see the entry for 'remedy, n.', in *OED Online*, last modified December 2023, last accessed 10 March 2024, https://doi.org/10.1093/OED/6942526268.

103 Claire Burridge, 'Incense in Medicine: An Early Medieval Perspective', *Early Medieval Europe* 28, no. 2 (2020): 219–55, https://doi.org/10.1111/emed.12394.

are counted; as a result, the total number of recipes in some manuscripts is significantly higher than might be expected based on their recipe collections' contents lists. When more than one recipe is listed under a single heading, each recipe after the opening example tends to be prefaced by *item*, 'likewise', marking the start of a distinct recipe for the same issue. There are, however, several grey areas, such as whether to include material that has only partially survived due to lost or damaged folia (e.g., a recipe might end prematurely due to the loss of the following page). In cases of partial survival, I have incorporated these recipes in the analysis only when a substantial amount of information has been preserved.

Finally, what information is recorded in the recipes themselves? As noted above in relation to the differences between simple and compound medicines, recipes can vary widely in their presentation, complexity, and level of detail. The division between *simplicia* and *compositiones*, for example, highlights that the number of active ingredients and targeted ailments ranges across a broad spectrum: a simple recipe might involve a single substance and be intended to treat one disease, whereas a complex antidote could list over fifty ingredients and aim to help scores of different illnesses, wounds, aches, and pains. In addition to these basic differences, there is also great variation with respect to the inclusion of instructions and, when included, level of detail. Some recipes provide guidance on the processes involved in the preparation, production, and administration of the treatment in question, defining, for example, the best time to collect the ingredient(s), specifying ingredient quantities or ratios, and recommending when and how long to administer the treatment. Conversely, other recipes record no more than a list of ingredients.

With this overview of recipes and recipe collections, it is possible to turn to the present study's selected manuscripts.

3.2 *The Manuscript Sample*[104]

The analyses in the following chapters are based on my transcriptions of recipes from a sample of twenty-four manuscripts (see Table 1 below for the list of codices). These manuscripts are today located in the Stiftsbibliothek St. Gallen (eleven manuscripts), Bibliothèque nationale de France (eight manuscripts), and Biblioteca Apostolica Vaticana (five manuscripts). These three libraries not only house many of the most important collections of early medieval manuscripts and charters but, within their collections, they each contain large concentrations of early medieval medical manuscripts. Augusto Beccaria's

104 For a more detailed review of the twenty-four manuscripts, see Appendix 1.

catalogue includes approximately eighty manuscripts containing medical writings produced in the eighth and ninth centuries and Ernest Wickersheimer identified a number of additional codices in French collections, bringing this total to roughly 100 codices.[105] As such, the twenty-four manuscripts under analysis represent a significant body of the surviving corpus of recipe literature. Moreover, not all of the manuscripts catalogued by Beccaria and Wickersheimer contain the types of recipes analysed in this study: some of the codices included in their catalogues do not contain any pharmaceutical writings while others only feature texts more closely linked to the classical and late antique canon. However, of the twenty-four codices, three in St Gall (codd. sang. 397, 550, and 899) and one in the Biblioteca Apostolica Vaticana (BAV pal. lat. 187), were not recorded in the earlier catalogues and it is important to remember that new cataloguing initiatives are increasing the number of manuscripts known to contain medical texts.[106] That being said, collectively, these four manuscripts contributed less than fifty recipes to the analyses: three of the four are not 'medical manuscripts', meaning that their contents primarily cover non-medical material, while the one predominantly medical codex of the group, BAV pal. lat. 187, is mostly dedicated to a known late antique pharmaceutical treatise, the *Alphabet of Galen*, and only contains a single page of 'miscellaneous' recipes. Despite their relatively minor contributions to the volume of surviving medical writings, these manuscripts do offer meaningful insights into the extent to which the knowledge of medical texts was spread and the ways in which it moved.

Overall, these twenty-four codices under consideration thus present a substantial sample of the extant manuscript evidence concerning recipes outside the established canon. Nevertheless, it is also essential to consider the selected manuscripts' representativity with respect to their chronological range, geographic distribution, and contents. In terms of dating, the earliest manuscripts under analysis, including cod. sang. 217 and BnF lat. 11218, are thought to have been produced in the late eighth or early ninth centuries, whereas the latest manuscripts, such as codd. sang. 752 and 899, have been dated to *c.* 900.[107] Recipes have also been added over time in many of the codices, including those that can be described as 'medical manuscripts' as well as those which focus on non-medical material. Where recipe additions appear to have been incorporated by *c.* 900, such as in the cases of BAV reg. lat. 598 and BnF lat.

105 Beccaria, *I codici*; Wickersheimer, *Les manuscrits*.

106 The new research has been led by the CEMLM cataloguing project; see Chapter 1, n. 39.

107 For more specific information and references regarding these manuscripts and those described below, see Appendix 1.

TABLE 1 Summary of manuscripts (including number of recipes in each manuscript)

Library	Manuscript	# of recipes
Bibliothèque nationale de France	lat. 2849A	54
	lat. 2858	2
	lat. 5543	65
	lat. 6882A	61
	lat. 7021	1
	lat. 9332	9
	lat. 11218	803
	lat. 11219	121
	Library subtotal	*1116*
Stiftsbibliothek St. Gallen	cod. sang. 44	917
	cod. sang. 217	316
	cod. sang. 397	2
	cod. sang. 550	3
	cod. sang. 751	1187
	cod. sang. 752	15
	cod. sang. 759	451
	cod. sang. 761	46
	cod. sang. 878	17
	cod. sang. 899	42
	cod. sang. 1396	118
	Library subtotal	*3114*
Biblioteca Apostolica Vaticana	pal. lat. 187	2
	pal. lat. 1088	835
	reg. lat. 598	12
	reg. lat. 1143	312
	vat. lat. 5951	1
	Library subtotal	*1162*
Total		5392

11219, this material has been included in the present study; later additions, such as the eleventh- and twelfth-century Old High German material seen in cod. sang. 878 and BnF lat. 11219, respectively, have not been considered in the analysis (though they provide insights into the long-term histories of several manuscripts). The majority of manuscripts, including codd. sang. 44, 751, and BAV pal. lat. 1088, have been dated to the ninth century, with some date ranges fairly broad, i.e., to the first or second half of the ninth century, and others more precise. For example, codd. sang. 397 and 878, the handbooks of Grimald, Abbot of St Gall (841–72), and Walahfrid Strabo, respectively, were produced in the decades when these scholars were active, while BnF lat. 5543 has been dated to around the year 847.

Regarding geographic distribution, these codices were written in centres of manuscript production across continental western Europe, including in ecclesiastical communities at the heart of Carolingian intellectual developments, such as St Gall and Reichenau, as well as at sites on the peripheries of the Frankish Empire, such as centres in northern Italy and Brittany (see the map for sites with known connections to a number of individual manuscripts under consideration as well as, in the cases where localisation remains regional, probable locations of production). Many of the manuscripts located in St Gall today, such as codd. sang. 752 and 899, appear to have originated within this community, while others, including codd. sang. 217 and 751, appear to have arrived not long after they were produced. These two codices, along with the medical half of cod. sang. 44, are thought to have been written in northern Italy and illustrate the connections between northern Italian sites of manuscript production and Alpine monastic centres. Indeed, despite their distance from the Frankish heartlands, northern Italian writing centres, such as Bobbio, Nonantola, and Verona, were deeply embedded within Carolingian ecclesiastical and intellectual networks, and the movement of several of the manuscripts involved in this study bears witness to these connections.[108] Moreover, a general survey of extant early medieval medical texts suggests that centres in northwest Francia and northern Italy were especially active in the production and dissemination of manuscripts containing medical writings during this period.[109] With this in mind, it is therefore worth noting that a significant proportion of the manuscripts in the sample are thought to have been produced and were circulating in these regions; codices that can be linked to more western Frankish intellectual centres include, for example, BnF lat. 2858, 5543, and 9332.

Lastly, the sample also contains a variety of manuscript types. Many of the manuscripts, including codd. sang. 751, 759, BAV pal. lat. 1088, reg. lat. 1143, BnF

108 On the movement of manuscripts and links between writing centres, including a number of those featured in this review, see Bernhard Bischoff, *Manuscripts and Libraries in the Age of Charlemagne*, trans. Michael M. Gorman (Cambridge: Cambridge University Press, 2007), 33, 122, and 147–8.

109 Leja, 'The Sacred Art', 4; Beccaria, *I codici*; Wickersheimer, *Les manuscrits*.

lat. 11218, and 11219, can be classed as medical manuscripts given their primary, if not exclusive, focus on writings concerning health and medicine. However, the sample also features more mixed manuscripts that contain texts on other topics, such as the aforementioned handbooks codd. sang. 397 and 878; cod. sang. 899, which is primarily a poetry anthology; and BnF lat. 2858, which contains the letters of Lupus of Ferrières. This assortment thus centres on medical manuscripts while also featuring codices in which medicine is but an element within a wider assemblage, reflecting the diverse codicological contexts in which medicine appears.

Based on the sample's a) inclusion of multiple manuscript types, b) varied geographic distribution that simultaneously emphasises regions associated with the production of medical manuscripts, and c) chronological spectrum spanning *c.* 775–900, this study considers a representative selection of early medieval Latin manuscripts that contain medical texts. The sample is also particularly well-suited, both chronologically and geographically, to the osteological evidence addressed in Part 2, a topic covered in Chapter 6. Table 1 summarises the distribution of recipes within the manuscript sample; the total number of recipes from the manuscript sample comes to 5392, with roughly three-fifths of the recipes found in the eleven manuscripts from St Gall and one-fifth found in the manuscripts of both the Biblioteca Apostolica Vaticana and Bibliothèque nationale de France, respectively. Given the uneven distribution of recipes between manuscripts—BnF lat. 7021 contains just one recipe whereas cod. sang. 751 includes over 1000—certain codices are referred to more frequently in the following chapters than others.

Building on this background to the texts and manuscripts, it is time to investigate the ingredients recorded in their folia.

CHAPTER 3

Impossible Imports or Available Exotics?

A Study of Non-local Materia Medica

1 Introduction: the Exotic Ingredients of an Antidote

> A 'sacred' antidote of colocynth. This is the recipe: eryngium roots, polypody roots, balsam bark, Nepal cardamom, long pepper, spignel, ginger, gentian, savin, costus, spikenard, cassia, agaric, sweet flag, colocynth: 2 *drachmae* each. Rustyback fern, wall germander, camphor: 1.5 ounces each. Aloe, saffron, rhubarb, mastic, cinnamon, scammony, dodder, hazelwort, peony: 1 ounce each. You make all this into a powder; add sufficient skimmed honey.[1]

The above ingredient list, found on f. 90r of BAV pal. lat. 1088, names the substances (and their respective amounts) needed to prepare the *Antidotum gira deacoloquintidis*, 'A 'sacred' antidote of colocynth'. A fairly typical antidote, the scribe claims that it treats roughly two dozen different conditions, from head pains to gout—and seemingly everything in between. The scribe even asserts that, in addition to curing present infirmities, it will defend against future maladies: *non solum presentes infirmitates curat, sed futuras egritudines defendit.* While this catch-all approach to treatment raises important questions regarding the practicality and applicability of antidotes more generally, here, I shall explore the *materia medica* listed within the antidote. Like the large number of conditions it supposedly treats, the recipe also incorporates a host of different ingredients—twenty-eight to be specific. Nearly all of these ingredients are derived from plants; honey (*mel*) and agaric (*agarico*), a mushroom, are the only exceptions. Where did these twenty-six different plants grow? Could a

1 BAV pal. lat. 1088, f. 90r: *Antidotum gira deacoloquintidis… Recipit hęc eringio radices, polopodię radices, sirobalsamo, amomo, piper longum, meu, gingiber, gentiana, brathea, costo, spico, casia, agarico, agaro, interiones, ana dragmas II, scolopendria, camitrius, cafora, ana untia I et dimidia, aloę, croco, reopontico, masticę, cinamo, diagridiu, epithimo, asaro, pionia, ana unt I, omnia pulueraem facis, adde mel dispumatum quod sufficit.* Only the recipe's ingredient list is included in the opening quotation; the full entry begins with the conditions the antidote treats and ends with instructions for its preparation; for the entire recipe, see Appendix 2, entry 16.26.

Carolingian individual, such as Walahfrid Strabo tending his monastic garden, have produced or foraged for these ingredients?

Ten of the twenty-eight products could have been grown or produced in northern and western Europe; these include eight plants native to the region—eryngium (*eringio*), polypody (*polopodię*), spignel (*meu*), gentian (*gentiana*), savin (*brathea*), rustyback fern (*scolopendria*), dodder (*epithimo*), and hazelwort (*asarum*)—as well as honey (*mel*) and the fungus agaric (*agarico*). Five plant ingredients, including sweet flag (*agaro*), colocynth (*interiones*), wall germander (*camitrius*), scammony (*diagridiu*), and peony (*pionia*), are generally native to the southern and/or eastern Mediterranean. Although these are not endemic to the territories under Frankish control, they could have been growing in neighbouring regions or perhaps cultivated in protected gardens, though Walahfrid Strabo does not record them in his poem on his own 'little garden', nor are they included in the diagram of the medicinal garden within the *Plan of St Gall*.[2] The remaining thirteen ingredients, balsam bark (*sirobalsamo*), Nepal cardamom (*amomo*), long pepper (*piper longum*), ginger (*gingiber*), costus (*costo*), spikenard (*spica*), cassia (*casia*), camphor (*cafora*), aloe (*aloe*), saffron (*croco*), rhubarb (*reopontico*), mastic (*mastice*), and cinnamon (*cinamo*), are from much further afield. While this three-tiered classification system is relative and some of the more Mediterranean plants may have been growing within the Carolingian world (had sweet flag, for example, been introduced to western European wetlands and riversides by this period? Were peonies being cultivated in aristocratic and monastic gardens, even if they were unrecorded by Walahfrid or the *Plan*?), it reveals that the antidote relies on ingredients of varying levels of localness—or, conversely, exoticness.[3] Secondly, despite this spectrum in localness/exoticness, it is apparent that, if this antidote were used in practice, a significant number of the ingredients, such as pepper, ginger, and camphor, would have travelled very long distances to reach any part of the Frankish Empire.

Many recipes present a picture similar to the antidote above, combining a mixture of potentially local and definitely non-local products. John Riddle's analysis of one of the recipe collections involved in the present study, the first collection in cod. sang. 44 (pp. 228–55), provides a useful example.[4] Using Henry Sigerist's 1923 transcription, he identified 361 different ingredients in the

---

2 Voigts, 'Anglo-Saxon Plant Remedies'; Walahfrid Strabo, *Hortulus*; Horn and Born, *The Plan of St. Gall*, 181–3.

3 Voigts, 'Anglo-Saxon Plant Remedies', 261–3.

4 Riddle, 'The Introduction and Use of Eastern Drugs', 185–98.

recipes of this collection.[5] Some of these ingredients, such as fennel and rose, are also recorded in the texts relating to gardens mentioned in Chapter 2, whereas others, including camphor and ambergris, appear to have been unknown to classical physicians. After eliminating ingredients used largely as emollients, flavouring agents, or solvents, such as honey, wine, and wax, Riddle delineates the twenty most frequently recorded ingredients: aloe (*aloes*), gum ammoniac (*ammonicum*), Nepal cardamom (*amomum*), parsley or celery seeds (*apium semen*), cinnamon (*cassia*), cumin (*ciminum*), colophony resin (*colofonia*), saffron (*crocus*), fenugreek (*fenugrecum*), frankincense (*libanus*), flax (*linum*), mastic (*mastice*), myrrh (*murra*), parsley (*petroselinum*), pitch (*picea*), pepper (*piper*), scammony (*scamonia*), storax (*storace*), terebinth (*terebintina*), and ginger (*zinziber*).[6] While seven of these ingredients could have grown locally, the remaining thirteen, nearly two-thirds of the ingredients in question, are not native to northern and western Europe. Like the opening antidote, there is a range of exoticness among the non-local products; a number of these ingredients, such as scammony and terebinth, can be found in the southern and eastern Mediterranean, though others, including cinnamon, pepper, and ginger, are grown in southeast Asia. Is it probable (or even possible) that such non-local ingredients were available in the Carolingian world? Is there evidence that reflects the movement and trade of these particular spices, gums, resins, and woods? Or are there signs suggesting that the Franks, like Cynehard, encountered difficulties in obtaining exotic ingredients?

This chapter will explore the question of practicality through the lens of non-local *materia medica*. After first reviewing evidence for the movement of exotic ingredients through gift exchange, trade, and even illicit means, I return to Riddle's study. Riddle and others, such as Michael McCormick, have highlighted the appearance of camphor, ambergris, and several other substances from southeast Asia in early medieval recipes. They argue that their use as *materia medica* in this period reflects the arrival of new pharmaceutical knowledge. Using my significantly larger sample of recipes, I expand on their work, identifying not only additional examples of camphor and ambergris, but also the occurrence of a cluster of new products that, within the recipe literature, appear to have travelled together as a distinct unit of information. By analysing the manuscript contexts in which this ingredient cluster is located and examining additional evidence concerning the trade of exotic substances, I present potential routes for the dissemination and spread of this pharmaceutical

---

5 *Studien und Texte*, ed. Sigerist, 78–99.
6 Riddle, 'The Introduction and Use of Eastern Drugs', 187–9.

information and suggest that it was, in fact, linked to the movement of the substances themselves. I argue that recipes incorporating such ingredients offer a window into dynamic centres of manuscript production where scribes integrated 'cutting edge' information and updated their recipe collections with new pharmaceutical knowledge. It must be remembered, however, that these non-local products would have been available only sporadically, in limited quantities, and at great expense. Recipes including these substances were not, therefore, practical in that they involved readily available ingredients that suited local conditions, but their inclusion reflects a scribal environment actively engaging with new ingredients and information. The findings of this case study suggest that such recipes were intended to be used if and when the necessary ingredients could be obtained.

2 Evidence for the Movement of Non-local *Materia Medica*

The example of Cynehard presented in Chapter 2 indicates that access to non-local ingredients was a major challenge in some parts of northwest Europe in the early Middle Ages. In this case, Cynehard, bishop of Winchester (d. *c.* 778), asked Lull, archbishop of Mainz (d. 786), to send some of the more exotic *materia medica* listed in recipes since many of these products were unavailable (and even unknown) in early medieval England.[7] The fact that he asked his Frankish colleague for help in supplying these ingredients does, however, suggest that the Carolingian world had better access to these types of ingredients—or at least that Cynehard thought this was the case. Surviving epistolary evidence supports this idea: as noted in Chapter 2, Lull, acting with two other English missionaries, Denehard and Burchard, sent a small selection of *exotica* as a gift to Abbess Cuneburg in England, and, as discussed below, Lull's predecessor as archbishop of Mainz, Boniface (*c.* 675–754), is recorded as having received similar gifts from Rome.[8] Perhaps Cynehard knew of—and wanted to partake in—this network of gift-giving among the ecclesiastical elite.

The early medieval Insular world provides another example that highlights the difficulty of procuring these types of non-local substances. Willibald (*c.* 700–89), an English missionary and later bishop of Eichstätt, travelled to the Holy Land in the early eighth century. In the *Hodoeporicon*, the record of his life

7 Wallis, *Medieval Medicine*, 110–11; 'Epistula 114', in *Die Briefe des heiligen Bonifatius und Lullus*, ed. Tangl, 247.

8 'Epistula 49', in *Die Briefe des heiligen Bonifatius und Lullus*, ed. Tangl, 78–80; 'Epistula 62', 127–8.

that, according to the preface, he dictated to the nun Huneberc, he describes smuggling balsam out of Tyre by concealing it inside a reed plugged with petroleum hidden inside a calabash.[9] Willibald and his companions were arrested and their baggage examined, but they were eventually released when the search turned up nothing more than a calabash smelling of petroleum.[10] Had the balsam been discovered, Willibald claims that the punishment for smuggling out such a valuable product was death. If the story is true, it reveals not only the high price and difficulty of obtaining balsam, but also its importance to Willibald: why else would he have risked his life for this substance? While it is not recorded if this balsam was intended for medical, perfuming, or incense purposes (or a combination of these functions), balsam (*balsamum*), as well as its sap (*opobalsamum*), bark (*xilobalsamum*), and fruits (*carpobalsamum*), is recorded with some frequency in recipes.[11]

Returning to the continent, there are a number of non-medical texts that record the exchange of some of the exotic substances listed in recipes within elite networks. While the written sources introduce a bias towards the literate elite, the expensive nature of these items would suggest that any circulation was limited to individuals operating within well-endowed ecclesiastical, aristocratic, and royal networks. As noted above, epistolary evidence indicates that Boniface, archbishop of Mainz, was sent spices and resins as gifts from Roman clergy on three occasions. In one case, Cardinal Deacon Gemmulus sent four ounces of cinnamon, four ounces of costus, two pounds of pepper, and one pound of cozumber (a derivative of storax detailed below).[12] While it is unknown how long Boniface's supplies would have lasted, perhaps the movement of such products from Rome into the missionaries' territory helps to explain Lull's access to frankincense, pepper, and cinnamon (his gifts to Cuneburg) as well as Cynehard's letter to Lull requesting *exotica*. Did he know that such products had been sent to Mainz at an earlier date? Even if Boniface's gifts were no longer present, it is possible that news of the (past) existence

9 Huneberc, *Vitae Willibaldi et Wynnebaldi*, ed. O. Holder-Egger, *MGH SS* 14.1 (Hanover: Hahn, 1887), 80–117; Huneberc, *Hodoeporicon*, in *The Anglo-Saxon Missionaries in Germany*, trans. Charles Hugh Talbot (London: Sheed and Ward, 1954), 170. On Huneberc, see Bernhard Bischoff, 'Wer ist die Nonne von Heidenheim?' *Studien und Mitteilungen zur Geschichte des Benediktinerordens und seiner Zweige* 49 (1931): 387–8; Peter Dronke, *Women Writers of the Middle Ages: A Critical Study of Texts from Perpetua (†203) to Marguerite Porete (†1310)* (Cambridge: Cambridge University Press, 1984), 1–35.

10 Huneberc, *Hodoeporicon*, 170.

11 Cf. entries for these products in Carmélia Opsomer, *Index de la pharmacopée du I*[er] *au X*[e] *siècle*, 2 vols. (Hildesheim: Olms-Weidmann, 1989).

12 'Epistula 62', in *Die Briefe des heiligen Bonifatius und Lullus*, ed. Tangl, 127–8.

of these substances in Mainz had spread and/or that the networks between Rome and Frankish ecclesiastical centres resulted in the sporadic distribution of these ingredients in the Rhineland.

A letter in the *Collectio sangallensis* from the second half of the ninth century suggests that access to these types of non-local substances increased in the years following Gemmulus' gifts to Boniface. In this case, the letter records that a bishop, probably Salomon II of Constance, sent Louis the German exotic goods, including fine textiles, an ivory comb, and foreign fruits and spices, in an attempt to appease him.[13] Although there is no reference to medicine, many of the fruits, spices, gums, and resins listed in the letter, such as dates, figs, pomegranates, cinnamon, galangal, pepper, cloves, and mastic, appear as ingredients in medical recipes. Regardless, this text suggests that ecclesiastical and aristocratic elites may have had access to a wider range of foreign products by the middle of the ninth century: Salomon's gifts contained a much more diverse spread.

However, predating Salomon's peace offerings to Louis the German, there is also evidence for an even richer collection of eastern products entering the Latin west. First described by the *Royal Frankish Annals* and then later mentioned by Notker the Stammerer (*c.* 840–912), Harun al-Rashid, the Abbasid caliph (r. 786–809), sent gifts to Charlemagne in 802 and 807.[14] The largesse displayed by Harun al-Rashid was extraordinary, a clear signal of his wealth and power; indeed, among the most remarkable of his gifts was an elephant, the famous Abul Abbas. Other products named include luxurious linens and silks, a water clock, two enormous brass candlesticks, and, most importantly for this study, 'perfumes and ointments and balsam' (*odores atque unguenta et balsamum*).[15] While the *Royal Frankish Annals* do not describe the ingredients of the perfumes and ointments, it is highly probable that they were composed

13 *Collectio Sangallensis*, ed. Karl Zeumer, MGH *Formulae* (Hanover: Hahn, 1886), 29, at p. 415, lines 15–19: *Palliolum coloris prasini et aliud polimitum, spatulas palmarum cum suis fructibus, cynamomi, calangani, cariofili, masticis et piperis fasciculum, Caricas ficorum, malogranata, pectinem elefantinum, vermiculos, cicadas, aves psitacos, merulam albam et longissimam spinam de pisce marino*; Michael McCormick, *Origins of the European Economy: Communications and Commerce, A.D. 300–900* (Cambridge, 2001), 710.

14 *Annales regni Francorum inde ab a. 741 usque ad a. 829 qui dicuntur Annales laurissenses maiores et Einhardi*, ed. Friedrich Kurze, MGH SS *Rer. Germ.* 6 (Hanover: Hahn, 1895). Abul Abbas is first mentioned in the entry for 801 (in transit); for the arrival of these gifts in 802, see p. 117; for 807, see pp. 122–5. Notker, *Gesta Karoli Magni Imperatoris*, ed. Hans F. Haefele. MGH SS *Rer. Germ. N. S.* 12. (Berlin: Weidmann, 1959), 62–5.

15 *Annales regni Francorum*, ed. Kurze, 123–4.

of eastern resins, gums, and spices, including, perhaps, many of the individual substances named in the examples above.

Although these records do not directly link the non-local products involved in elite gift-giving to medical uses, the connection between exotic substances and medicine is more explicit in other sources.[16] The annual purchase of honey and spices, *pigmenta*, for the treatment of sick monks recorded in the *Gesta* of the Abbey of Fontenelle offers one such example. The abbot Ansegisus (*c.* 770–*c.* 833) allocated a pound of silver per year for this purpose.[17] The use of the term *pigmenta* is somewhat ambiguous as the word could refer to a range of products including paints, pigments, and their composite parts as well as spices and medicaments.[18] In this case, it makes sense to read *pigmenta* as spices due to the direct link with medical practice; these substances, however, may have been intended for multiple purposes given that medical recipes share many ingredients in common with paints and pigments.[19] The particular products the abbot intended to buy remains unknown.

A final example offers more specificity while continuing to blur the lines between substances intended for medicinal, artisanal, and ecclesiastical uses: a ninth-century list from Corbie details various items the monks intended to buy at the market in Cambrai—if they had sufficient funds (*si pretium habemus*).[20] A diverse range of products are named, from fairly humble goods, such as wax, to imported spices and resins, including pepper and mastic. While many of these items, such as bandages and leeches, were clearly destined for medical

16 The ointments recorded by the *Royal Frankish Annals* for the year 807 present a partial exception: while their purpose is not stated, it seems likely that they were intended for medical uses.

17 *Chronique des Abbés de Fontenelle (Saint-Wandrille)*, ed. and trans. Pascal Pradié (Paris: Belles Lettres, 1999), 13.8, at p. 188: *Ad infirmorum curam mel et pigmenta libram I.* See also McCormick, *Origins of the European Economy*, 709.

18 Jan Frederik Niermeyer, *Mediae Latinitatis Lexicon Minus*, 2nd ed. (Leiden: Brill, 2002), 796.

19 For more on ink and paint production, see Dominique Cardon, *Natural Dyes: Sources, Tradition, Technology and Science* (London: Archetype, 2007) and, for the early medieval context, McKitterick, *The Carolingians and the Written Word*, 241–6 and Adriano Caffaro, *Scrivere in oro: Ricettari medievali d'arte e artigianato (secoli IX–XI). Codici di Lucca e Ivrea* (Naples: Liguori, 2003). For the multipurpose nature of these substances more generally, see also Hilary Becker, 'Pigment nomenclature in the ancient Near East, Greece, and Rome', *Archaeological and Anthropological Sciences* 14 (2022), https://doi.org/10.1007/s12520-021-01394-1; and Nicholas Everett, 'The Manuscript Evidence for Pharmacy in the Early Middle Ages', in *Writing the Early Medieval West*, ed. Elina Screen and Charles West (Cambridge: Cambridge University Press, 2018), 115–30.

20 *Polyptyque de l'abbé Irminon ou dénombrement des manses, des serfs et des revenus de l'abbaye de Saint-Germain-des-Prés sous le règne de Charlemagne*, ed. Benjamin Edme Charles Guérard, 2 vols. (Paris: Imprimerie royale, 1844), vol. 2, 336.

purposes, others could have served a variety functions. The mineral products named, such as sulphur and orpiment, are often associated with the production of inks and paints but are also listed as ingredients in recipes; likewise, many of the exotic spices, resins, roots, and other plant products could have been used to prepare incense or medications—or the incense could have been used for medical purposes, as it, too, appears as an ingredient in medical recipes.[21] Overall, nearly all of the goods recorded in this list could have been used in a pharmaceutical context, thereby offering a glimpse into the range of non-local *materia medica* that was being commercially traded—or at least that the monks expected to be available for purchase—at Cambrai in the ninth century. Intriguingly, the quantities requested for each of the exotic products vary significantly: some substances, such as pepper, were to be bought in bulk (120 pounds), whereas much smaller amounts were named for others, including galangal, spikenard, and cozumber (ten pounds for galangal, five for both spikenard and cozumber). While this could reflect the volume of each product needed by the monastic community, it may also relate to the prices of these individual substances and/or indicate that some products were circulating in smaller quantities.

Before examining non-local *materia medica* in recipes, it is important to consider what these records suggest about the potential availability of exotic ingredients in the Carolingian world. First, given that relatively few non-medical sources document these types of substances, it is likely that access to such products, whether acquired through trade, gift exchange, or even illicit means, would have been extremely limited. The handful of references reviewed above do, however, indicate that at least a number of the many non-local ingredients listed in recipes *did* appear in the Frankish Empire during this period.

Nonetheless, although these items made appearances, the length of time they would have lasted, in terms of both quantity and quality, also deserves consideration. The texts suggest that exotic products did not typically move in large volumes: take the ounces and pounds recorded in the letter to Boniface or the five pounds of spikenard and cozumber in Corbie's 'shopping list'. The large amount of pepper named in this source is an exception, but even 120 Carolingian pounds, roughly equivalent to forty kilograms today, is not a vast sum, depending on how long it was intended to last and/or how widely it was

21 For example, *thymiama* appears as an ingredient in *Ad cadiuo homine* of BAV reg. lat. 1143 (f. 109r); see Appendix 2, entry 18.3. For more on the topic of incense in medicine, see Burridge, 'Incense in Medicine'. Also noted by Henry Sigerist in passing; see Henry E. Sigerist, '"The Sphere of Life and Death" in Early Medieval Manuscripts', *Bulletin of the History of Medicine* 11, no. 3 (1942), 292–303, at p. 296.

expected to be distributed.[22] While the record of gift-giving among elites suggests only the sporadic arrival of these items in the west, the 'shopping list' from Corbie and the annual supply of *pigmenta* documented by the *Gesta* of the Abbey of Fontenelle point to more regular trade in spices. Moreover, as noted above, these records only present evidence of elite communities—royal, aristocratic, and ecclesiastical—partaking in the giving, receiving, and buying of exotic substances. The presence of *exotica* at Cambrai's market, however, reveals that individuals outside of or on the peripheries of these elite networks may have been able to acquire such products, too. Yet, even taking the biases of the sources into account, it seems unlikely that these non-local substances circulated widely among the majority of the population given their expense and relative rarity.

With this review of the general movement and potential availability of a selection of foreign products, let us examine their appearance as ingredients in recipes.

3 Exotic *Materia Medica*

Defining what constitutes 'non-local' presents a number of challenges.[23] At the most fundamental level, given the size of the Frankish Empire, the variety of (micro-)climates within its borders, and its influence into neighbouring regions, where does 'local' end and 'non-local' begin?[24] A monk in St Gall

22 Jean Lestocquoy gives fifteen Carolingian pounds as roughly equivalent to five kilograms; see Jean Lestocquoy, 'Épices, médecine et abbayes', in *Études mérovingiennes. Actes des journées de Poitiers, 1er-3 mai 1952* (Paris: A. et J. Picard, 1953), 179–86, at pp. 184–5. On pepper's comparatively 'mundane' nature among *exotica*, see, for example, Kasper Grønland Evers' study of ancient trade between the Indian subcontinent and Roman Empire, *Worlds Apart Trading Together: The Organisation of Long-Distance Trade Between Rome and India in Antiquity* (Oxford: Archaeopress, 2017), 72–4. Likewise, on pepper's status as a 'necessary luxury' (though focused on the later Middle Ages), see Paul Freedman, 'Spices and Late-Medieval European Ideas of Scarcity and Value', *Speculum* 80, no. 4 (2005): 1209–27, https://doi.org/10.1017/S0038713400001391. See also Zohar Amar and Efraim Lev, *Arabian Drugs in Early Medieval Mediterranean Medicine* (Edinburgh: Edinburgh University Press, 2017).

23 On one approach to defining gradations of localness, see Bernhard Zeller, Charles West, Francesca Tinti, Marco Stoffella, Nicolas Schroeder, Carine van Rhijn, Steffen Patzold, Thomas Kohl, Wendy Davies, and Miriam Czock, *Neighbours and Strangers: Local Societies in Early Medieval Europe* (Manchester: Manchester University Press, 2020), xiv-xv.

24 As noted in Chapter 1, Linda Ehrsam Voigts has also considered the potential impact of past climatic conditions on the cultivation of medicinal plants in the Insular world, pointing to another important dimension to take into account when investigating this

would have had relatively easy access to alpine plants but perhaps encountered difficulties in procuring Mediterranean products. On the other hand, an aristocratic household in Septimania might have experienced the opposite situation. While this points to the difficulty of assessing ease of access within the Carolingian world, what about products that would have been imported from outside of the Empire? Would goods sent from the eastern Mediterranean be considered exotic beyond the Alps but more readily available in Rome, Ravenna, and sites that maintained a greater level of contact with the Byzantine world? Even non-local substances, therefore, are subject to varying degrees of accessibility and exoticness. That being said, non-local *materia medica* that were native to the lands beyond the Mediterranean basin, such as southeast Asia, would have travelled extremely long distances—and required significant financial backing—to reach any part of the Carolingian world. These types of substances, including a number of the gums and resins already noted, are unambiguously non-local. This chapter therefore concentrates on *materia medica* that would have been grown or collected far beyond north-western Europe and the Mediterranean region, such as animal products from the Himalayas and spices, resins, and woods from the Maluku Islands.

3.1 *What's in a Name? The Challenge of Identifying Ingredients and Their Origins*

When attempting to understand the relative localness of *materia medica*, geographic descriptors attached to an ingredient's name may seem to provide especially valuable insights. Attic honey, African snails, and Illyrian irises—all recorded as ingredients in recipes—each link a product to a particular location, but do they really indicate their source? It may be useful to consider modern parallels: French fries are not inherently French, nor are Belgian waffles necessarily Belgian, though these geographic labels may provide insights into consumers' perceptions. In some cases, such as *fenugrecum* or *reopontico* (terms for fenugreek and rhubarb, respectively), the geographic descriptor appears to have become integrated into the name of the product itself. On the other hand, as Hilary Becker has noted with respect to the terminology used for pigments in ancient sources, such labels could be used to differentiate between 'discrete varieties', reflecting whence these products originated historically rather than at the time the authors were writing.[25] Moreover, Becker cautions that this nomenclature may not convey the substances' actual points

topic. Voigts, 'Anglo-Saxon Plant Remedies', 261–3. See also Pilsworth, *Healthcare in Early Medieval Northern Italy*, 80.

25 Becker, 'Pigment nomenclature in the ancient Near East, Greece, and Rome'.

of origin and could instead document another location along the journey to their final destination.[26] Given these ambiguities, the ingredients selected for analysis in the present chapter do not contain geographic descriptors as standard elements within their names.

More fundamentally, however, the identities of many ingredients continue to be debated given the challenges posed by translating and interpreting ancient and medieval terms for *materia medica*.[27] Consider, for example, Jerry Stannard's thorough investigation into 'the plant called Moly' that unpacks the many varied modern identifications (at least a dozen) that have been proposed for the plant(s) in question and the convoluted textual puzzle presented by the Greek and Latin sources involved in the 'moly tradition'.[28] Stannard's detective work revealed not only that 'many of the attempts to identify moly have gone astray', but also that 'in the Greek tradition, moly designates at least three different plants', which resulted in further confusions in Latin translations and the descendants of these texts.[29] Stannard found that one of the major turning points in this nomenclatural enigma stemmed from a misinterpretation of a section of Dioscorides' *De materia medica*: just before describing moly, which, in Dioscorides' case, most likely refers to an *Allium* species, the text addresses wild rue.[30] Dioscorides reports a resemblance between the two plants based on their shared colours and explains that, as a result, the Cappadocians also call the former 'moly'.[31] This mention of synonymy appears to have confused later writers, who then interpreted moly as referring to both an *Allium* and wild rue; simultaneously, some authors conflated moly with plants with similar-sounding names (e.g., Galen's 'mylē'), and the range of synonyms for each these plants added further layers of complexity.[32] Becker, too, highlights the importance of regional name variation, while the multiple linguistic traditions on which medical texts drew introduced additional variables.[33]

Yet, as Gavin Hardy and Laurence Totelin note, 'despite all these difficulties, scholars since Antiquity have attempted to identify plants named in 'older' authorities', and, following the development of Linnaean binomial nomenclature, there has been a strong emphasis on species-specific identification.[34]

26 Ibid.
27 Gavin Hardy and Laurence Totelin, *Ancient Botany* (London: Routledge, 2016), 93–104.
28 Jerry Stannard, 'The Plant Called Moly', *Osiris* 14 (1962): 254–307.
29 Stannard, 'The Plant Called Moly', 254.
30 Stannard, 'The Plant Called Moly', 259–63; Dioscorides, *De materia medica*, 3.46–7.
31 Dioscorides, *De materia medica*, 3.46–7.
32 Stannard, 'The Plant Called Moly', 263–6.
33 Becker, 'Pigment nomenclature in the ancient Near East, Greece, and Rome'.
34 Hardy and Totelin, *Ancient Botany*, 94–5.

However, given that the terms for *materia medica* were unstable and variable (across languages, time, and space), it is often necessary to take a broader and more cautious approach to the identification of ingredients. In fact, it must be remembered that multiple, distinct species can be used to produce a single ingredient. The spice known as 'cinnamon', for example, can be harvested from several different species within the *Cinnamomum* genus, including *C. cassia*, *C. burmannii*, *C. loureiroi*, and *C. verum*.[35] While the early medieval Latin terms *cinnamomum* and *cassia* (and their orthographic variants) are each commonly identified with only one species, it seems more appropriate to classify both as plants potentially related to all those that are today considered to represent 'cinnamon'. Although it may appear problematic that the various species belonging to the *Cinnamomum* genus are native to a vast region, from Sri Lanka to China to Indonesia, it is evident that, regardless of which species is concerned, the tree would have grown in south, east, or southeast Asia and, for the purposes of this study, fall into the category of unambiguously non-local ingredients.[36] The following case study therefore focuses on a select group of ingredients whose origins were, without question, extremely far from Francia.

3.2 *From Ambergris to Zedoary*

The aforementioned work of John Riddle and Michael McCormick offers a useful entry point into an investigation of non-local *materia medica* unrecorded in classical and late antique medical writings. In the first recipe collection of cod. sang. 44 (pp. 228–55), Riddle highlights the appearance of two new products: camphor, an aromatic extract from the wood of the camphor laurel, and ambergris, a pungent substance produced in the digestive tract of sperm whales.[37] In Riddle's analysis of recipes from several manuscripts beyond this study's manuscript sample, he also notes galangal and zedoary, both

35 Pei Chen, Jianghao Sun, and Paul Ford, 'Differentiation of the Four Major Species of Cinnamons (*C. burmannii, C. verum, C. cassia,* and *C. loureiroi*) Using a Flow Injection Mass Spectrometric (FIMS) Fingerprinting Method', *Journal of Agricultural and Food Chemistry* 62, no. 12 (2014): 2516–21, https://doi.org/10.1021/jf405580c.

36 Chen, Sun, and Ford, 'Differentiation of the Four Major Species of Cinnamons'. For a helpful visualisation, see Figure 9 in Weiwei Wang, Khanh Trung Kien Nguyen, Chunguang Zhao, and Hsiao-Chun Hung, 'Earliest curry in Southeast Asia and the global spice trade 2000 years ago'. *Science Advances* 9, no. 29 (2023): https://doi.org/10.1126/sciadv.adh5517.

37 Riddle, 'The Introduction and Use of Eastern Drugs', 190–1. See also Bruno Laurioux, 'Parfums d'Orient. La science des épices au Moyen Âge', in *Parfums et odeurs au Moyen Âge. Science, usage, symboles*, ed. Agostino Paravicini Bagliani (Florence: SISMEL Edizioni del Galluzzo, 2015), 61–87.

rhizomes in the ginger family, as similarly newly recorded *materia medica*.[38] McCormick comments on the appearance of *azarum*, camphor, and ambergris in cod. sang. 44 and mentions further examples of camphor in the *Lorscher Arzneibuch*; Glasgow, University Library, Hunter 96; and a section of cod. sang. 217 that is not part of the sample of recipes involved in this study.[39] Both Riddle and McCormick argue that the appearances of camphor, ambergris, and the other ingredients they each identified in the recipe literature reflect the arrival of these products in the Latin west during this period.[40] While it is impossible to prove this without further evidence, such as archaeological finds or additional textual sources (e.g., the record of gift exchanges noted above) that directly confirm the importation of these substances, the linked movement of knowledge and goods will be reconsidered below. The names of these substances—derived, in both medieval Latin and modern English, from

38 Riddle's examples of zedoary and galangal (which he terms 'galingale') come from London, British Library, Harley MS 585; Glasgow, University Library, Hunter 96 (*olim* T.4.13); and Karlsruhe, Badische Landesbibliothek, Aug. perg. 120. These findings are based on his assessment of the published transcriptions of recipe collections in *Studien und Texte*, ed. Sigerist, and Grattan and Singer, *Anglo-Saxon Magic and Medicine* (note: the text of the recipe collection analysed in London, BL Harley MS 585, the *Lacnunga*, is written not in Latin but in Old English). It must also be noted that there is some debate regarding the timing of zedoary's arrival in the west: Heinrich Zörnig claims that it appears in the works of Paul of Aegina and Aetius of Amida, but Riddle suggests that this is a later interpolation. See Riddle, 'The Introduction and Use of Eastern Drugs', 191–2 and Heinrich Zörnig, *Arzneidrogen als Nachschlagebuch für den Gebrauch der Apotheker, Ärzte, Veterinärärzte, Drogisten und Studierenden der Pharmazie*, 2 vols. (Leipzig: Klinkhardt, 1909), vol. 1, 558.

39 McCormick, *Origins of the European Economy*, 714, nn. 83–4. For the manuscripts in question, see Bamberg, Staatsbibliothek, Msc. Med. 1 and Glasgow, UL Hunter 96. Although McCormick suggests that *azarum* was introduced to western Europe during the Carolingian period, I suggest that *azarum* represents an alternative spelling of *asarum*, hazelwort, a plant native to Europe and known in Antiquity. This seems to make more sense in the contexts in which I have seen the term. In the recipes containing *azarum* in cod. sang. 44 (all of which appear within a few folia of each other in one of the manuscript's recipe collections: pp. 345, 351–3), the other ingredients are all locally available products, including beer, a substance highlighted in Chapter 4 in relation to adaptations made to suit local conditions. In one of these recipes, the juice of the ingredient in question (*azari sucum*) is recommended, strengthening an identification with hazelwort rather than a resin. For examples, see Appendix 2, entries 5.18.3 and 5.22.

40 McCormick, *Origins of the European Economy*, 714–15; Riddle, 'The Introduction and Use of Eastern Drugs', 190–6; Riddle also highlights zedoary and galangal as new ingredients, though his references to these substances appear in other manuscripts, including Glasgow, UL Hunter 96 and London, BL Harley MS 585. On camphor and ambergris, see also Amar and Lev, *Arabian Drugs in Early Medieval Mediterranean Medicine*, and especially Chapter 3, '"Arabian' Substances', 129–227 (camphor is discussed in detail on pp. 144–8, and ambergris on pp. 148–52).

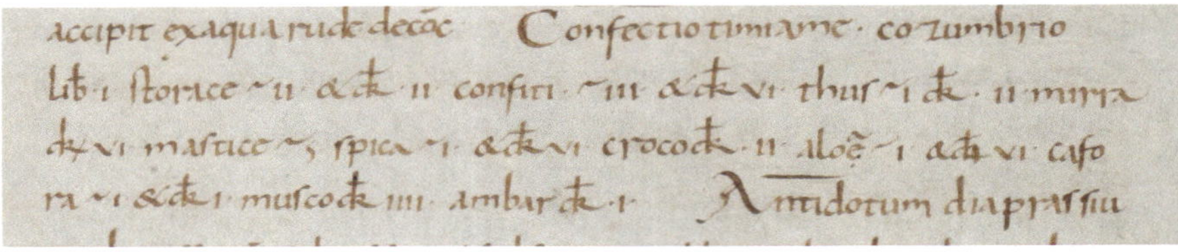

FIGURE 3 *Confectio timiame* in St. Gallen, Stiftsbibliothek, cod. sang. 44 (p. 247), an early medieval composite manuscript, the second half of which contains medical texts and was written in northern Italy in the ninth century (https://www.e-codices.unifr.ch/de/csg/0044/247)

Arabic terms, though often originally stemming from other languages such as Malay—do point to their eastern origins and immediately support the idea that Islamicate trade networks were central to their westward diffusion.[41] Are there additional examples of ambergris, camphor, galangal, or zedoary found in within the manuscripts under analysis? Is there evidence to suggest that knowledge of these products spread within the Frankish Empire?

3.3 *The* Confectio Timiame*: Camphor, Ambergris, and Other Non-local* Materia Medica

Despite highlighting the newness of camphor and ambergris and their appearances in the same manuscript, cod. sang. 44, neither Riddle nor McCormick point out that these two products actually appear in the very same recipe in this manuscript, the *Confectio timiame*, as shown in Figure 3 and detailed below:

> A preparation of incense. Cozumber, 1 pound; storax, 2 ounces and 2 *denarii*; confita, 3 ounces and 6 *denarii*; frankincense, 1 ounce and 2 *denarii*; myrrh, 6 *denarii*; mastic, ½ ounce; spikenard, 1 ounce and 6 *denarii*; saffron, 2 *denarii*; agarwood, 1 ounce and 6 *denarii*; camphor, 1 ounce and 1 *denarius*; musk, 4 *denarii*; ambergris, 1 *denarius*.[42]

41 Camphor, for example, can be traced to the Malay *kāpūr*; Hūšang A'lam, 'Camphor', in *Encyclopædia Iranica*, edited by Ahmad Ashraf, Nicholas Sims-Williams, Mahnaz Moazami, Mohsen Ashtiany, Christopher J. Brunner, Manouchehr Kasheff, and Habib Borjian. Vol. 4/7 (1990): 743–7, https://iranicaonline.org/articles/camphor-npers; Riddle, 'The Introduction and Use of Eastern Drugs', 190–2. On camphor, see also Amar and Lev, *Arabian Drugs in Early Medieval Mediterranean Medicine*, 144–8.

42 Cod. sang. 44, p. 247: *Confectio timiame. Cozumbrio lib I, storace ~ II et dr II, confiti ~ III et dr VI, thus ~ I dr II, mirra dr VI, mastice ~ s, spica ~ I et dr VI, croco dr II, aloa ~ I et dr VI, cafora ~ I et dr I, musco dr IIII, ambar dr I.* See Appendix 2, entry 5.7.

Although this is a recipe for incense and does not include a list of ailments it intends to treat, its appearance within a recipe collection and listing of many ingredients that are frequently named in treatments suggest that it was intended for use in a medical context. Its simple presentation is not unlike many of the recipes for composite ingredients, such as oxymel (a mixture of vinegar, honey, and sometimes additional components) or mixed oils (rose oil (*oleo roseo*), cedar oil (*oleo cedrinum*), myrtle oil (*oleo mirtino*), and so on), that would have required advance preparation before they could have been used in recipes. Finally, as noted above, incense appears as an ingredient in recipes, confirming that it could have been used for both pharmaceutical and liturgical functions.[43]

A review of this recipe's twelve ingredients, cozumber (*cozumbrio*), storax (*storace*), confita (*confiti*), frankincense (*thus*), myrrh (*mirra*), mastic (*mastice*), spikenard (*spica*), saffron (*croco*), agarwood (*aloa*), camphor (*cafora*), musk (*musco*), and ambergris (*ambar*), reveals its total reliance on non-local products: not a single ingredient is native to northern and/or western Europe. Most of the ingredients are aromatic gums and resins, although ambergris and musk stand out as animal-based substances.

While Riddle and McCormick emphasised the newness of only ambergris and camphor, the appearance of three other ingredients in this incense recipe, cozumber, confita, and musk, is similarly noteworthy. McCormick does make a passing reference to cozumber, classifying it as an 'exotic substance' and noting that its 'derivation … is unclear'; confita, on the other hand, is mentioned by neither author.[44] According to Carmélia Opsomer's *Index de la pharmacopée du Ier au Xe siècle*, these ingredients do not occur in classical sources, though both terms are listed in later medical texts, such as the *Alphita*, a thirteenth-century medico-botanical glossary.[45] This text records that the two substances are related to each other (*cozimbrum* is described as *fex confite*) and represent derivatives of storax, an identification which fits within the context of an incense recipe.[46] In Alejandro García González' commentary on this glossary,

43 Burridge, 'Incense in medicine'; Henry E. Sigerist, '"The Sphere of Life and Death" in Early Medieval Manuscripts', 296.

44 McCormick, *Origins of the European Economy*, 708.

45 *Cozimbrium* is recorded six times in *Index de la pharmacopée du Ier au Xe siècle* (see Opsomer, *Index de la pharmacopée*, vol. 1, 222) in non-classical texts, while there is no entry for *confita*. *Alphita*, ed. Alejandro García González (Florence: SISMEL Edizioni del Galluzzo, 2007). Sigerist describes cozumber as a 'precious kind of aromatic gum' and notes that confita is usually found 'in connection with gums', although he was 'not sure what it actually is'; Sigerist, '"The Sphere of Life and Death" in Early Medieval Manuscripts', 296.

46 *Alphita*, ed. García González: *confita*, entry C4 (at p. 174), and *cozimbrum*, C114 (at p. 184).

he identifies 'confita' as a 'deformation of the Greek γομφίτης', thereby linking it more specifically to a gum resin derived from storax, *Styrax officinalis*.[47] The linguistic origins of cozumber, however, remain uncertain (though the *Alphita*'s entry for storax again refers to this substance as a derivative product).[48]

Excepting medical contexts, I have seen cozumber mentioned in only two other contemporary sources, both addressed at the beginning of this chapter: it is recorded in a) the letter to Boniface as one of the gifts sent by Gemmulus, and b) the Corbie 'shopping list' as one of the *pigmenta* the monks were expected to buy at the Cambrai market.[49] The lack of cozumber and confita in classical texts, their appearance in early medieval recipes and, in the case of cozumber, two non-medical records, as well as their continued presence in later medical writings strongly support the argument that these two products, at least in these specific forms, first arrived in western Europe in the eighth century. The documentation of cozumber in non-medical sources, moreover, adds weight to the argument put forward by Riddle and McCormick that both the substances themselves *and* information about them arrived in the Frankish world during this period. While it should not be assumed that cozumber is representative of all of the newly recorded ingredients, the Corbie list also includes galangal and zedoary.[50] The appearance of multiple previously unrecorded non-local substances in this context suggests that these products, and quite possibly other *exotica*, were circulating in the Latin west at this time—if only in small quantities and at great expense. Indeed, since the abbot's instructions only represent a *pigmenta* 'wish list', it remains unknown what substances were *actually* available for purchase at the Cambrai market; that the Corbie monks *expected* to be able to buy these products, however, is significant.

While galangal and zedoary are both named as new ingredients by Riddle and McCormick, and while additional examples can be found in the present recipe sample, neither appear in the *Confectio timiame*.[51] Let us return to this

47 Ibid, 400–1: '*Confita* < deformación del gr. γομφίτης ... designa la gomorresina del 'estoraque', una planta identificada con la estiracácea *Styrax officinalis L.*'

48 Ibid, 403, 551. For the entry on storax, see S46 (at pp. 290–1).

49 'Epistula 62', in *Die Briefe des heiligen Bonifatius und Lullus*, ed. Tangl, 127–8; *Polyptyque de l'abbé Irminon*, ed. Guérard, vol. 2, 336.

50 *Polyptyque de l'abbé Irminon*, ed. Guérard, vol. 2, 336.

51 Galangal is listed as ingredient twice in BnF lat. 11218: first in the *Pocio mirabilis contra omnes infirmitates* (f. 99r) and secondly in a recipe for which the title has faded and is no longer legible (f. 124v, following the *Antidotum de peretro* and preceding the *Pocio ad apostema*). Both galangal and zedoary are named as ingredients in BnF lat. 11219: galangal appears in the *Puluera ad epaticos* (f. 221vb) and in a recipe for those who cannot urinate, *Ad eos qui urinam facere non possunt* (f. 225va); zedoary is listed in the *Potio ad*

incense recipe and consider one final ingredient, musk, that appears to represent a reintroduced substance in the Latin west—though likely entirely new to the Frankish world. In Latin, the first attestation of this substance, a secretion of the musk deer, occurs in Jerome's (d. 419) *Adversus Iovinianum*.[52] Musk then disappears from the written record in the west, though it is mentioned by a handful of Greek sources, such as Paul of Aegina (fl. seventh century), during the following centuries.[53] The next Latin references to musk come from Carolingian medical texts, such as this incense recipe, suggesting that it was reintroduced to western Europe during this period. Most significantly from a medical perspective, musk appears in neither classical medical writings nor late antique Latin medical texts, revealing that even if musk had been known in earlier periods, it was not recorded in relation to medicine in the west.[54]

The existence within a single recipe of a cluster of five newly introduced (or reintroduced) non-local ingredients is particularly striking. While the recipe's exclusive reliance on foreign, imported substances adds to its overall exoticness, its listing of a variety of new products is most noteworthy. By incorporating substances unrecorded in classical and late antique medical texts, it becomes clear that not only were multiple sources used in the creation of this recipe collection, but that some of these sources included information beyond the classical canon. Furthermore, this recipe's inclusion within a recipe collection indicates that at least one site of manuscript production had access to non-classical medical information and, crucially, was open to recording it. In this collection, the incense recipe appears to be fully integrated within the composition; information from non-classical and non-local sources is not segregated from the rest of the material or distinguished in any way.

Riddle and McCormick consulted transcriptions of recipe collections from a number of other manuscripts not analysed in the present study, finding

carbunculum (ff. 223va–233vb). For these recipes see Appendix 2, entries 3.10, 3.16, 4.1, 4.6, and 4.2, respectively.

52 Anya H. King, *Scent from the Garden of Paradise: Musk and the Medieval Islamic World* (Leiden: Brill, 2017); Amar and Lev, *Arabian Drugs*, again, see Chapter 3, "Arabian' Substances', 129–227 (musk is discussed on pp. 157–62).

53 King, *Scent from the Garden of Paradise*, see especially pp. 133–6 for late antique references to musk.

54 Amar and Lev, *Arabian Drugs*, 157–62. Although galangal is generally thought to have been newly introduced to the west during this period, it may have followed a similar trajectory; cf. Dioscorides, *De materia medica*, 1.4–5. For the standard interpretation, see Amar and Lev, *Arabian Drugs*, 110–12; for the idea that it was introduced in the thirteenth century, see Carlo Battisti, 'Ripercussioni lessicali del commercio orientale nel periodo giustinianeo', in *Moneta e scambi nell'alto medioevo, 21–27 aprile 1960*, Settimane 8 (Spoleto: Fondazione Centro italiano di studi sull'alto medioevo, 1961), 627–82, at p. 639.

additional examples of recipes with their highlighted ingredients (ambergris, camphor, galangal, and zedoary). This indicates that knowledge of these ingredients was not limited to a single centre of manuscript production, namely, the northern Italian site in which cod. sang. 44 was copied, but rather that this information was spreading within the Latin west. Yet, given that the studies of Riddle and McCormick were based on a more limited sample of recipe collections from the Carolingian period (i.e., the transcriptions of Sigerist, Jörimann, and Stoll), their work only scratched the surface of the so-called 'miscellaneous' recipe literature. Indeed, McCormick notes, 'I have not had the leisure to undertake the exhaustive philological and historical study these treatises—and their MSS—deserve: they may still hold some surprises'.[55] By considering a larger sample of recipes, what can now be said about the dissemination of this knowledge?

3.4 *The Recurrent Cluster: Parallels Among Incense Recipes*

Each of the five newly introduced ingredients found in the *Confectio timiame* (ambergris, camphor, confita, cozumber, and musk) appears in additional recipes within the sample. In nine recipes, one or two of these newly recorded ingredients are listed alongside typical *materia medica*, both local and exotic. This chapter's opening example, the *Antidotum gira deacoloquintidis*, which included camphor among its ingredients, represents one of these nine recipes. Nineteen additional recipes, however, have been identified as closely related variants within an incense recipe tradition—a tradition to which the *Confectio timiame* also belongs. I shall first review the spread of this family of incense recipes with its unique group of ingredients before exploring the appearance of these ingredients individually.

The manuscript evidence suggests that knowledge of this incense preparation was rapidly disseminated. As shown in Table 2, I have identified variants of it in five other manuscripts. Four of these codices are today located in the Stiftsbibliothek St. Gallen (codd. sang. 752 and 761 each contain one recipe, cod. sang. 878 preserves two, and cod. sang. 899 lists three), though they were produced in several different, if closely connected, writing centres (St Gall, Fulda, Reichenau, and St Gall, respectively).[56] A manuscript in the Bibliothèque nationale de France, BnF lat. 11219, adds a further twelve recipes

55 McCormick, *Origins of the European Economy*, 714, n. 84.

56 Cod. sang. 752, p. 82; Cod. sang. 761, p. 66; cod. sang. 878, p. 334; cod. sang. 899, p. 137; see Appendix 2, entries, 10.3, 12.5, 13.2.1–2, and 14.3.1–3, respectively.

that are also based on this core group of ingredients.[57] These numerous recipe variants and their constituent parts deserve a more detailed examination.

The titles of the recipes in codd. sang. 752 and 761, *Thymiama paltgrimi* and *Thimiama*, respectively, leave no doubt that these, too, are preparations for incense. The two recipes in cod. sang. 878, representing the only material written on p. 334, lack such an obvious reference to incense: the first recipe, labelled 'cod. sang. 878 (a)' in the tables, is missing a title, while the second recipe, 'cod. sang. 878 (b)', is listed as *Item aliter*, 'likewise in another way'. It can be assumed, however, that these recipes also concern incense given the parallels they share with the other recipes and the absence of this particular combination of ingredients in other contexts. Like cod. sang. 878, the groups of incense recipes in cod. sang. 899 (see Figure 4) and BnF lat. 11219 are clustered together on individual folia and represent the only material on the pages in question. In both manuscripts, titles explicitly link these recipes to incense.[58]

As seen in Table 2, the twenty recipes, despite containing a variety of different ingredients, centre around a primary group of five substances (i.e., ingredients that appear in at least ninety percent of the recipes), and these almost perfectly parallel the five newly recorded ingredients. The five core ingredients are agarwood, confita, cozumber, camphor, and musk, meaning that ambergris is the only newly recorded product that is listed less consistently. Of the five primary ingredients, agarwood appears in all twenty recipes, confita and cozumber in nineteen (ninety-five percent), and camphor and musk in eighteen (ninety percent). Notably, agarwood, the fragrant wood of aquilaria trees, is both the only ingredient to appear in every recipe and, despite its similarly exotic origins, the only ingredient within the core group that was already recorded in the west in Antiquity.[59] Table 2 reveals that, in addition to these five most frequently named ingredients, frankincense, storax, cloves, and cinnamon are listed in the majority of recipes, while ambergris, spikenard, saffron, myrrh, mastic, and galingale appear in half of the recipes or less. Although these twenty recipes are evidently related and share many similarities, very few present exactly the same group of ingredients and none is perfectly identical; that is, even though several preparations, such the second recipe of cod. sang. 899 and seventh recipe of BnF lat. 11219, contain the same ingredients, they are arranged differently and/or name varying quantities.

57 BnF lat. 11219, ff. 227r–227v; see Appendix 2, entries 4.8–19.

58 Note: while all twelve incense recipes in BnF lat. 11219 are found on f. 227v, the title of this section occurs on the preceding page, f. 227r.

59 Arlene López-Sampson and Tony Page, 'History of Use and Trade of Agarwood', *Economic Botany* 72 (2018): 107–29, https://doi.org/10.1007/s12231-018-9408-4.

TABLE 2 Incense recipes containing the ingredient cluster

Ms	**Cod. sang. 899 (a)**	**Cod. sang. 878 (b)**	**BnF lat. 11219 (h)**	**Cod. sang. 44**	**BnF lat. 11219 (e)**	**BnF lat. 11219 (i)**	**BnF lat. 11219 (a)**	**Cod. sang. 899 (b)**	**BnF lat. 11219 (g)**	**BnF lat. 11219 (j)**
Recipe title	*Confectio timiamatis*	*Item aliter*	*Confectio timiamatis*	*Confectio timiame*	*Confectio timiamatis ad gragantum*	*Item timiamatis confectio*	*Timiama*	*Item alia timiamatis confectio*	[untitled]	*Item*
Ingredients	cozumber	cozumber	cozumber	cozumber	cozumber	cozumber	cozumber	cozumber	cozumber	cozumber
	confita	confita	confita	confita	confita	confita	confita	confita	confita	confita
	agarwood	agarwood	agarwood	agarwood	agarwood	agarwood	agarwood	agarwood	agarwood	agarwood
	camphor	camphor	camphor	camphor	camphor	camphor	camphor	camphor	camphor	camphor
	musk	musk	musk	musk	musk	musk	musk	musk	musk	musk
	ambergris	ambergris	ambergris	ambergris	ambergris	ambergris	ambergris			
	frankincense	frankincense	frankincense	frankincense	frankincense	frankincense	frankincense	frankincense	frankincense	frankincense
	storax	storax	storax	storax	storax	storax	storax	storax	storax	storax
	cloves	cloves	cloves		cloves	cloves	cloves	cloves	cloves	cloves
	cinnamon	cinnamon	cinnamon		cinnamon	cinnamon	cinnamon	cinnamon	cinnamon	
	spikenard	spikenard	spikenard	spikenard	spikenard	spikenard		spikenard	spikenard	spikenard
	saffron	saffron	saffron	saffron						saffron
	myrrh	myrrh	myrrh	myrrh						
	mastic	mastic	mastic	mastic						
	galingale	galingale	galingale							

Note: the order of the ingredients in each recipe has been rearranged to illustrate their parallels more clearly; recipes are ordered from most complex to simplest

TABLE 2 Incense recipes containing the ingredient cluster (*cont.*)

Ms	**Cod. sang. 899 (c)**	**BnF lat. 11219 (c)**	**BnF lat. 11219 (f)**	**BnF lat. 11219 (d)**	**Cod. sang. 878 (a)**	**Cod. sang. 761**	**Cod. sang. 752**	**BnF lat. 11219 (l)**	**BnF lat. 11219 (k)**	**BnF lat. 11219 (b)**
Recipe title	*Item alia*	*Item Alia*	[untitled]	*Alia*	[untitled]	*Thimiama*	*Thymiama paltgrimi*	*Confectio timiama*	*Item*	*Tymiamum*
Ingredients	cozumber	cozumber	cozumber	cozumber	cozumber	cozumber	cozumber	cozumber	confita	cozumber
	confita	confita	confita	confita	confita	confita	confita	confita		
	agarwood	agarwood	agarwood	agarwood	agarwood	agarwood	agarwood	agarwood	agarwood	agarwood
	camphor	camphor	camphor	camphor	camphor	camphor	camphor	camphor		
	musk	musk	musk	musk	musk	musk	musk		musk	
					ambergris	ambergris			ambergris	
	frankincense	frankincense	frankincense	frankincense				frankincense	frankincense	frankincense
	storax	storax	storax	storax	storax			storax		
	cloves	cloves	cloves	spikenard				cloves		cloves
	cinnamon	cinnamon	cinnamon					cinnamon		cinnamon
	saffron									

Note: the order of the ingredients in each recipe has been rearranged to illustrate their parallels more clearly; recipes are ordered from most complex to simplest

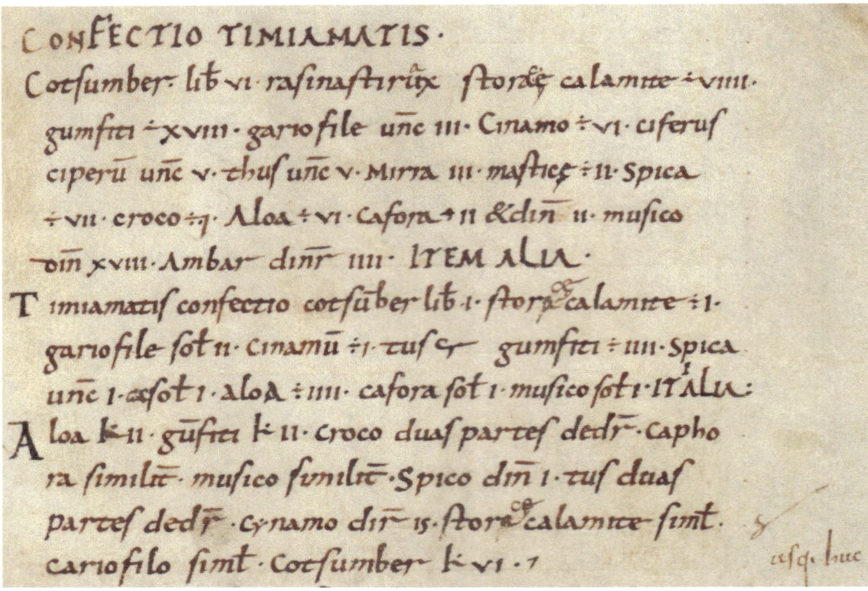

FIGURE 4 Three incense recipes in St. Gallen, Stiftsbibliothek, cod. sang. 899 (p. 137), a poetry manuscript that also includes several sections of recipes (https://www.e-codices.unifr.ch/de/csg/0899/137)

Overall, the consistency of the five core ingredients, all exotic and the majority newly recorded in the west, suggests that an incense recipe tradition from the east arrived in the west during this period. To investigate how this knowledge spread, it is essential to consider when and where the manuscripts containing these recipes were produced.[60] Codd. sang. 761 and 878 represent the earliest of the six manuscripts that contain this distinctive cluster of ingredients, with Bischoff dating both to the first half of the ninth century. Regarding cod. sang. 878, Walahfrid Strabo's *vademecum*, Bischoff has identified the hand on p. 334 as Walahfrid's own and has categorised it as belonging to his penultimate script phase, thereby dating it to the second quarter of the ninth century.[61] In contrast, cod. sang. 44 was composed in the second half of the ninth century and cod. sang. 752 has been dated to the very end of the century,

60 See Appendix 1 for full descriptions of the manuscripts.

61 Bischoff, *Katalog der festländischen Handschriften*, vol. 3, no. 5862; Bernhard Bischoff, 'Eine Sammelhandschrift Walahfrid Strabos (Cod. Sangall. 878)', in *Mittelalterliche Studien. Ausgewählte Aufsätze zur Schriftkunde und Literaturgeschichte*, ed. Bernhard Bischoff, vol. 2 (Stuttgart: Hiersemann, 1967), 34–51.

c. 900.[62] Cod. sang. 899 and BnF lat. 11219 were traditionally dated to the late ninth or early tenth centuries (with some individual hands dated even later), but more recent analyses have dated the hands responsible for these recipes to the late ninth century.[63] The page of incense recipes in the latter codex, f. 227v, is particularly striking: the varied scripts indicated that the twelve recipes were written by at least six different individuals, the implications of which will be revisited below.

Codd. sang. 752, 761, 878, 899, and BnF lat. 11219 were written at centres north of the Alps (St Gall, Fulda, Reichenau, St Gall, and 'western Francia', respectively), whereas the medical half of cod. sang. 44 was produced in northern Italy and then moved to St Gall shortly after its composition.[64] Despite being among the later manuscripts in this group, the movement of cod. sang. 44 illustrates a possible route for the transmission of this recipe and parallels the known movement of cozumber based on the gifts sent to Boniface. With this in mind, I suggest that the new incense tradition may have been first included in Latin medical texts in the Italian peninsula. Links between intellectual centres in northern Italy and present-day Switzerland and Germany, such as St Gall, Reichenau, and Fulda, then resulted in the dissemination of this recipe within the Carolingian world.[65] Indeed, Florence Eliza Glaze has drawn attention to the movement of manuscripts with medical texts between several monastic centres in this region, including Reichenau, St Gall, and Murbach, though the codices in which these incense recipes are located were not addressed.[66]

The high degree of subtle variation seen between all twenty incense recipes suggests that individuals may have been experimenting with using these newly introduced ingredients, learning what ratios produced the desired result, and trialling with which other substances they worked well in combination. The creation of variants may also reflect ad hoc adaptation responding to the

62 Bischoff, *Katalog der festländischen Handschriften*, vol. 3, nos. 5530 and 5845; Bernhard Bischoff, 'Italienische Handschriften des neunten bis elften Jahrhunderts in frühmittelalterlichen Bibliotheken ausserhalb Italiens', in *Il libro e il testo: Atti del Convegno Internazionale, Urbino, 20–23 Settembre 1982*, ed. Cesare Questa and Renato Raffaelli (Urbino: Università degli Studi di Urbino, 1984), 169–94.

63 My thanks to Rosamond McKitterick and Anna Dorofeeva for their reassessments of the scripts in these manuscripts.

64 Bischoff, *Katalog der festländischen Handschriften*, vol. 3, nos. 5845, 5847, 5862, 5865, 4670–1, and 5530, respectively; Bischoff, 'Eine Sammelhandschrift Walahfrid Strabos', pp. 34–51; Bischoff, 'Italienische Handschriften', 177–8.

65 Bischoff, *Manuscripts and Libraries in the Age of Charlemagne*, trans. Gorman, 33, 122, 147–8.

66 Glaze, 'The Perforated Wall', 73–5, 92–8; Contreni, 'Masters and Medicine', 267–82.

fluctuating availability of ingredients. Given that the vast majority of the substances listed in these recipes represent unambiguously non-local products (whether newly recorded or long known), ingredient access may have been highly unstable and uncertain. The page of incense recipes in BnF lat. 11219 offers a remarkable window onto an evolving body of knowledge: as noted above, a new palaeographical assessment of f. 227v suggests that these twelve incense recipes were written by at least half a dozen different scribes.[67] Most significantly, the scripts appear to be closely related, possibly representing a series of teachers and students. These scribal relationships suggest that the individuals responsible for the different recipe variants were all working at the same writing centre and added to the manuscript over the course of a few generations, building up a collection of distinct yet related incense recipes in the decades around the year 900. Ultimately, this growing corpus of incense recipes bears witness to an active scriptorium where scribes continued to engage with and add to manuscripts over time, recording the latest iterations of this incense tradition.

To contextualise this family of incense recipes, it is important to investigate whether alternative, unrelated incense recipes circulated in the Carolingian period. My analysis of the recipe sample uncovered two additional incense recipes, the *Conpositio thymiamatis* and *Tymiama simplex*, both located in cod. sang. 759.[68] Despite sharing titles similar to those seen above, these two recipes, as seen in Table 3, contain none of the core ingredients observed in the twenty other incense recipes reviewed above and appear to derive from an entirely distinct tradition. They do, however, share some ingredients with the longer incense recipes, such as myrrh and storax, and generally rely on similar types of substances—namely, non-local gums, resins, and spices—but all of their ingredients represent products that were recorded in the classical and late antique west. It should also be noted that, although these two recipes in cod. sang. 759 are the only other incense recipes found within the sample, the contents list of a lost collection in BnF lat. 6882A parallels the list of the collection in which the two recipes occur in cod. sang. 759.[69] Therefore, while BnF lat. 6882A no longer includes incense recipes, its contents list indicates that this alternative incense recipe group circulated more widely than the surviving recipes would suggest.[70]

67 My thanks to Anna Dorofeeva for her palaeographical analysis of this material.

68 Cod. sang. 759, p. 89: *Conpositio thymiamatis*; and p. 91: *Tymiama simplex*; see Appendix 2, entries 11.20–1.

69 Cod. sang. 759, pp. 53–8; BnF lat. 6882A, ff. 1v–8v.

70 BnF lat. 6882A, f. 7r; the titles are listed here as *Conpositio timiamatis* and *Timiama simplex*.

TABLE 3 Ingredients in incense recipes from cod. sang. 759

Recipe title	*Conpositio thymiamatis*	*Tymiama simplex*
Ingredients	myrrh	myrrh
	storax	storax
	ungiculas marinas	*ungellas*
	bdellium	
	cinnamon	
	ladanum	
	iris	
	saffron	
	Nepal cardamom	
	wine	
	honey	
		mastic
		rose

Several further points may help to shed light on how and why the incense recipes containing newly introduced ingredients and those in cod. sang. 759 differ. First, the ingredients listed in the latter manuscript appear to have much in common with biblical recipes for incense.[71] Exodus XXX.34, for example, offers the following instructions: 'And the Lord said to Moses: Take unto thee spices, stacte, and onycha, galbanum of sweet savour, and the clearest frankincense, all shall be of equal weight'.[72] Although the recipes in cod. sang. 759 record neither galbanum nor frankincense, both list spices, myrrh (stacte), and possibly onycha, paralleling the biblical incense recipe.[73] Secondly, Bischoff dated both manuscripts to the first half of the ninth century, suggesting that

71 On the reception of recipes in Exodus, see especially Béatrice Caseau, 'La parfum de Dieu', in *Parfums et odeurs au Moyen Âge. Science, usage, symboles*, ed. Agostino Paravicini Bagliani (Florence: SISMEL Edizioni del Galluzzo, 2015), 3–22 and Iolanda Ventura, '"Sume tibi aromata prima": Profumi ed aromi nell'esegesi ad *Ex. 30*', in *Parfums et odeurs au Moyen Âge. Science, usage, symboles*, ed. Agostino Paravicini Bagliani (Florence: SISMEL Edizioni del Galluzzo, 2015), 349–428.

72 Exodus XXX.34: *Dixitque Dominus ad Moysen: sume tibi aromata, stacten et onycha, galbanen boni odoris, et tus lucidissimum; aequalis ponderis erunt omnia.*

73 The terms *unguiculas* and *ungellas* may be linked with onycha, but the interpretation of all three words is debated; for more on this debate, see Harold J. Abrahams, 'Onycha,

cod. sang. 759 was written in Brittany whereas BnF lat. 6882A was written in southwest France.[74] These origins not only place the manuscripts on the early end of the spectrum of those considered in this study but also outside of the northern Italian-transalpine network noted above. While it is true that BnF lat. 11219, the manuscript containing the largest number and range of incense recipes with newly introduced ingredients, is also thought to have been produced at a site outside of this network, it represents one of the latest manuscripts included in the study. Taking these factors into consideration, it seems plausible that knowledge of the 'new' incense recipe family (i.e., the recipes containing the newly recorded ingredients) had not reached the centres that produced cod. sang. 759 and BnF lat. 6882A by the early ninth century. The gradual accumulation of recipes in BnF lat. 11219 demonstrates that this situation changed over time: the new tradition was widely diffused and further expanded during the ninth century and beyond. Based on the evidence of the manuscripts' origins as well as the lack of newly recorded ingredients in the recipes of cod. sang. 759, it appears that this codex preserved an older incense tradition, and possibly one with biblical influences.[75] Finally, that the recipe collection in cod. sang. 759 was based on an earlier exemplar (since the same collection was once part of BnF lat. 6882A, too) adds further weight to the age of this incense recipe. Given that two early ninth-century manuscripts produced in different (and distant) writing centres are known to derive from this lost exemplar, it seems likely that the original collection was compiled no later than *c.* 800, though it could be considerably earlier. As such, these recipes could predate the earliest surviving recordings of the newly introduced ingredients, such as the letters that document the eighth-century gifts of cozumber to Boniface, and their physical presence in the Latin west.

Before turning to evidence for the arrival of these substances in the Carolingian world, and how this relates to the practicality of the recipes that record them, the appearance of the newly introduced ingredients in recipes *independent* of preparations for incense must also be considered.

3.5 *Moving Beyond Incense: the Spread of Knowledge*

As noted above, this chapter's opening recipe, the *Antidotum gira deacoloquintidis* of BAV pal. lat. 1088, already confirms that at least one of these ingredients, camphor, can be found in other pharmaceutical prescriptions and was

Ingredient of the Ancient Jewish Incense: An Attempt at Identification', *Economic Botany* 33, no. 2 (1979): 233–6.

74 Bischoff, *Katalog der festländischen Handschriften*, vol. 3, nos. 5846 and 4419, respectively.

75 Amar and Lev, *Arabian Drugs*, 129–227.

not exclusively associated with incense. In total, the sample contains a single non-incense recipe with ambergris, two with camphor (including the aforementioned *Antidotum gira deacoloquintidis*), two with confita, three with cozumber, and three with musk (see Table 4).[76] These eleven references represent only nine recipes since two recipes, both in cod. sang. 44, include two newly introduced ingredients: the *Confectio saponi Constantini* lists both confita and musk and the second recipe under the entry titled *Potio maniacis siue gutta catiua* contains confita and cozumber.[77] While it must be recognised that the appearance of these products within the recipe sample remains very limited overall, it is significant that *each* of these substances are named in at least one non-incense recipe. In fact, as discussed below, I suggest that their limited distribution is central to understanding the dissemination of these eastern *materia medica* and the knowledge regarding their uses.

Although cod. sang. 44 and BAV pal. lat. 1088 contain the bulk of the examples, with both including four instances of newly recorded ingredients, three other manuscripts, cod. sang. 751, BAV vat. lat. 5951, and BAV reg. lat. 1143, each include an additional example of one of these ingredients in a recipe.[78] Musk and cozumber appear most frequently and exhibit the widest spread among manuscripts, each occurring three times and in three separate manuscripts. Notably, only one of these manuscripts, cod. sang. 44, contains an incense recipe. This is also the only manuscript to record recipes that use multiple newly introduced ingredients in a single preparation. Two recipes, the *Potio muscata ad omne infirmum* of BAV vat. lat. 5951 and the *Medicamentum ad maculas oculorum et ad caliginem* of BAV pal. lat. 1088 have been inserted in the margins, representing slightly later but near contemporary additions.[79]

---

76 While further examples of galangal and zedoary have also been identified (see above), the following section concentrates on the appearances of the ingredient cluster connected to the incense recipe tradition given the chapter's primary focus.

77 Cod. sang. 44, p. 282: *Confectio saponi Constantini*; and p. 285: *Potio maniacis siue gutta catiua*; see Appendix 2, entries 5.14 and 15. On the wider tradition of the *Sapone Constantini*, see Innocenzo Mazzini, 'Il sapone di Costantino', in *Costantino il grande: dall'Antichità all'umanesimo: colloquio sul Cristianesimo nel mondo antico, Macerata, 18–20 Dicembre 1990*, ed. Giorgio Bonamente and Franca Fusco (Macerata: Università degli studi di Macerata, 1992–3), vol. 2, 693–9. The recipes in the manuscripts Mazzini consulted do not contain these ingredients.

78 In cod. sang. 44 and BAV pal. lat. 1088, two ingredients are repeated, such that only three different substances within the cluster are found in these manuscripts.

79 BAV vat. lat. 5951, f. 1r: *Potio muscata ad omne infirmum*; BAV pal. lat. 1088, f. 34v: *Medicamentum ad maculas oculorum et ad caliginem*; see Appendix 2, entries 19.1 and 16.1, respectively.

TABLE 4 Newly introduced exotics outside of incense recipes

	Manuscripts					
Ingredients	**Cod. sang. 44**	**Cod. sang. 751**	**BAV vat. lat. 5951**	**BAV pal. lat. 1088**	**BAV reg. lat. 1143**	**Total**
Ambergris	-	1	-	-	-	1
Camphor	-	-	-	2	-	2
Confita	2	-	-	-	-	2
Cozumber	1	-	-	1	1	3
Musk	1	-	1	1	-	3
Total	4	1	1	4	1	11

By reconsidering the origins of the five manuscripts containing examples of newly introduced *materia medica* outside of (or in addition to) incense recipes, it is possible to assess the spread of medical knowledge from another perspective and compare these findings to the distribution of manuscripts containing incense recipes. As noted above, cod. sang. 44 appears to have been written in northern Italy in the second half of the ninth century, before moving to St Gall shortly after its composition; cod. sang. 751 followed the same trajectory.[80] The early ninth-century BAV vat. lat. 5951 has been located to either Italy or Burgundy while BAV pal. lat. 1088 has been linked to Lyon in the middle or second half of the ninth century.[81] Finally, Bischoff suggested that BAV reg. lat. 1143 was written in Mainz in the early ninth century.[82] With this context in mind, three features stand out. First, codd. sang. 44 and 751 fit with the pattern observed above: evidence such as the letter to Boniface indicates that, at least in some cases, these eastern substances moved north into the Frankish Empire from the Italian peninsula. These two manuscripts, which together contain recipes listing ambergris, confita, cozumber, and musk (not to mention the full suite of ingredients included in the incense recipe of cod. sang. 44), followed a

80 Bischoff, *Katalog der festländischen Handschriften*, vol. 3, no. 5844.
81 Ibid, nos. 6927 and 6574.
82 Ibid, nos. 6766–7.

similar path, moving from northern Italy to St Gall and helping to disseminate information about these new products.

Secondly, the single instance of one of the newly recorded exotic products in BAV reg. lat. 1143 is particularly interesting when considered in view of its origins. In this case, the recipe *Ciraturiu artriticus opotatricus a parlasensis*, found on ff. 187r–187v, records cozumber as its thirty-fifth ingredient (out of an astounding list of sixty-four ingredients).[83] This relatively early manuscript was composed in Mainz, the seat of Boniface, who, as noted above, received exotic gifts from Rome—and these gifts included cozumber. While it may be tempting to connect the existence of cozumber at Mainz to its subsequent inclusion in a medical recipe, this is a fairly large leap to make given that the manuscript was composed roughly two or three generations after Boniface's death. It should not be assumed, therefore, that there is a direct link between the appearance of cozumber in a recipe and the gifts received by Boniface, though this possibility, or that Mainz was known to have had access to these products, is an attractive hypothesis, especially in the light of Lull's gifts to Cuneburg and Cynehard's request for exotic *materia medica*.

The possible Burgundian origins of BAV vat. lat. 5951 and BAV pal. lat. 1088 suggest another direction in which this knowledge and these products travelled. Like cod. sang. 44, BAV pal. lat. 1088 contains four references to the newly introduced products but, in contrast to cod. sang. 44, these represent four separate recipes (cod. sang. 44 only contains two recipes with new ingredients since each recipe lists two of the substances in question).[84] The relatively high number of newly recorded ingredients listed in BAV pal. lat. 1088, combined with its later date, supports the idea that the number of available exotics, or at least an awareness of them, increased throughout the Carolingian period. The origins of this codex also call to mind BnF lat. 11219, the manuscript that contains the highest number of incense recipe variants. As the latter manuscript is thought to have been produced in western Francia at the very end of the ninth century, it demonstrates that knowledge of these newly recorded products had spread far beyond the northern Italian-transalpine network by *c.* 900, extending into the heartlands of Frankish territories and beyond. It is also important to remember that the Corbie monks' shopping list for the Cambrai market indicates that at least some of these substances themselves were circulating

83 BAV reg. lat. 1143, ff. 187r–187v: *Ciraturiu artriticus opotatricus aparlasensis*; see Appendix 2, entry 18.10.

84 As noted above, for both manuscripts, the four references to newly recorded ingredients refer to three separate ingredients (confita is mentioned twice in cod. sang. 44 and camphor is recorded twice in BAV pal. lat. 1088).

in this part of the Empire in the ninth century. The individuals compiling the recipes that contain references to these specific ingredients may have acquired first-hand knowledge of these products by this time (or were only a few steps removed from first-hand knowledge).

With this in mind, and by comparing the frequency of incense recipes to non-incense recipes with individual newly introduced ingredients, it becomes possible to consider how pharmaceutical information about these *materia medica* spread within the Carolingian world. Although cod. sang. 44—the only manuscript to contain both an incense recipe *and* unrelated recipes that include newly introduced ingredients—represents an exception, I suggest that the dissemination of the incense recipe tradition and of pharmaceutical information concerning the individual ingredients took separate, if at times intersecting and ultimately converging, paths.

The diffusion of the incense recipe appears to reflect a rapid process, and one in which a core unit of knowledge—the five primary ingredients—was consistently transmitted over time and between sites. Although I have focused on the use of incense in medical contexts, its primary role was liturgical, and I propose that this burst of incense recipe interest was underpinned by wider developments in the Carolingian world, namely, that the legislation promulgated by the court brought about an increased use of incense in the liturgy.[85] Although, as noted in Chapter 2, normative evidence does not necessarily reflect smooth transitions on the ground, the liturgical use of incense does appear to have expanded during this period.[86] The provision of sufficient quantities of incense thus became an urgent matter in terms of both spiritual and corporeal health.[87]

The arrival of this new incense recipe tradition would have offered an alternative to the older, possibly biblical recipes, such as those recorded in cod. sang. 759 and BnF lat. 6882A. By relying on different ingredients, the new recipe would have provided more options for sourcing the components of incense, thereby allowing for greater overall production or for the creation of a substitute if certain ingredients were unavailable. The recording of so many variants

85 Burridge, 'Incense in Medicine'. On the symbolic significance of incense, perfumes, and odour, and especially in relation to the Church, see selected chapters in Agostino Paravicini Bagliani, ed., *Parfums et odeurs au Moyen Âge. Science, usage, symboles* (Florence: SISMEL Edizioni del Galluzzo, 2015), including Rémi Corbineau and Patrice Georges-Zimmermann, 'Le parfum de la mort. Plantes et aromates pour la préparation des corps (Moyen Âge et période moderne)', 161–80 and Martine Ostorero, 'L'odeur fétide des démons: une preuve de leur présence corporelle au sabbat', 259–88.

86 McCormick, *Origins of the European Economy*, 716–19.

87 Leja, *Embodying the Soul*.

that use different combinations and/or ratios of ingredients likewise would have offered alternatives that could have augmented these monastic communities' abilities to produce enough incense to satisfy both pharmaceutical and ecclesiastical purposes.

Returning to the non-incense recipes that incorporate individual newly recorded ingredients, the introduction of these particular *materia medica* seems to have occurred for different, though ultimately related, reasons. Several key patterns emerge: first, these recipes do not appear in the same manuscripts as the incense recipes themselves, with the exception of cod. sang. 44. Secondly, as noted initially, the spread of this knowledge seems to have been fairly limited given that these ingredients are found in only nine recipes across six manuscripts. That being said, it is diverse: unlike the incense recipes, none of these recipes represents a variant of another, which is a particularly interesting finding given that cod. sang. 44 and BAV pal. lat. 1088 share a substantial number of recipes. Critically, the recipes are often located in manuscripts that were produced in areas (or even at specific sites, such as Mainz) in which these ingredients appear to have circulated. This correlation between the recorded knowledge and the appearance of the substances themselves suggests that individuals within this milieu may have encountered some of these ingredients directly (or perhaps had heard of earlier gifts of the substances, knew someone who saw the range of products available at the Cambrai market, etc.). Taking account of these factors, I suggest that the individual inclusion of newly recorded ingredients reflects these encounters: while the scribes responsible for the surviving recipes may not have been the individuals who received, purchased, and/or used these substances, they have documented the experiences of someone who did. This slow spread of knowledge—a case-by-case diffusion based on access to expensive, rare substances—contrasts with the rapid dissemination of the incense tradition, where a core unit of information was transmitted with relative speed due to the urgency of incense production. Both patterns of movement appear to be linked to the arrival of the substances themselves and reveal that individuals in the Carolingian world were open to adopting and adapting new sources of knowledge and novel *materia medica* to suit their needs.

Due to the overarching importance of incense, this recipe tradition blossomed in an atmosphere receptive to new information about its production. This openness to previously unknown substances, as well as the knowledge of how to use them, laid the groundwork for the spread of these newly introduced ingredients both alongside and independent of the incense recipe tradition. The particular cultural and intellectual environment and the needs of monastic communities thus links the two discrete patterns of dissemination highlighted in this case study.

4 The Practicality of Non-local *Materia Medica*: Putting the Case Study in Perspective

On the basis of this analysis, what can now be said about the practicality of these ingredients? And what are the implications of this case study for assessing the recording of non-local ingredients more generally?

The above review of a selection of newly recorded *materia medica* has highlighted the movement of both knowledge *and* ingredients. The correspondence between the arrival of pharmaceutical information regarding these previously unrecorded ingredients and the physical substances themselves points to the practical nature of these recipes, though a number of important caveats must be addressed. First, while it is true that sources beyond the medical literature bear witness to the existence of exotic substances in the west in this period—and, of particular note, include several of the key ingredients analysed in this chapter—it must be remembered that much of this evidence, such as records of diplomatic gifts, registers exceptions rather than norms. That is, not only did such exchanges occur sporadically, but the surviving records emphasise the movement of especially noteworthy goods within very elite networks. Therefore, while this evidence remains immensely valuable, caution is needed.

On the other hand, the Abbey of Fontenelle's annual supply of *pigmenta* or the shopping list from Corbie do suggest more regular trade in these types of imported substances. Still, these sources only paint a partial picture of the situation on the ground. They reveal what these communities *intended* to buy and not what was actually available. Ultimately, the documentary evidence indicates that some unambiguously non-local products, including newly introduced *materia medica*, were circulating in the Carolingian world. This circulation, however, was limited. Even if certain *exotica* were available at the market at Cambrai, for example, it is likely that most non-local items were present in relatively small quantities (though the 120 pounds of pepper suggests that larger amounts of some substances may have been available) and, given their expense, restricted to an elite clientele. In short, evidence for the occasional existence of these ingredients should not be read as evidence for their regular availability.

Nevertheless, I would suggest that recipes including newly recorded ingredients were practical in a limited way. Although the ingredients in question would have been far from local, the recipes that include them appear to demonstrate some degree of familiarity with these substances, if only indirectly. Such recipes would have provided blueprints for possible preparations *when* these ingredients were available. This is particularly relevant when considering the rapid dissemination of the new incense recipe: its addition to existing western incense traditions opened up multiple options for incense production depending on the availability of ingredients; having a range of options may have been necessary for these communities given their increasing incense needs and the variable availability of the ingredients involved. Overall, although the evidence for the existence of these substances in the Latin west is sporadic and should not be understood as reflecting their sustained presence, the sources reveal the possibility of their availability within the Frankish Empire. The repeated inclusion of the five newly recorded exotics in medical recipes can therefore be seen as practical information that was ready to be deployed when a need arose and when the ingredients were on hand: this is 'latent knowledge'.

Finally, the wider implications of this case study must be considered: to what extent can we extrapolate from these findings? Are these newly recorded ingredients representative of non-local *materia medica* more generally? While it would be dangerous to use this case study as a proxy for all exotic ingredients, it is notable that a significant number of non-local ingredients that were known in classical Antiquity, such as pepper, ginger, and cinnamon, not only continue to appear in the recipe literature but are also named in the non-medical sources examined above. The monks of Corbie, for example, intended to buy these three products, among a number of other foreign goods, at the Cambrai market. This combination of medical and other documentary sources therefore suggests that many exotic substances, not unlike the newly recorded ingredients, may have been practical in that they stored this latent knowledge—information that was by no means always or even consistently useable, but that offered options when the conditions were right. It must be noted, however, that previously known ingredients present a more challenging group to study: since they have long been recorded in pharmaceutical prescriptions, their individual appearance in recipes, in contrast to the newly introduced ingredients, cannot be used to trace the dissemination of knowledge and its possible connection with the presence of the physical substances themselves.

Despite this general picture of practicality, there are counter examples that challenge this finding. The case of silphium presents one such case: this plant is thought to have become extinct during Antiquity and yet continues to appear in later recipes.[88] Within the sample analysed in this study, it is recorded over

88 Ken Parejko, 'Pliny the Elder's Silphium: First Recorded Species Extinction', *Conservation Biology* 17, no. 3 (2003): 925–7.

twenty times. Although it is possible that the term may have been used to refer to a different, related plant in the early Middle Ages or that scribes continued to copy it without knowing it had gone extinct (or perhaps with the hope that it might be identified in the future) or that they were simply unsure (and wanted to record it, again, in case of possible future use), the surviving evidence does not provide additional information. Instead, the inclusion of recipes that rely on substances that would have been impossible to obtain suggests that, in some cases, older authorities may have been copied without a consideration of the possible practicality of the information they contained *or* that they were preserved for other reasons.[89] While the silphium example represents a very small percentage of the total number of recipes, it is a useful reminder that, despite the strong evidence for practicality on the basis of latent knowledge, the situation remained highly complex and variable.

5 Conclusion

This chapter offers just a glimpse of the vast range of non-local *materia medica* recorded in early medieval recipes. The analysis of a cluster of newly introduced ingredients speaks to the arrival and distribution of this knowledge within northwest Europe. Tracing the distribution of incense recipes containing these core ingredients as well as the appearance of each of these ingredients individually has uncovered patterns in the diffusion of this information and related this diffusion to the movement of the substances themselves. The need for increasingly large amounts of incense appears to have been a key factor underpinning the spread of the new incense recipe. Simultaneously, the entry of the substances themselves allowed for their gradual application in medical contexts. While these patterns are grounded in the evidence provided by the recipes and the manuscripts in which they are located, non-medical texts have offered important insights into the movement of the ingredients, as well. By bringing together these varied types of evidence, it becomes possible to see the *potential* practicality of recipes that incorporate non-local *materia medica*.

89 For example, a number of rough parallels can be found with treatments listed in Marcellus' *De medicamentis liber*. A recipe for *Sales catarticos* in cod. sang. 751 (p. 418) that uses *silfiu* is similar to several preparations in Book 30 of *De medicamentis liber*, including recipes 51 (*Confectio salis cathartici*) and 52 (*Liquamen catharticum*); see Marcellus, *De medicamentis liber*, ed. Liechtenhan and Niedermann, trans. Kollesch and Nickel, 30.51–2 (pp. 532–5); see Appendix 2, entry 9.21.

The findings presented in this chapter connect to several major debates. In particular, while some scholars argue that the Mediterranean (and beyond) was still a zone of connectivity during this period, others hold a more minimalist view.[90] This debate has major implications for understanding the degree to which, if at all, exotic goods were entering continental Europe and also relates to the question of whether trade can be used as a more general proxy for assessing networks of communication and exchange. The results of my analyses support a middle ground: while it appears that such non-local products were known in the west, they may not have been regularly available—and when they were available, these ingredients were probably only present in small quantities and, given their expense, accessible to a select few. As stated above, evidence for the existence of these substances should not be equated with their *regular* presence and widespread availability. The recipes that include such rare, expensive, non-local *materia medica* therefore represent latent knowledge: they offer additional options for treatments and/or liturgical incense use if and when the necessary ingredients were available.

Finally, although this chapter has focused on the spread of non-local *materia medica* within the Carolingian world, these developments represent only the very end point of movements on a much larger, global scale. While space does not permit me to examine these movements in detail, ingredients coming from as far away as the Himalayas and the Maluku Islands likely travelled west via multiple, intersecting networks. The Abbasid Caliphate's expanding power and trading connections during this period, especially in the east, must have played a particularly important role in introducing a greater range of products from southeast Asia in western Europe. Indeed, diplomatic exchanges, such as Harun al Rashid's gifts, exemplify the potential for direct links between the two empires. The Arabic origins of many of the terms for these substances (in both Latin and English) confirm that the trade networks of the Islamicate world

90 McCormick provides a useful overview of the maximalist-minimalist debate in the opening chapter of *Origins of the European Economy*, see pp. 1–24. Caroline Goodson has presented convincing evidence for a more minimalist interpretation (personal communication and 'Ingredients for Medicine in Early Medieval Italy', Goodson's paper at the Society for the Promotion of Byzantine Studies' 2019 Symposium, *Blood in Byzantium* (1 April 2019)). For more on this debate, see also the work of Chris Wickham, Richard Hodges, and Sauro Gelichi, including Chris Wickham, *Framing the Early Middle Ages: Europe and the Mediterranean, 400–800* (Oxford: Oxford University Press, 2005) and Sauro Gelichi and Richard Hodges, eds., *From One Sea to Another. Trading Places in the European and Mediterranean Early Middle Ages: Proceedings of the International Conference, Comacchio 27th-29th March 2009* (Turnhout: Brepols, 2012), with chapters from Gelichi, Hodges, McCormick, and Wickham.

were central to the movement of these products across Eurasia. Recent scholarship has also suggested the impact of simultaneous developments in Tang China on the diffusion of both knowledge and *materia medica*.[91]

Meanwhile, within the Mediterranean world, the spread of non-local substances may have also been facilitated by Byzantine connections and Radhanite traders.[92] That some of the newly recorded ingredients, such as confita, appear to reflect an evolving Latinisation of originally Greek terms suggests that Byzantine networks were involved in the introduction and spread of the incense recipe tradition. Considering the movement of information and substances between sites in the Italian peninsula and communities north of the Alps, intellectual, policital, and ecclesiastical centres with strong Byzantine connections, such as Rome and Ravenna, likely represent key nodes in the transmission of pharmaceutical knowledge and products, crucial gateways linking east and west.[93]

Ultimately, a combination of all these networks may have been involved in the introduction of the newly recorded ingredients, and further investigations into the dynamics underpinning this long-distance trade must be pursued in a future study. This chapter confirms McCormick's remark that the manuscripts 'may still hold some surprises'.[94] It is evident that these types of 'miscellaneous' recipes offer new insights into the evolution of medical knowledge and practice in the Carolingian world. To develop a more complete understanding of early medieval medicine, it is essential to explore this rich corpus in greater depth within both global and local frameworks, and the next chapter turns to the latter perspective.

---

91 Alain George, 'Direct Sea Trade Between Early Islamic Iraq and Tang China: From the Exchange of Goods to the Transmission of Ideas', *Journal of the Royal Asiatic Society* 25, no. 4 (2015): 579–624. https://doi.org/10.1017/S1356186315000231.

92 Amar and Lev, *Arabian Drugs*, 129–227. On Byzantine connections in the west, see, for example, T. S. Brown, 'Byzantine Italy, *c.* 680-*c.* 876', in *The New Cambridge Medieval History* II, *c. 700-c. 900*, ed. Rosamond McKitterick (Cambridge: Cambridge University Press, 1995), 320–48; Michael McCormick, 'Byzantium and the West, 700–900', in *The New Cambridge Medieval History* II, *c. 700-c. 900*, ed. Rosamond McKitterick (Cambridge: Cambridge University Press, 1995), 349–80.

93 Thomas S. Brown, 'Ravenna and Other Early Rivals of Venice: Comparative Urban and Economic Development in the Upper Adriatic c.751–1050', in *Byzantium, Venice and the Medieval Adriatic: Spheres of Maritime Power and Influence, c. 700–1453*, ed. Magdalena Skoblar (Cambridge: Cambridge University Press, 2021), 173–87.

94 McCormick, *Origins of the European Economy*, 714, n. 84.

CHAPTER 4

Medicine and the Mead Hall?

Using Alcoholic Beverages to Explore Potentially Local Materia Medica

1 Introduction: a Snapshot From Cod. Sang. 752

The frequency with which alcoholic beverages are mentioned in medical texts is noteworthy. Various alcoholic drinks, including wine, beer, and mead, appear in many dietetic works detailing the foods and drinks best suited to balancing the humours or, conversely, those to be avoided. Recipes, too, make frequent use of these beverages and others, such as mixtures of wine with honey or water. Of the fifteen recipes from cod. sang. 752 included in this study, the first, fifth, and fifteenth recipes each include wine as an ingredient, while the fourteenth recipe notes both beer and mead (see Figure 5 for the fourteenth and fifteenth recipes):

> On Melancholy. To get rid of black bile, a purgative that purges cold and dry humours: dodder, 10 denarii; dried mint, 10 pounds, 2 scruples; pepper, 1 ounce; grind these together finely and then give the entire potion, 10 scruples, or half potion, 5 scruples, with half a cup of old wine. Do this frequently, it is most useful.[1]

> For paralysis: juice of the herb sage, 6 *denarii*; juice of savin, 4 *denarii*; skimmed honey, 2 *denarii*; wine, 1 ounce. The fasting [patient] should drink [this]; it heals wonderfully.[2]

> On improving haemorrhoids: take plantain and the sour herb, which by another name is named *gundereba*, and tallow from mutton, this is *unslit*, and these three ingredients should be beaten in a mortar and then roasted in a small pan. And in this way, the fasting [patient] should

1 Cod. sang. 752, p. 5: *De melancolicis ad fel nigrum deponendum purgatorium quod deponit umores frigidos et siccos. Epitimo đ x, menta sicca lib x ℈ ii, piper ℈ i, hęc conteres subtilissime et dabis exinde integra potione ℈ x et media potione ℈ v cum uino uetere medio calice. Faciat hoc frequenter, utilissimum est*. For a transcription of the recipe, see Appendix 2, entry 10.1.

2 Cod. sang. 752, p. 5: *Ad paralisin. Sucum erbę saluie đ vi, sucum sauine đ iiii, mel dispumatum đ ii, uino ℈ i. Ieiunus bibat, mirifice sanat*. See Appendix 2, entry 10.2.

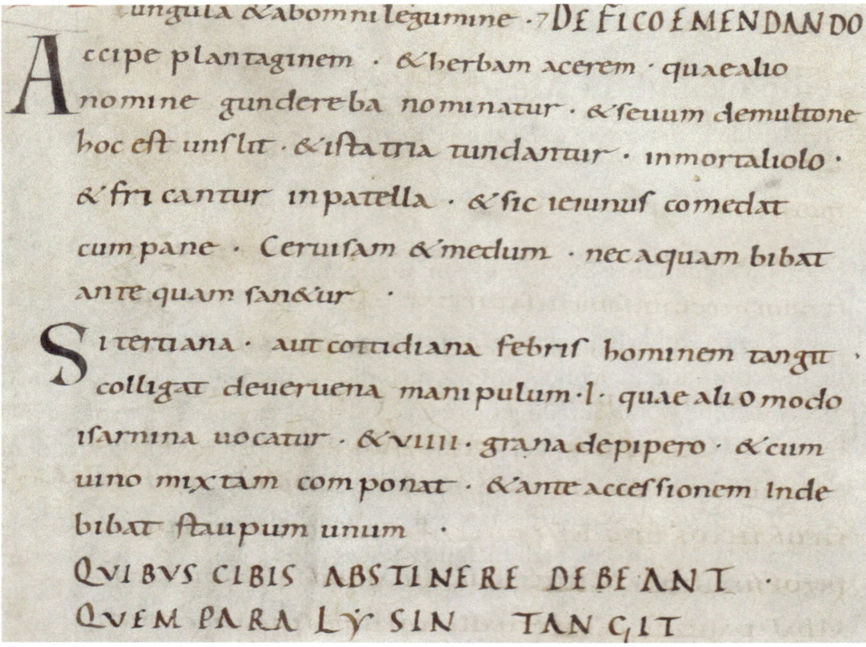
ungula & ab omni legumine · 7 DE FICO EMENDANDO
Accipe plantaginem · & herbam acerem · quae alio
nomine gundereba nominatur · & seuum de multone ·
hoc est unslit · & ista tria tundantur · in mortaliolo ·
& fricantur in patella · & sic ieiunus comedat
cum pane · Ceruisam & medum · nec aquam bibat
ante quam sanetur ·
Si tertiana · aut cottidiana febris hominem tangit ·
colligat de ueruena manipulum · I · quae alio modo
isarnina uocatur · & VIIII · grana de pipero · & cum
uino mixtam componat · & ante accessionem inde
bibat staupum unum ·
QUIBUS CIBIS ABSTINERE DEBEANT ·
QUEM PARALYSIN TANGIT

FIGURE 5 Two recipes in St. Gallen, Stiftsbibliothek, cod. sang. 752 (p. 158), a manuscript compilation with the *Medicina Plinii*, Gargilius Martialis' *Medicinae ex oleribus et pomis*, the *Oxea et chronia passiones Yppocratis, Gallieni et Urani*, etc. and additional medical recipes, such as those pictured (https://www.e-codices.unifr.ch/de/csg/0752/158)

eat [this] with bread. [They] should drink beer and mead but not water before [they] are healed.[3]

If a tertian or quotidian fever strikes a person: [they] should collect a handful of vervain, which in another way is called *isarnina*, and nine grains of pepper, and mix them together with wine. [They] should drink one *staupus* [of this mixture] before the onset of the fever.[4]

3 Cod. sang. 752, p. 158: *De fico emendando. Accipe plantaginem et herbam acerem, quae alio nomine gundereba nominatur, et seuum de multone, hoc est unslit, et ista tria tundantur in mortaliolo et fricantur in patella, et sic ieiunus comedat cum pane. Ceruisam et medum nec aquam bibat antequam sanetur*. See Appendix 2, entry 10.4.

4 Cod. sang. 752, p. 158: *Si tertiana aut cottidiana febris hominem tangit. Colligat de ueruena manipulum i, quae alio modo isarnina uocatur, et viiii grana de pipero, et cum uino mixtam componat, et ante accessionem inde bibat staupum unum*. See Appendix 2, entry 10.5.

After the final recipe on p. 158, there is a short text that describes certain foods and drinks from which to abstain if suffering from paralysis, *Quibus cibis abstinere debeant quem paralysin tangit*. Bread, various meats (beef, pork, and goat), fish, most legumes, and unrefined olive oil are to be avoided, as are all drinks that have the potential to cause inebriation.[5] The author of this passage, however, makes several exceptions, noting three alcoholic beverages that would be acceptable to drink: thin white wine, thin mead, and thin, light beer.

Within this manuscript's fifteen remedies under analysis in the present study, four—nearly a third of the total—include alcoholic beverages. All three of the alcohols that appear in these recipes are also noted in the dietary guidelines that follow one of the manuscript's recipe clusters. The sheer prevalence of alcohol in medical texts, and especially as ingredients in recipes (even if their primary function was as a liquefying agent rather than an active pharmacological component), demands a closer look. The traditional stereotypes attached to each of these beverages, moreover, add another dimension to this investigation into alcoholic drinks' relationship(s) with medicine and connect to this book's core questions regarding practicality.

In this chapter, I shall first review the attitudes towards and roles played by various alcohols in classical and late antique medicine before turning to the early medieval evidence. In contrast to classical medical texts, which promote the use of wine but regard beer as unhealthy, my analysis of eighth- and ninth-century recipes has uncovered treatments that list beer as an ingredient. Simultaneously, I have tracked the spread of a Germanic term for mead, *medus*, in medical contexts. The appearance of these two alcohols in recipes and related medical writings (such as accompanying dietary advice), often listed together, indicates that classical and late antique medical knowledge was not passively received; rather, early medieval scribes actively engaged with and added to this material. Supported by non-medical sources that document beer and mead production in the Carolingian world, I argue that the inclusion of beer and *medus* reveals adaptations made to suit local conditions. Such changes reflect another aspect of the practicality of the recipes involved in this study and bear witness to an evolving body of medical literature.

5 Cod. sang. 752, pp. 158–9: *Quibus cibis abstinere debeant quem paralysin tangit*. See Appendix 2, entry 10.6.

2 Wine, Beer, and Mead in the Classical Mediterranean

Beer, ale, and mead tend to be portrayed as having northern European origins; these alcohols are seen in Germanic contexts and as drinks consumed by rowdy barbarians. Wine, in contrast, is more often associated with the classical, Mediterranean world. The stereotypes persist today: beer remains the everyman's drink while wine tends to be more expensive and perceived as more sophisticated. These stereotypes depend, at least in part, on the narrative of a 'clash of cultures' that resulted in a sharp break between classical Antiquity and the barbaric 'Dark Ages'. Modern scholarship has, thankfully, revised the notion of decline and fall, highlighting instead the vibrant, flourishing intellectual cultures of the early Middle Ages as well as many continuities between the Roman Empire and its successors.[6] Nevertheless, with the exception of craft brewing, the contrasting images of less refined (barbarian) beer and sophisticated (classical) wine have largely endured. The divide can be seen along geographic lines, as well, with northern and western Europe known for its production of beer whereas southern, Mediterranean Europe is famed for its vines. Is this divide purely due to the environmental and climatic conditions needed to produce each beverage or have cultural factors played a role? Is the separation between beer- and wine-drinking areas a more modern concept that has been inappropriately applied to the past?

The north-south division of alcoholic beverages in a European context has been explored extensively in recent scholarship.[7] The fact that there were (and are) many areas in Europe where both cereals and grapes can grow

---

6 See, for example, Rosamond McKitterick's work on literacy, scholarship, and culture in the Carolingian period, such as McKitterick, 'The Carolingian Renaissance of Culture and Learning'; McKitterick, 'Eighth-Century Foundations'; Rosamond McKitterick, ed., *Carolingian Culture: Emulation and Innovation* (Cambridge: Cambridge University Press, 1994); or McKitterick, *The Carolingians and the Written Word*. On the wider political, economic, and social dynamics of this period, see also the outputs from the ESF project 'Transformation of the Roman World' (mentioned in Chapter 2), including Hansen and Wickham, eds., *The Long Eighth Century*; Corradini, Diesenberger, and Reimitz, eds., *The Construction of Communities*; and Theuws and Nelson, eds., *Rituals of Power*.

7 Ruth C. Engs, 'Do Traditional Western European Drinking Practices Have Origins in Antiquity?' *Addiction Research* 2, no. 3 (1995): 227–39, https://doi.org/10.3109/16066359509005208, at pp. 228–31; Max Nelson, 'The Geography of Beer in Europe from 1000 BC to AD 1000', in *The Geography of Beer: Regions, Environments, and Societies*, ed. Mark Patterson and Nancy Hoalst-Pullen (Dordrecht: Springer, 2014), 9–21, at pp. 9–10; Benjamin Wayens, Isabelle van den Steen, and Marie-Eve Ronveaux. 'A Short Historical Geography of Beer', in *Food and Environment: Geographies of Taste*, ed. Armando Montanari (Rome: Società Geografica Italiana, 2002), 93–114, at pp. 93–4.

immediately challenges the strict partition of drinking cultures along geographic lines. North-south theories are both misleading and outdated, reducing a highly complex situation to a simple dichotomy.[8] Yet these stereotypes, despite their inaccuracies, have a long history and understanding their development is crucial to unpicking the changing roles of various alcohols in western medical traditions.

Both written sources and the archaeological record speak to the ancient origins of humankind's relationship with alcoholic substances. At present, the earliest archaeological evidence for fermentation in Europe has been dated to the Bronze Age.[9] The alcoholic beverages produced at this time appear to have been of a mixed nature, potentially combining fermented cereals, fruits, and honey. This blend of substances blurs the distinctions between beer, wine, and mead, providing no evidence to support a geographic divide in the initial stages of alcohol production. Early textual sources, however, relate the development of particular traditions in different regions, with winemaking centred in the south, brewing in the north, and many areas of overlap between the two. The information and biases passed down in these texts, at first largely written by Greek authors, became orthodoxy, establishing the stereotypes on which later writers would continue to build.

The earliest surviving negative depictions of beer in Greek sources come from the plays of Aeschylus, written in the early fifth century BC. Further examples can be seen in the works of Cratinus (fifth century BC) and Antiphanes (fourth century BC). By charting the portrayal of beer, *zūthos* (ζῦθος), in Greek drama, Nelson shows that beer is repeatedly seen as an unmanly product of Thrace and Egypt. He explains that 'the drinking of beer continued to be made fun of, particularly with regard to its effeminate qualities'.[10] These negative stereotypes were not restricted to the stage, but rather maintained and expanded by writers in other fields, including medicine.

Although no references to beer appear in the Hippocratic corpus, Galen comments on *zūthos*, mentioning it in relation to the 'Alexandrian diet', thereby continuing to associate beer-drinking with Egypt and to see it as a foreign

8 Nelson, 'The Geography of Beer', 10.

9 Andrew Sherratt, 'Alcohol and its Alternatives: Symbol and Substance in Pre-Industrial Cultures', in *Consuming Habits: Global and Historical Perspectives on How Cultures Define Drugs*, ed. Jordan Goodman, Paul E. Lovejoy, and Andrew Sherratt, 2nd ed. (London: Routledge, 2007), 11–45, at p. 25.

10 Max Nelson, *The Barbarian's Beverage: A History of Beer in Ancient Europe* (London: Routledge, 2005), 25, 32.

peculiarity.[11] He writes that the beverage causes flatulence and bad humours.[12] These two qualities were also noted earlier by Dioscorides in *De materia medica*. Dioscorides' vast work, as mentioned in Chapter 2, addresses the medical properties of roughly 1000 different substances, and he includes two entries for beer, differentiating between *zūthos* and *courmi* (*κοῦρμι*). The former, made from barley, is 'especially hurtful to the membranes, it is apt to cause flatulence, to engender an unhealthy state of humors, and to cause elephantiasis'.[13] On *courmi*, made from either barley or wheat, he writes: it 'causes headaches, is unwholesome, and does damage to the sinewy parts'.[14] Dioscorides specifically links wheat beers to Spain and Britain.

In stark contrast, *De materia medica* contains roughly one hundred entries for different types of wines and other fruit-based alcohols, honey-based alcohols, and alcohols made up of both honey and fruit, nearly all of which highlight the potential medicinal values of these types of drinks. At this point, it is important to note that the definitions of the various alcohols under consideration have changed over time and the situation is more complicated than a simple tripartite division between wine, beer, and mead. For the purposes of this discussion, I use the term 'wine' to mean any fermented beverage produced from fruit. Grapes are generally, but by no means exclusively, the fruit in question.[15] The term 'beer' represents fermented beverages made from malted cereals, including wheat, barley, and other grains. Finally, 'mead' refers to fermented beverages produced from honey. As will be discussed below, there is some overlap and ambiguity between the categories of wine and mead due to blends of the two substances and mixtures of wine with honey. Many modern translations are perhaps overzealous in their use of 'mead', deploying it in cases where a term like 'honeyed-wine' might be more appropriate. However, as Nelson notes, 'the distinction between those substances which were meant to ferment and those simply added to, or macerated in, a fermented beverage for flavour can rarely be determined either from archaeological remains or from the information in our written sources'.[16] I shall revisit the question

11 Galen, *In Hippocratis Aphorismos*, 2.20. In *Claudii Galeni Opera Omnia*, ed. Karl Gottlob Kühn, 20 vols. (Leipzig: Carl Cnobloch, 1821–33), see specifically XVIIb.492.14–493.5.

12 Galen, *De simplicium medicamentorum temperamentis ac facultatibus*, 6.6.3. In *Claudii Galeni Opera Omnia*, ed. Karl Gottlob Kühn, 20 vols. (Leipzig: Carl Cnobloch, 1821–33), XI.379–892K and XII.1–377K, see specifically XI.882.5–8.

13 Dioscorides, *De materia medica*, 2.87.

14 Ibid, 2.88.

15 It will be noted if a fruit other than or in addition to grapes is used to produce a beverage.

16 Nelson, *The Barbarian's Beverage*, 2.

of terminology, especially with regard to mead, below, but first Dioscorides' comments on wine(s) and mead(s) must be considered.

Of the 162 entries in Book 5 of *De materia medica*, seventy-one of the first seventy-three entries concern grapes, wine, mead, and related products such as honey and vinegar; the two exceptions are entries for water and sea water. The rest of Book 5, excluding entry 114 on wine lees, addresses mineral products. While the entry on wine itself (entry 6), does mention some potentially harmful effects caused by overindulging in the beverage, from flatulence to drunkenness, the passage emphasises wine's beneficial qualities: 'its use is recommended both in health and in sickness'.[17] According to Dioscorides, all pure and unmixed wine is nutritious and wholesome; counters poisons, bites, and stings; improves 'distention and loosening of the stomach or bowel'; and helps 'people who perspire and are weakened'.[18]

Moving to the blended beverages, wine prepared with honey, termed *melitites* (*μελιτίτης*), 'is given in cases of chronic fevers to those who have a weak stomach … and it is suitable for arthritics, nephritics, and for those of weak constitution'.[19] Dioscorides defines *melitites* as a mixture of must, honey, and salt, and differentiates this from *oinomeli* (*οἰνόμελι*), a combination of dry wine and a little honey. On mead, known as either *melicraton* (*μελίκρατον*) or *hydromeli* (*υδρόμελι*), Dioscorides writes that it is useful for people 'who are sickly, who cough, who have lung inflammations, and who are weakened from perspiration' as well as 'those with stomach problems or rheums or [those] who have no appetite'.[20] Dioscorides then continues with the descriptions of wines made from a range of different fruits, including quinces, pears, pomegranates, dates, and figs, and flavoured with various additives, such as resins, pine cones, or particular herbs and spices. He provides instructions for their preparation and information on their properties. Several entries focus on wines made exclusively for a particular medical purpose, such as entries 55, 'wine for headcolds', and 67, 'abortifacient wine'.[21]

Wine, mead, and combinations of the two were therefore seen as substances fundamentally linked to health: while too much could result in unpleasant side effects, these beverages, when consumed in moderation, were understood to have many medicinal properties. Dioscorides' prolix commentary on fruit- and honey-based alcohols certainly contrasts with his brief and highly negative

17 Dioscorides, *De materia medica*, 5.6.
18 Ibid.
19 Ibid, 5.7.
20 Ibid, 5.9.
21 Ibid, 5.55 and 67.

presentation of the two types of beer noted above. His descriptions of all of these beverages, and the general attitudes they represent, appear to have influenced later Greek and Latin medical authors alike.

Prejudice against beer and beer-drinkers can also be seen in other types of writing, reinforcing and repackaging the stereotypes about foreigners and their odd tastes. Tacitus, a Roman senator and historian active in the late first and early second centuries, composed an ethnographic work on the Germanic peoples living beyond the empire, *Germania*. In Chapter 23, Tacitus describes their drinking habits, writing that 'for drink they use the liquid distilled from barley or wheat, after fermentation has given it a certain resemblance to wine'.[22] He also records that some tribes buy wine from their Roman neighbours and notes their overindulgence when it comes to alcohol: 'if you humour their drunkenness by supplying as much as they crave, they will be vanquished through their vices as easily as on the battlefield'.[23] While Tacitus' comments on beer itself are not overly negative, the barbarians' intemperance is presented as inferior to the 'civilised' Roman approach to alcohol.

Pliny, too, records information on beer and beer-drinkers in his encyclopaedic *Natural History*. Noting that 'the nations of the west also have their own intoxicant, made from grain soaked in water', he highlights Spain, Gaul, and Egypt as specific regions that produced beer.[24] Like Tacitus, his basic presentation of beer remains neutral, but the character of those who drink this alcohol is again critiqued, noting that 'in no part of the world is drunkenness ever out of action, in fact they actually quaff liquors of this kind neat and do not temper their strength by diluting them, as is done with wine ... Alas, what wonderful ingenuity vice possesses! A method has actually been discovered for making even water intoxicated!'[25] Thus, in contrast to the medical texts, which found problems with the substance of beer itself, writings outside of the medical

22 Tacitus, *Germania*, in *Agricola. Germania. Dialogue on Oratory*, trans. M. Hutton and W. Peterson (Cambridge, MA: Harvard University Press, 1914), 166–7: *Potui humor ex hordeo aut frumento, in quandam similitudinem vini corruptus.*

23 Tacitus, *Germania*, trans. Hutton and Peterson, 166–7: *si indulseris ebrietati suggerendo quantum concupiscunt, haud minus facile vitiis quam armis vincentur.*

24 Pliny, *Natural History*, ed. Rackham, vol. 4, 14.149: *Est et occidentis populis sua ebrietas e fruge madida, pluribus modis per Gallias Hispaniasque, nominibus aliis sed ratione eadem. Hispaniae iam et vetustatem ferre ea genera docuerunt. Aegyptus quoque e fruge sibi potus similis excogitavit.*

25 Pliny, *Natural History*, ed. Rackham, vol. 4, 14.149: *nullaque in parte mundi cessat ebrietas; meros quippe hauriunt tales sucos nec diluendo ut vina mitigant ... heu, mira vitiorum sollertia! inventum est quemadmodum aquae quoque inebriarent.*

arena instead seem to take issue with the beer-drinkers, disapproving of their apparent tendency to overindulge in alcohol.

As noted in Chapter 2, Pliny recorded a vast amount of medical advice, including hundreds of recipes, in his encyclopaedia. Despite this extensive corpus of medical material, he never refers to beer in a medical context, neither addressing its potential medical properties nor including it as an ingredient in recipes. Just as with Dioscorides, the treatment of beer starkly contrasts with the information provided for wine, mead, and mixed alcoholic beverages. While Pliny, like Dioscorides, does not hide the potential dangers of consuming these drinks in excess, he frequently recommends their use in treatments, and there are hundreds of references to mead and/or honey-wine in the *Natural History*. The terms used by Pliny include *mulsum*, *aqua mulsa*, *hydromel*, *melitites*, and *thalassomeli* (a mixture of seawater, rainwater, and honey, possibly fermented). Most of these cases represent the use of these substances in recipes, though some are full descriptions of the particular substance in question. In Book 24, for example, Pliny writes that 'if [fenugreek] is boiled down with mallows, and honey wine [*mulso*] be afterwards added, a draught is praised as a preeminent remedy for troubles of the uterus and intestines'.[26] He advises that 'for pain of the kidneys or liver, [bugloss] is taken in hydromel [*aqua mulsa*], should there be fever, otherwise in wine'.[27]

Notably, although beer was not deemed by Pliny to have medical properties, other cereal-based products were recorded in treatments. Regarding bread, for example, he writes that 'in hydromel [*aqua mulsa*], it is very soothing to indurations'.[28] Thus, in Pliny's eyes, beer was seen to be useless, whereas other cereal-based products as well as alcohols derived from fruits and honey possessed beneficial medicinal properties or could serve as neutral components within a recipe (e.g., as a liquefying agent). This particular disapproval of beer, whether it was seen as an actively harmful substance or as related to uncouth barbarians, left its mark for centuries and continues to influence the stereotypes surrounding beer- and wine-drinking today.

---

26 Pliny, *Natural History*, ed. Jones, vol. 7, 24.187: *si vero cum malva decoquatur postea addito mulso, potus ante cetera vulvis interaneisque laudatur.*

27 Pliny, *Natural History*, ed. Jones, vol. 6, 22.52: *et in dolore renium aut iocineris ex aqua mulsa, si febris sit, sin aliter, e vino bibitur.*

28 Pliny, *Natural History*, ed. Jones, vol. 6, 22.138: *ex aqua mulsa duritias valde mitigat.*

3 Changing Tastes in Late Antiquity?

Although beer may have been looked down on as an inferior drink consumed by foreigners, many of those 'foreigners', such as Gauls and Egyptians, actually lived within the bounds of the Roman Empire. The Germanic tribes mentioned by Tacitus, while they mostly remained beyond the *limes* for a few more centuries, were a constant presence on the frontier and an increasing force within the army. Romans certainly would have had contact with beer-drinking communities or, indeed, could have belonged to both drinking cultures. The increasing visibility of beer appears to have resulted in a softening of some of the extreme views of earlier writers, though some sources indicate that many Romans continued to disapprove of it. To be clear, although beer seems to have achieved some degree of acceptability in the provinces, it was not perceived as on par with wine.[29] Medicine is a field in which this changing attitude can be discerned, if only slightly: in contrast to Dioscorides' description of the harmful properties of beer and Pliny's disregard for the drink from a medical perspective, a handful of late antique Latin authors do comment on beer in medical contexts.

The *Medicina Plinii*, noted in Chapter 2 as an example of the late antique reworking of existing texts, is made up of three books of recipes. As its name suggests, much of the material is derived from Pliny's *Natural History*, though other influences can also be seen.[30] Book 3 contains a chapter on scrofulous, swollen glands; the tenth and final recipe of this chapter recommends that the leaves of elder be ground up and mixed with the dregs of beer and then applied with a linen cloth.[31] It is important to remember the size of this work: the three books making up the *Medicina Plinii* contain hundreds of recipes. The use of beer dregs to help scrofulous swellings is the single reference to beer in the entire text, meaning that beer appears in less than one percent of the text's remedies. Wine, in contrast, appears very regularly; it is one of the standard liquifying agents recorded in recipes. Despite this seemingly insignificant representation of beer, the sheer fact that it is included in a recipe is significant, marking a departure from earlier Mediterranean medical writings and

29 Nelson, *The Barbarian's Beverage*, 74.

30 *Plinii Secundi Iunioris qui feruntur De medicina libri tres*, ed. Önnerfors; *The* Medicina Plinii, trans. Hunt; Doody, 'Authority and Authorship in the Medicina Plinii', 93–105; Doody, *Pliny's Encyclopedia*.

31 *Plinii Secundi Iunioris qui feruntur De medicina libri tres*, ed. Önnerfors, 3.6.10: *ebuli folia conteruntur et mixta cum faece ceruisiae super additis foliis eiusdem ebuli in linteolo alliga<n>tur*. See also *The* Medicina Plinii, trans. Hunt, 3.6.10.

confirming that sources other than Pliny's *Natural History* were incorporated in the *Medicina Plinii*.

Marcellus of Bordeaux, the Gallo-Roman statesman active in the late fourth and early fifth centuries, and his large pharmaceutical collection, *De medicamentis liber*, were also introduced in Chapter 2.[32] While he cites both 'Plinies', meaning Pliny the Elder's *Natural History* and the *Medicina Plinii*, as sources for his work, it is clear that a wider range of material influenced the text.[33] In particular, the local, Gallic environment appears to have left a strong imprint, both in terms of Marcellus' writing style and with respect to the medical information he recorded.[34] Remembering that many classical sources associated beer-drinking with Gaul, it is perhaps unsurprising to see this beverage appear alongside wine, mead, and mixed alcohols. Beer is listed in two treatments, and both are distinct from the single instance recorded in the *Medicina Plinii*. First, in Chapter 16, on coughs and lung conditions, Marcellus suggests drinking a potion of salt dissolved in beer.[35] Chapter 28, on worms and intestinal issues, provides the second example, where beer appears to be a liquefying agent in which a compound medicine is soaked.[36] Of particular note in the second recipe is that Marcellus comments on what to do if the reader finds him- or herself in a province in which beer is not available: in this case, they are instructed to use water in which myrtle has been cooked.[37] While these two recipes double the total seen in the *Medicina Plinii*, *De medicamentis liber* contains over 2000 recipes. Consequently, beer appears in less than 0.1% of recipes.

Given the extremely low frequencies with which beer is mentioned, these examples of late antique medical authors recording beer in their recipes may seem trivial, barely representing an increase over their classical predecessors. Slight as this increase is, however, it still indicates a change, moving from

32 Marcellus, *De medicamentis liber*, ed. Liechtenhan and Niedermann, trans. Kollesch and Nickel; Stannard, 'Marcellus of Bordeaux', 47–53.

33 Doody, *Pliny's Encyclopedia*, 138.

34 Stannard, 'Marcellus of Bordeaux', 49.

35 Marcellus, *De medicamentis liber*, ed. Liechtenhan and Niedermann, trans. Kollesch and Nickel, 16.33: *Salis quantum intra palmam tenere potest qui tussiet in potionem ceruisae aut curmi mittat et calidum bibat, cum dormitum uadit, neque postea loquatur, sed tacitus somnum capiat; cito sanabitur, si hoc uel triduo fecerit.*

36 Ibid, 28.13: … *Facies pilulas magnitudine ea, qua ano inici possint, ipsasque factas infundes in ceruesiae nouae sextariis duobus et mellis cyatho.*

37 Ibid: *Quod si in ea prouincia faciendum fuerit hoc medicamentum, in qua ceruisia non est, ex aqua dabis, in qua myrta cocta sit, ad sextarios duos aut cum sapae mixtae sextariis duobus atque ex eo temperabis potionem et dabis bibendam.*

the outright disapproval of beer to a (very) limited application. In the case of Marcellus, the provincial environment in which he was writing may have played an important role in his acceptance, however small, of the medicinal qualities of beer. These initial inclusions of beer in medical writings appear to have paved the way for early medieval medical writers active in the west.

4 The Rise of Beer and *Medus* in the Early Middle Ages

The opening examples from cod. sang. 752 suggest that the changing attitudes towards alcohols seen in late Antiquity continued to develop over the following centuries. Four aspects of this example stand out, marking a departure from the classical and late antique medical writings reviewed above. First, and perhaps most obviously, the increasing proportion of references to beer is noteworthy: it is mentioned twice in this small selection of material. The first example comes from the fourteenth remedy, where it is recommended that beer and mead be consumed during the patient's recovery. Beer is then noted as an exception in the list of foods and drinks to avoid if suffering from paralysis: light beer is considered acceptable. While beer is not recorded as an ingredient in recipes in this manuscript, its appearance in two types of dietary guidelines still places it within a medical environment. Secondly, the references to beer, mead, and wine are presented neutrally and beer sits as an equal with wine and mead. Furthermore, where mead is recorded in these recipes, it is written as *medus* as opposed to any of the terms noted above, such as *mulsum*, *aqua mulsa*, *melicraton*, or *melitites*. Finally, all of the references to alcohols come from medical material found outside of established classical and late antique pharmaceutical writings given the selection criteria involved in this study. Therefore, although neither beer nor *medus* is named as an ingredient in these recipes, the references to these beverages are highly significant.

Turning to the rest of the manuscript sample, additional examples of beer and *medus*, both in dietary guidelines and as ingredients within recipes, suggest an increasing acceptance of beer as well as several other linked developments. In total, I have recorded forty references to beer and sixteen references to *medus* within the texts under analysis. From these examples, beer appears as an ingredient in twenty-six recipes and as a drink recommended for consumption or avoidance in fourteen dietary guidelines accompanying recipes, while *medus* appears as an ingredient in five recipes and in dietary guidelines eleven times. I shall review the beer examples first.

4.1 *Beer*

Of the twenty-six early medieval recipes that include beer as an ingredient within the sample, none appears to have been derived from the few recipes with beer found in the *Medicina Plinii* and *De medicamentis liber*. Within these twenty-six cases, however, several recipes are repeated, suggesting the existence of shared sources that have not survived or the inheritance of a common tradition. Codd. sang. 44, 751, and BAV pal. lat. 1088, for example, all present a treatment intended to expel 'serpents and other worms' that uses the juice of wild cucumber mixed with fresh beer.[38] An earlier recipe in cod. sang. 751 offers the same instructions, too, but is labelled as a cure for haemorrhoids, *Ad fico*; perhaps the combination of wild cucumber and beer was recorded as a treatment for multiple maladies or perhaps the scribe added the wrong recipe or title at this point in the manuscript (or was copying an exemplar in which this error had already occurred).[39] Another case of parallel treatments can be seen in cod. sang. 44 and BAV pal. lat. 1088: a recipe intended to help with 'hardness of the stomach' combines flax seeds and honey in beer.[40] Taking the repeated material into account, the manuscript sample features twenty-one distinct recipes that include beer as an ingredient. These twenty-one recipes are unknown in classical and late antique sources and represent a substantial increase in the recording of beer in recipes when compared to the previous periods.

These examples must be contextualised within the full sample of recipes. The transcribed texts produced over five thousand individual recipes, meaning that the twenty-six prescriptions listing beer as an ingredient still form but a very small percentage of the total. Indeed, the frequency with which beer is mentioned may look fairly similar to the late antique examples addressed above: as seen in Table 5, beer appears in less than one percent of the recipes

---

38 Cod. sang. 44, p. 364: *Ad serpentes uel alios uermes de homine expellendos. Potio probata. Ius de cocurbita saluatica, nuce plena cum nouella ceruisia, ieiuno dabis bibere luna decurrente*. Cod. sang. 751, p. 423: *Ad serpentes uel alios uerme de ominem expellendum, potio probata. Ius de cocurbita siluatica, nucae plena cum nouella ceruisa, ieiuno bibere dabis luna decurrente*. BAV pal. lat. 1088, f. 37r: *Ad serpentes uel aliorum uermes de homine expellendum, potio probata. Sucum de cucurbita siluatica, nuce plena cum nouella ceruisa, ieiuno dabis bibere luna decursa*. See Appendix 2, entries 5.28.1, 9.23.1, and 16.5.1, respectively.

39 Cod. sang. 751, p. 413: *Item* [*Ad fico*]. *Cucurbita saluatica, nuce plena cum molle ceruisa, dabis diebus supra dictis*. See Appendix 2, entry 9.16.2.

40 Note: the recipe collections in which these two recipes are located, though not identical, are based on the same tradition; see Appendix 1 for more details. Cod. sang. 44, p. 366: *Item ad duritiam uentris. Lino semen cum mel tritum in ceruisa ieiunus bibat, mirum est*; BAV pal. lat. 1088, f. 40v: *Item ad duritiam uentris. Lini semen cum mel tritum in ceruisia ieiunus bibat, mirum est*. See Appendix 2, entries 5.30.6 and 16.7.5, respectively.

TABLE 5 The appearance of beer as an ingredient (general)

	# of recipes with beer	% of recipes with beer
Classical medical writings	0	0.0%
Marcellus, *De medicamentis liber*	2	0.1%
Medicina Plinii	1	0.2%
Recipe sample under analysis	26	0.5%

in all cases, occurring in 0.5% of the recipes from the manuscript sample, 0.1% of the recipes of Marcellus, and 0.2% of the recipes from the *Medicina Plinii*. Yet, as insignificant as these numbers may seem, it is notable that the percentage of early medieval medical recipes mentioning beer more than doubles the percentages seen in the late antique texts.

A more detailed examination of the distribution of recipes that list beer nuances this general picture, revealing that, although beer is rarely recorded overall, its appearance in recipes is often concentrated. As Table 6 illustrates, the spread of the twenty-six recipes that name beer as an ingredient is far from uniform. Not only are these recipes found in only seven of the twenty-four manuscripts under analysis (codd. sang. 44, 751, 550, 759; BAV pal. lat. 1088; and BnF lat. 11218 and 11219), but the distribution is uneven even *within* these manuscripts. Cod. sang. 44 contains just over forty percent of the recipes that list beer as an ingredient (eleven of twenty-six), while cod. sang. 550 and BnF lat. 11219 each include a single instance of a recipe with beer. This analysis can be taken further by looking at the spread of recipes within cod. sang. 44, a manuscript with three separate large recipe collections. Do the individual texts within this manuscript parallel the uneven distribution pattern seen among the manuscript sample as a whole? This tendency is confirmed, with nine of cod. sang. 44's eleven recipes with beer located within the manuscript's second major recipe collection found on pp. 337–54. More specifically, three recipes with beer appear on p. 345, one on p. 347, two on p. 350, one on p. 351, and two on p. 353, revealing the that the nine recipes form a fairly tight cluster within the collection, too. Indeed, the three recipes on p. 345 all come under the same heading, *Potio ad nescia*, 'Potion for hip pain', and, in each case, act

TABLE 6 The appearance of beer as an ingredient within the recipe sample under analysis (ordered by %)

	# of recipes with beer	% of recipes with beer
Cod. sang. 550	1	N/A[a]
BAV pal. lat. 1088	2	0.2%
Cod. sang. 751	4	0.3%
BnF lat. 11218	4	0.5%
Cod. sang. 759	3	0.7%
BnF lat. 11219	1	0.8%
Cod. sang. 44	11	1.3%

Note:

a Cod. sang. 550 does not provide a large enough sample of recipes for comparison (three total for the manuscript). All of the other manuscripts containing recipes with beer include over 100 recipes and thus present comparable datasets.

as the potion's liquefying agent.[41] The nine recipes with beer in this collection reflect a marked increase in the frequency with which beer appears: given that the collection contains 247 recipes, beer occurs as an ingredient in 3.6% of the recipes in the collection. This percentage is significantly higher than any of those previously noted (again, see Tables 5 and 6), representing a roughly twenty-fold and fifty-fold increase (by percentage) when compared to the *Medicina Plinii* and *De medicamentis liber*, respectively.

What are the implications of this unequal distribution? The diversity of recipes combined with their irregular spread within the sample suggests that these recipes stem from multiple sources. That these recipes include beer already indicates that they incorporate information from beyond the classical canon. Yet, it is their distribution and diversity that signify that these recipes draw on a *variety* of non-classical sources: within this study's recipe sample, unique examples of treatments that list beer as an ingredient can be seen in five of the seven different manuscripts. Moreover, even though all four instances of beer in cod. sang. 751 have parallels in other manuscripts, the parallel recipes are found in cod. sang. 44, BAV pal. lat. 1088, and BnF lat. 11218, thereby revealing that cod. sang. 751 could not have drawn exclusively on one of these others as an

41 Cod. sang. 44, p. 345: *Potio ad nescia*; see Appendix 2, entries 5.18.2–4.

exemplar. On the other hand, the shared recipes of BAV pal. lat. 1088 and cod. sang. 44 are located in a collection of recipes linked to the *Tereoperica* family of recipe collections that is found in both codices. Though not identical, these collections are closely related, as these recipes that record beer illustrate.[42] In fact, in cod. sang. 44, these two recipes correspond to the only beer-containing recipes outside of its primary cluster of recipes that list beer as an ingredient on pp. 345–53. Overall, given the varied origins of the manuscripts under analysis, it is not surprising that their texts contain information from different traditions and were shaped by multiple, if often shared, influences. Before considering these non-classical sources, the availability of beer in the Carolingian world, and how this information can shed light on the question of practicality, it is useful to examine the evidence for *medus* in the recipe literature.

4.2 *Mead and* Medus

As noted above, all references to mead in the selected sections of cod. sang. 752 use the term *medus*, and classical Latin and Latinised Greek terms for various potentially alcoholic honey-based (or at least honey-containing) beverages, including *mulsum*, *aqua mulsa*, *hydromel*, *oenomel*, and *melitites*, are absent. The *Etymologiae* of Isidore of Seville provides information on a variety of alcohols containing honey and represents one of the earliest written sources to use the term *medus*.[43] Isidore first distinguishes between *hydromel* and *oenomel*, classifying the former as a combination of honey and water and the latter as a mixture of honey and wine.[44] *Mulsum* and *melicratum*, on the other hand, seem to be more variable in their composition: *mulsum*, for example, is recorded as both 'wine mixed with honey' and 'a drink made from water and honey'.[45] In contrast, *medus* alone is said be made from honey with no comments referring to the addition of other liquids.[46] This suggests that, unlike many of the other beverages listed above which may represent honey-wine or mead-wine mixtures, *medus* may have been a honey-based alcohol more similar to a modern

42 Three versions of a series of recipes to expel serpents and other worms, *Ad serpentes uel alios uermes de homine expellendos*, are found codd. sang. 44 (p. 364), 751 (p. 423), and BAV pal. lat. 1088 (ff. 37r–37v), while versions of a cluster of recipes under the heading *Ad uentris dolorem* are found in cod. sang. 44 (p. 366) and BAV pal. lat. 1088 (f. 40v). See Appendix 2, entries 5.28, 9.23, and 16.5 for the former; see entries 5.30 and 16.7 for the latter.

43 Additional early examples of the use of *medus* can be seen in the writings of Venantius Fortunatus and Anthimus, both active in the sixth century; Anthimus' letter on diet is considered later in this chapter.

44 Isidore, *Etymologiae*, 20.3.11–12.

45 Ibid, 20.3.10.

46 Ibid, 20.3.13.

understanding of mead. Indeed, the word *medus* is related to the English word 'mead', as both stem from a proto-Germanic root; 'mead' was known as *me(o)du* in Old English and *metu* in Old High German, while the modern equivalents in Dutch and German are *mee* and *Met*, respectively.[47] Thus, while it is unclear if the term *medus* documents an alternative type of honey-based alcohol, the term itself can be connected to a Germanic linguistic tradition distinct from the terms used in classical and late antique sources.

The presence of *medus* in medical contexts did not result in the disappearance of the other terms for alcohols involving honey: I recorded twenty-three examples of *hydromel*, one example of *melicratum*, 150 examples of *mulsum* or *aqua mulsa*, and two examples of *oenomel* in the recipe sample. Indeed, the word for 'mead' in many Romance languages has descended from one of the classical terms, *hydromel*.[48] Eventually, however, this classical vocabulary would be largely lost from Germanic languages, as the modern English, Dutch, and German terminology reveals.

Within the sample under analysis, eleven of the sixteen references to *medus* (68.7%) occur within dietary guidelines, such as the examples already seen in cod. sang. 752, and only five recipes (32.2%) include *medus* as an ingredient. This breakdown is roughly the opposite of what was found for beer: the latter served as a recipe ingredient in two-thirds of its recorded occurrences. Of the five recipes where *medus* is listed as an ingredient, two are found in cod. sang. 751 while the remaining three are located in BnF lat. 11218. On p. 305 of cod. sang. 751, for example, *medus* is recommended as part of a treatment for groin or bladder pain and difficulty urinating; later in the same manuscript, it is also listed as an ingredient in a potion intended to expel worms and other sources of harm, *maleficia*.[49] In BnF lat. 11218, the three recipes occur within just a few folia (ff. 115v–122v). In the first instance, mead is used in a treatment for jaundice, whereas the final two examples are found in two different recipes under the same heading, *Ad ueretrum suscitandum*, a treatment for what would probably be known today as erectile disfunction.[50]

47 Angus Stevenson, ed., *Oxford Dictionary of English*, 3rd ed. (Oxford: Oxford University Press, 2010).

48 Consider, for example, the terms used for 'mead' in Spanish, French, Italian, Portuguese, and Catalan: *hidromiel*, *hydromel*, *idromele*, *hidromel*, and *hidromel*, respectively.

49 Cod. sang. 751, p. 305: *Item ad ilii dolorem uel uesicae et difficultatem urinae*; p. 413: *Potio ad oua colobrina*. See Appendix 2, entries 9.1.4 and 9.17, respectively.

50 BnF lat. 11218, ff. 115v–116r: *Ad prugine qui uocatur morbus regio*; f. 122v: *Ad ueretrum suscitandum*; f. 122v: *Item ad ipsum suscitandum*. See Appendix 2, entries 3.13 and 3.15.1–2, respectively.

The relative frequency with which *medus* is included in dietary guidelines (as opposed to its use as an ingredient in recipes) is noteworthy not only in comparison to beer but also with respect to the other terms relating to honey-based beverages. In contrast to *medus*, these words—*mulsum*, *aqua mulsa*, *melitites*, *oenomel*, and *hydromel*—are always listed as ingredients within recipes or, given that they represent complex ingredients that needed to be prepared before they could be used, presented as recipes themselves. Cod. sang. 759, for example, provides two recipes that offer instructions on how to make *hydromel*.[51] The separate contexts in which these words are found suggest a difference between their uses and/or sources.

Also of note, *medus* is consistently recorded alongside beer. The two beverages are paired in all eleven of the dietary guidelines with *medus*. In fact, the five recipes that use *medus* are the only occasions in which it is mentioned without a simultaneous reference to beer, and all but three of the dietary guidelines involving beer, or nearly eighty percent, also include *medus*. While some of these guides appear as part of treatments, such as the opening example in cod. sang. 752 that lists the foods from which to abstain if suffering from paralysis, other guides were of a more preventative nature and advocated for the avoidance or consumption of specific foods and drinks at certain times of the year in order to maintain health. Within the manuscript sample, calendrical guides to diet linking beer and *medus* can be found in cod. sang. 759, BnF lat. 2849A and 11218.[52] In the entry for the month of May, BnF lat. 2849A suggests that beer and *medus* should be avoided, but recommends drinking beverages made from wormwood and fennel.[53] For August, cod. sang. 759 likewise instructs its readers to avoid beer and *medus*, though the text does not provide alternatives.[54] Cod. sang. 759 also includes one of the three instances in which beer appears in a dietary guide without the accompanying *medus*, though it must be noted that this recommendation (that beer should be avoided in June), has been inserted into the text; given the tight spacing of the interlinear addition, perhaps the scribe simply ran out of room to include a reference to *medus*, as well.[55]

51 Cod. sang. 759, p. 66: *Confectio ydromellis*; pp. 88–9: *Confectio ydromellis*. See Appendix 2, entries 11.12 and 11.19, respectively.

52 On dietary calendars in the early medieval west, see 'Die frühmittelalterlichen lateinischen Monatskalendarien. Text, Übersetzung, Kommentar', ed. and trans. Frank-Dieter Groenke (Diss., Freie Universität Berlin, 1986).

53 BnF lat. 2849A, f. 23v: *Ceruisa nec metus non bibat, absentio et faniculo bibat.*

54 Cod. sang. 759, p. 8: *ceruissa et metus non bibat.*

55 Cod. sang. 759, p. 8: *aqua bibere \ceruissa non bibere/ nisi pusca usitare, lactucas manducare, acetum bibere.*

The consistent pairing of the two beverages may reflect their original connection in an earlier dietary treatise that has since been lost. Alternatively, while classical texts offer no information on a possible link between the two substances, a late antique letter on diet, Anthimus' *De observatione ciborum*, may shed light on the topic. Anthimus, a Byzantine physician active in the sixth century, was exiled to the west during a period of political intrigue in Constantinople. While acting as an ambassador of Theodoric, king of the Ostrogoths (r. 493–526), Anthimus composed a letter on diet in honour of his host Theuderic, king of the Franks (r. 511–34) in the area around Metz.[56] The letter fuses Greek, Roman, and Frankish cultural and dietary traditions, offering the reader advice on how to maintain good health through the observance of a healthy diet. In Chapter 14, for example, Anthimus reports on the medicinal powers of raw bacon according to Frankish medical traditions. He writes, 'as for raw bacon which, so I hear, the Franks have a habit of eating, I am full of curiosity regarding the person who showed them such a medicine as to obviate the need for other medicines … Look at what power there is in raw bacon, and see how with it the Franks heal what doctors try to cure with drugs or with potions'.[57] While bacon may seem entirely unrelated to the beverages under consideration, the location of this discussion is significant: the description of the particularly Frankish bacon-eating and medicating traditions occurs immediately before the entry detailing beer and mead. On these beverages, Anthimus comments that 'beer, plain mead and spiced mead are absolutely fine for drinking by almost everyone. Beer that is well brewed possesses goodness and surpasses expectation … Mead that is well brewed is very beneficial, provided that the honey is good'.[58] Like the references to mead in the dietary guidelines assessed in the manuscript sample, Anthimus uses the term *medus*. His use of the term also predates Isidore's usage in the *Etymologiae*, offering the earliest surviving witness and making it particularly meaningful that it occurs within this Frankish context.

---

56 Mark Grant, 'Introduction', in Anthimus, *On the Observance of Foods*, ed. and trans. Mark Grant, 2nd ed. (Totnes: Prospect, 2007), 12.

57 Anthimus, *De observatione ciborum*, ed. and trans. Liechtenhan, Chapter 14 (at pp. 9–10): *De crudo uero laredo, quod solent, ut audio, domni Franci comedere, miror satis, quis illis ostendit talem medicinam, ut non opus habeant alias medicinas … ecce quale beneficium in laredo crudo, ut, quod medici in medicamentis uel potionibus temptant sanare uel inplastris uulnera curare, de laredo crudo Franci sanantur.*

58 Ibid, Chapter 15 (at p. 10): *ceruisa bibendo uel medus et aloxinum quam maxime omnibus congruum est ex toto, quia ceruisa, qui bene facta fuerit, beneficium prestat et rationem habet … Similiter et de medus bene factum, ut mel bene habeat, multum iuuat.*

Indeed, *De observatione ciborum*, through its detailed depiction of certain Frankish practices and references to oral traditions (such as the medicinal properties of bacon), indicates that Anthimus picked up this information through personal experience. The paired description of beer and *medus* may therefore reflect that these beverages were traditionally viewed as linked in Frankish customs and help to explain their continued coupling in Carolingian writings on diet. On the other hand, Anthimus may have initiated the association of these two alcohols, and their consistent linkage in later texts may simply reflect the influence of *De observatione ciborum* on eighth- and ninth-century authors.[59]

4.3 *Summary*

Ultimately, these results suggest that a subtle but significant shift occurred in the early medieval west. The recipes and other medical writings analysed above document an increased presence of beer in medical contexts as well as the use of the term *medus* for mead. That beer, mead (under any name), and wine appear to be treated similarly, or at least without prejudice, also marks a notable change. The medical knowledge recorded in eighth- and ninth-century manuscripts must now be considered within the wider context and related to the question of practicality.

5 Contextualising Beer and Mead in Early Medieval Europe

While classical sources suggest that beer was being produced in parts of western Europe in Antiquity, is there evidence confirming its continued production in the Carolingian period? Writings like Isidore's *Etymologiae* point to brewing as an alternative to wine in regions that could not sustain viticulture.[60] Since much of the Frankish Empire covered areas that could support both grape and cereal production, do non-medical texts suggest that multiple beverages coexisted or that, just as in the classical world, a particular class of alcoholic beverages was privileged over others? Documentary evidence, such as the *Capitulare de villis*, can help to address these questions.

59 According to Beccaria's catalogue, copies of or extracts from Anthimus' letter have survived in eight early medieval manuscripts, including two involved in the present study, codd. sang. 751 and 878; see Beccaria, *I codici*, nos. 133 and 139.

60 Isidore, *Etymologiae*, 20.3.17–18.

Composed in the late eighth century, the *Capitulare de villis* concerns the management of royal estates.[61] The seventy chapters of the text cover a wide range of topics, from the administration of justice to the care of horses and hounds, and the production of beer and wine is addressed in several places. Chapter 8, for example, focuses exclusively on wine, detailing the care of vineyards as well as the production and shipping of wine and its general supply on royal estates.[62] The maintenance and cleanliness of wine-presses is also mentioned in Chapters 41 and 48. The significance of brewing is expressed in Chapter 61, which states that master-brewers should be attached to stewards, following their movements while on service to ensure that good beer was readily available.[63] Brewers are also classed among the essential workmen to have in each district; other professions listed include shoemakers, carpenters, blacksmiths, and fishermen.[64] Although the production of mead and the keeping of bees is not explicitly described by the capitulary, both mead and honey are mentioned in several chapters, including Chapter 34, which asks that particular care is taken when making products to eat or drink, thereby confirming that mead and honey were being produced, as well.[65] Significantly, *medus* is the term used to describe mead.

61 *Capitulare de villis*, ed. Alfred Boretius, *MGH Capit.* 1 (Hanover: Hahn, 1883), no. 32; H. R. Loyn and John Percival, *The Reign of Charlemagne. Documents on Carolingian Government and Administration* (London: Edward Arnold, 1975), 64–73.

62 *Capitulare de villis*, ed. Boretius, no. 32, c. 8: *Ut iudices nostri vineas recipiant nostras, quae de eorum sunt ministerio, et bene eas faciant et ipsum vinum in bona mittant vascula et diligenter praevidere faciant, quod nullo modo naufragatum sit; aliud vero vinum peculiare conparando emere faciant, unde villas dominicas condirigere possint. Et quandoquidem plus de ipso vino conparatum fuerit quod ad villas nostras condirigendum mittendi opus sit, nobis innotescat, ut nos commendemus qualiter nostra fuerit exinde voluntas. Cippaticos enim de vineis nostris ad opus nostrum mittere faciant. Censa de villis nostris qui vinum debent, in cellaria nostra mittat.*

63 Ibid, no. 32, c. 61: *Ut unusquisque iudex quando servierit suos bracios ad palatium ducere faciat; et simul veniant magistri qui cervisam bonam ibidem facere debeant.*

64 Ibid, no. 32, c. 45: *Ut unusquisque iudex in suo ministerio bonos habeat artifices, id est fabros ferrarios et aurifices vel argentarios, sutores, tornatores, carpentarios, scutarios, piscatores, aucipites id est aucellatores, saponarios, siceratores, id est qui cervisam vel pomatium sive piratium vel aliud quodcumque liquamen ad bibendum aptum fuerit facere sciant, pistores, qui similam ad opus nostrum faciant, retiatores qui retia facere bene sciant, tam ad venandum quam as piscandum sive ad aves capiendum, necnon et reliquos ministeriales quos ad numerandum longum est.*

65 Ibid, no. 32, c. 34: *Omnino praevidendam est cum omni diligentia, ut quicquid manibus laboraverint aut fecerint, id est lardum, siccamen, sulcia, niusaltus, vinum, acetum, moratum, vinum coctum, garum, sinape, formaticum, butirum, bracios, cervisas, medum, mel, ceram, farinam, omnia cum summo nitore sint facta vel parata.*

The *Plan of St Gall*, a manuscript mentioned in Chapter 2 in relation to its gardens and spaces of medical care, also contains information on the production of alcohols in the Carolingian world. In particular, the diagram highlights the centrality of brewing within a monastic complex. Three separate breweries are depicted in the *Plan*, corresponding to individual brewing areas for the monks, distinguished guests, and pilgrims.[66] In the granary, storage areas for cleaned and malted cereal are recorded, while a drying kiln, mortars, and milling areas were all located nearby.[67] Conveniently, this brewing area was situated near the cooper, who would have been responsible for constructing the barrels in which the beer would have been kept.

The *Capitulare de villis* and *Plan of St Gall* therefore provide evidence for not only the presence of beer, mead, and wine during the Carolingian period but also their production within its territories. This indicates that all of the beverages addressed above could have been sourced within the Carolingian world. Notably, beer and *medus* appear in recipes in manuscripts produced at writing centres in the Frankish heartlands *and* in manuscripts written at sites newly under Frankish control, such as those copied in northern Italian centres. As discussed in Chapter 1, the movement of manuscripts and exchange of knowledge testifies to the deep-rooted connections between these areas despite the relatively recent conquest of Lombardy in 778. The presence of beer and *medus* in such manuscripts adds another dimension to this picture, confirming the existence of strong cultural and intellectual links: the recipe literature records shared cultural practices and medical knowledge.

6 Beer, Mead, and the Question of Practicality

The results presented above demonstrate several key features. First, a long-term transition towards the acceptance of beer for medical purposes can be seen through the changing portrayal of the beverage and its gradual increase in recipes. Secondly, the recipe literature documents the adoption of a new term for mead, *medus*, in medical contexts, paralleling the term's appearance in other early medieval sources. Third, these two developments appear to be linked, with beer and mead (specifically as *medus*) often found together. The relationship between the two beverages is further strengthened by their connections to Frankish traditions, highlighted by Anthimus' *De observatione*

66 Nelson, *The Barbarian's Beverage*, 103.

67 Ibid, 103–4.

ciborum. Fourth, although wine continues to occur more frequently than either beer or mead, it is important to recognise that these beverages are presented on equal terms: all three are recorded in recipes as well as in dietary guidelines. In contrast to classical sources, beer is not dismissed as unhealthy, uncouth, or otherwise unsuitable for medical purposes in this textual sample.

The significance of each of these changes must be considered in context. Although the recipes under analysis are strongly related to classical and late antique medical traditions, this chapter, like the previous one, reveals that they also contain influences *beyond* these traditions. In this case, I have identified ingredients that were unrecorded in classical and late antique recipes. The similarities seen across many manuscripts suggest that these additions should be viewed collectively as part of a larger pattern—a pattern linked to ingredient availability. The inclusion of these non-classical ingredients represents a widespread, practical development, i.e., the use of locally produced and readily available substances.

However, while non-medical texts, such as the *Capitulare de villis* and *Plan of St Gall*, support the idea that these beverages were expected to have been locally available in early medieval western Europe, it is important to avoid placing too much weight on the evidence of such normative texts. With this in mind, the pairing of beer and *medus* in dietary guidelines takes on greater significance: their frequent, linked appearance in the medical literature at this time—and specifically in the lists of substances that were either acceptable to consume or best to avoid—is noteworthy as these writings appear to reflect contemporary dietary and drinking habits. As such, dietary guidelines offer a more direct glimpse into Carolingian food and drink, highlighting the substances that likely featured in daily life. The evidence from a range of textual sources therefore indicates that beer and mead formed part of the standard 'dietary landscape' and their inclusion as ingredients in recipes thus documents a practical shift in medicine: their use as liquefying agents reflects adaptations made to suit local conditions.

7 Conclusion

The appearance of beer and *medus* in the recipe literature demonstrates an active engagement with and adaptation of medical knowledge during this period. By tracing the occurrence of these ingredients within the sample of recipes and comparing the results to classical and late antique texts, it has been possible to chart a transformation in pharmaceutical writings over time. In doing so, this chapter also showcases the importance of large sample sizes and in-depth textual analyses. Such detailed studies have the potential to identify significant patterns in the data that could be missed in studies with smaller textual samples, such as a single recipe collection. By analysing over 5000 recipes, it was possible to detect particularly significant data clusters. Following the large-scale analysis with more specific studies of the clusters and then investigating the patterns that emerged within manuscripts and their recipe collections accentuated the increasing frequency of references to beer. While this beverage was listed roughly 0.5% of recipes from the entire manuscript sample, it was included in nearly 2% of the recipes in cod. sang. 44. This percentage increased even further when its recipe collections were considered separately: nine of the recipes that record beer can be found in the collection on pp. 337–54, representing close to 4% of the 247 treatments contained within this collection. Therefore, as illustrated by, on the one hand, the observation of a general increase in references to beer and *medus*, and, on the other hand, the identification of a striking concentration of recipes involving beer in cod. sang. 44, the recipe sample involved in this study has the potential to reveal both large-scale patterns as well as very specific information.

Finally, it must be remembered that the texts in which the examples of beer and *medus* were identified continue to share many features with classical and late antique medical writings. The introduction of these ingredients cannot be said to mark a sharp break in intellectual traditions, but rather the gradual evolution of the medical knowledge in circulation. The developments noted above, though limited in scale, reflect two significant changes: a) that the compilers of recipe collections were open to incorporating non-classical information and traditions, and b) that these changes were of a highly practical nature. The supporting evidence, such as the *Capitulare de villis* and *Plan of St Gall*, indicates that the alcoholic beverages listed in recipes were being produced in, and therefore likely obtainable in, the Carolingian world. This picture is further strengthened by the frequent linking of beer and mead in dietary guidelines.

Ultimately, the addition of such practical ingredients supports the idea that these collections were intended to be used in the practice of medicine. The texts document changes to recorded medical knowledge, and these changes appear to reflect responses to the local environment, medical traditions, and/or available ingredients. While the individuals responsible for the composition of these texts worked with a body of knowledge largely descended from classical traditions, their adaptations and additions to the recipe literature suggest that they took into account practical considerations in an attempt to produce recipe collections intended for use in practice.

CHAPTER 5

Evidence for Practicality Beyond *Materia Medica*

1 Introduction: the Importance of Investigating Additional Elements Within Recipes

> A proven potion for abdominal disease: Take three handfuls of agrimony roots in a new bowl and add to it nine cups of wine. It should be cooked until there is a third remaining. [The patient] drinks it when it is necessary. [Also add] roots of butcher's broom; roots of caltrops; roots of asparagus; roots of angelica; roots of celery; roots of parsley; dried pennyroyal; 3 heads of garlic; dried seeds of mallow, 1 ounce; 4 leeks with their roots; betony with its roots, either dried or fresh; roots of violets; garden cress; wild rue or, if not available, cultivated; coriander; dill; and sufficient oil.[1]

The above potion recorded in BAV reg. lat. 1143, the *Potionem probata ad ilica passio*, offers an allegedly tried and tested treatment for those suffering from abdominal pains. The recipe presents a number of different features that argue for its practicality. The most eye-catching of these is the bold claim in the title: this is a *potionem probata*, a recipe that has been used. As seen in the case of Terenti(an)us, however, such statements need more careful scrutiny. Phrases that promote the 'tried and tested' nature of recipes appear frequently, usually either in the title or, most often, at the recipe's close. These efficacy clauses are best understood as advertisements for the treatment, representing a recurrent trope rather than a clear indicator of contemporary use. While it remains possible that the inclusion of a term like *probata* could reflect the scribe's personal experience (or knowledge of others' experiences), it would be inappropriate to assume this without further evidence. Indeed, as the example of Terenti(an)us showed, even recipes with detailed descriptions of use and

1 BAV reg. lat. 1143, ff. 185r–185v: *Potionem probata ad ilica passio. Agrimonia radices prinde manipulos tres, mitte in ulla noua et addis ibidem uinum staupos nouem et coquatur usque ad tertiam partem et bibit quando oporte fuerit. Radicem de rusco, radicem de tribulo, radicem de sparago, radicem de olisatro, radicem appio, radicem de petroselino, puleio siccum, allii capitinas iii, semen de malua sicca uncia una, porros iiii cum radicinas suas, bettonica cum radice sua siue sicca siue uiride, radicem de uiola, nasturtium, ruta siluatica, et si non domestica, coriandrum, anetum, oleum quod sufficit.* The recipe continues with simple instructions for preparing the potion with these ingredients; for the full transcription, see Appendix 2, entry 18.9.

what might, at first glance, seem to be convincing signs of personal experience may reflect information copied from an earlier source. Any first-person comments regarding the use of a recipe must always be read with great caution. Three other aspects of this recipe, however, may offer more direct insights into its potential practicality.

As seen in Chapters 3 and 4, an analysis of the *materia medica* listed in recipes offers a useful entry point into the question of practicality. In this case, does the *Potionem probata ad ilica passio* rely on products that could have been obtained within the Carolingian world? The recipe lists nearly twenty different ingredients, all of which are entirely plant-based and could have been grown or found within northwest Europe. These include agrimony roots cooked in wine; the roots of butcher's broom, caltrops, asparagus, angelica, celery, parsley, and violets; dried pennyroyal; three heads of garlic; one ounce of mallow seeds; four leeks with roots; betony, with its roots either dried or fresh; cress; wild rue or, if necessary, the cultivated variety; coriander; dill; and oil. The use of products that were likely available in Francia suggests that that this recipe was, at least with respect to its ingredients, highly practical.

Moving beyond the *materia medica*, two other features of the recipe stand out: a) the appearance of the term *staupus*, a unit roughly equivalent to a cup, to measure wine, and b) the recording of an ingredient substitution. Both of these topics deserve further analysis and will be addressed below. The use of the Latinised vernacular term *staupus* points to a changing linguistic environment. Is its appearance in this recipe a unique occurrence, perhaps reflecting a scribe unfamiliar with classical terminology, or is it part of a larger pattern? Should its use be viewed as a practical adaptation, or does it reveal potential linguistic barriers encountered by early medieval readers and writers attempting to engage with the pharmaceutical literature? Secondly, the substitution suggestion (in this case, the use of cultivated rue if wild rue was unavailable) offers a practical solution to sourcing ingredients, a backup plan if the desired ingredient could not be obtained. Is such advice a record of contemporary practices or, like the case of Terenti(an)us, information from an earlier source, such as the late antique pseudo-Galenic text, *Περὶ ἀντεμβαλλομένων*, *On substitute drugs*? This chapter focuses first on the unit *staupus*, before returning to the question of substitution instructions.

The exploration of these two features illustrates the importance of considering recipes in their entirety when investigating the question of practicality. The *Potionem probata ad ilica passio* serves as a useful segue from the previous chapters' focus on *materia medica* to the present analysis of other elements within recipes. In the former, practicality was considered with respect to useability, asking whether the recipes could have been put into practice based on their ingredients. This chapter turns to the question of design, considering whether certain features within recipes would have made them more or less useable—or understandable—to those engaging with the texts, and especially within the context of therapy. In sum, moving beyond *materia medica* to the additional information contained within recipes offers another perspective on the potential practicality of pharmaceutical writings and, complementing the findings of the preceding chapters, suggests that many recipes would have offered practical, useable information to those individuals with access to the texts.

2 *Staupus*: a Vernacular 'Intrusion'[2]

2.1 *Past Studies on* Staupus

Near the start of the *Potionem probata ad ilica passio*, the reader is instructed to cook agrimony roots in wine measured by the *staupus*. This unit, a Latinised Germanic term, is roughly equivalent to a cup, beaker, or goblet. While the use of this term has not been extensively studied, its appearance in early medieval texts has been noted by a number of scholars, generating a range of interpretations about its volume.[3] Benjamin Guérard, for example, suggested that the unit was just under a litre whereas Henry Sigerist interpreted it as a small cup and equivalent to one *cyathus*, approximately 50 mL.[4] More recently, Ulrich Stoll has described one *staupus* as comparable to one *hemina*, roughly 300 mL.[5] While these large differences indicate that a consensus has not been reached, attempting to define the unit with such precision seems anachronistic and inappropriate. For the present study, moreover, determining the exact volume of a *staupus* is not of great importance; rather, the word's origin is of interest as this reveals that a Germanic term for a unit of measurement was incorporated into Carolingian medical texts. Stemming from the proto-Germanic **staupa*, the word is related to the modern, though now archaic, German *Stauf* (beaker,

2 McCormick, *Origins of the European Economy*, 713; McCormick's comments on the unit *staupus* are addressed below.

3 For more general studies of weights and measures, see Henry E. Sigerist, 'Maße und Gewichte in den medizinischen Texten des frühen Mittelalters', *Kyklos* 3 (1930): 439–44 and Bernhard Bischoff, 'Maße und Gewichte zur Zeit Papst Hadrians I. (772–795)', in *Anecdota novissima. Texte des vierten bis sechzehnten Jahrhunderts*, ed. Bernhard Bischoff (Stuttgart: Hiersemann, 1984), 169–70. See also Isidore's sections on weights, measures, and their symbols in Book 16: Isidore of Seville, *Etymologiae*, 16.15–17.

4 *Polyptyque de l'abbé Irminon*, ed. Guérard, vol. 1, 188; *Studien und Texte*, ed. Sigerist, 175.

5 *Das Lorscher Arzneibuch*, ed. and trans. Stoll, 40.

cup) and English 'stoup' (a basin for holy water) as well as to a variety of terms for vessels in other Germanic languages, including Norwegian (*staup*), Swedish (*stop*), Danish (*støb*), Middle High German (*stouf*), and Old High German (*stou(p)f*).[6]

Moving beyond the debate regarding the volume of a *staupus* and its relationship to classical units, a number of scholars have also commented on its linguistic significance. Julius Jörimann, for example, makes a special note of its occurrence in the collections he transcribed and edited, despite the fact that the term only appears twice in this material. He highlights the Germanic influence indicated by the use of *staupus* when describing the practical nature of many of the recipes' measurements; other units he mentions as practical include simple, comparative measurements such as a 'handful' or an 'eggshell-full'.[7] Michael McCormick similarly comments on the 'intrusion of [this] vernacular Frankish term' in the *Lorscher Arzneibuch*, writing that the use of *staupus* indicated that 'the Lorsch physician composed or reformulated recipes which he actually used'.[8] While I agree with both scholars that the inclusion of this unit is noteworthy, I have reached a different conclusion regarding its significance based on the analysis of a much wider selection of material. If the unit *staupus* were only to be found in the recipes of the *Lorscher Arzneibuch*, the argument that it documents a *medicus* recording his own experiences of practice would be stronger (though still debateable), but, as the opening example of this chapter as well as Jörimann's comments make clear, the *Lorscher Arzneibuch* is not unique in its use of this unit. Instead, as the following analysis demonstrates, it is part of a much larger trend, and I argue that it is, in fact, the term's widespread appearance that makes it particularly significant. That is, the prevalence of the unit *staupus*—rather than its uniqueness—is not only striking but also especially relevant to consider when exploring the question of practicality.

2.2 *The Appearance of* Staupus *in the Recipe Sample*

The unit *staupus* occurs 139 times within the sample of recipes involved in this study (see Table 7). As the term may appear multiple times within a single recipe, this totals ninety-five recipes. These recipes are widely distributed among the manuscripts under analysis: the unit can be found in fifteen of the

6 Jacob Grimm and Wilhelm Grimm, eds., *Deutsches Wörterbuch*. 32 vols. (Leipzig: S. Hirzel, 1854–1961), vol. 17, 1169–74. My thanks, too, to Rosamond McKitterick for alerting me to the English term 'stoup'.

7 *Frühmittelalterliche Rezeptarien*, ed. Jörimann, 90.

8 McCormick, *Origins of the European Economy*, 713.

TABLE 7 An overview of the appearance of the unit *staupus*

Manuscript	Total # of *staupus* references	Total # of recipes including *staupus*
Cod. sang. 44	6	5
Cod. sang. 397	1	1
Cod. sang. 550	2	1
Cod. sang. 751	60	38
Cod. sang. 752	1	1
Cod. sang. 759	12	9
Cod. sang. 761	1	1
Cod. sang. 899	1	1
BAV pal. lat. 1088	2	2
BAV reg. lat. 1143	3	3
BnF lat. 2849A	14	9
BnF lat. 5543	3	2
BnF lat. 9332	1	1
BnF lat. 11218	30	19
BnF lat. 11219	2	2
Total	139	95

twenty-four codices. While the relative prevalence of *staupus* confirms that its use in the *Lorscher Arzneibuch* should not be read as a distinctive addition by the 'Lorsch physician', these findings may appear to be somewhat insignificant when considered against the backdrop of the entire recipe sample. The ninety-five recipes that record the unit *staupus* represent only about two percent (1.8%) of the recipes under analysis. It is, however, important to remember that many recipes do not specify any units, or any detailed instructions for that matter, offering only lists of *materia medica*. With this in mind, the appearance of *staupus* nearly 150 times is highly significant. Building on this general perspective, it is essential to examine the contexts in which *staupus* is found in more detail.

A recipe in BnF lat. 5543 offers a useful example to begin reviewing how *staupus* is deployed and what it is used to measure. In this manuscript, the sixth entry within a group of recipes titled *Cura ad omnes apostomas*, a cure for all abscesses, offers the following instructions:

> Likewise [a cure for all abscesses]: horehound juice, 3 cups; celery, 3 [cups]; betony, similarly; honey, similarly; old wine, 9 cups [glossed with *staupos*]; cook on a fire slowly in an earthen pot until 12 cups [remain].[9]

The first ingredient, horehound juice (*marrubio ius*), is given as three cups, using the classical Latin word *calyx*. The next three ingredients do not list a unit as they all involve the same amount: celery (*apio*) is paired simply with '*III*', while betony (*betonica*) and honey (*mel*) are listed as *similiter*. Nine cups of the final ingredient, old wine (*uinum uetus*), is written out again with the classical term. An interlinear gloss above *calices*, however, adds *staupos*, indicating that this word is a synonym for *calices*. Crucially, unlike many of the glosses seen in the manuscripts under analysis, it is written in the same hand as the main text and is not a later addition. Indeed, the scribe may have thought that glossing *calyx* at this point was necessary since the recipe then ends with the newly introduced unit: the mixture should be cooked until twelve *staupos* remain. Was the switch from *calyx* to *staupus* made to help readers who were less familiar with the classical unit? Was the gloss added by the scribe for Latin/Romance speakers who might not know the Germanic *staupus*? Or was it simply to clarify that the two units should be read as equivalent in this recipe since the scribe changed words, whether intentionally or accidentally, in the middle of the recipe?

Regardless of the underlying rationale for providing the gloss, it represents a user-friendly addition to the text that would have helped readers to understand the instructions. Such a clarification, though it could be linked to an educational context and the study of vocabulary, is also particularly suited to a practical setting. The ingredients in this recipe may be fairly safe and an incorrect measurement would have been unlikely to do much harm; many other treatments, however, involve highly toxic substances and, if they were consulted in practice, a misunderstanding regarding the amount of an ingredient to use or a dose to administer could have had serious consequences.

This recipe in BnF lat. 5543 also illustrates two of the three main types of liquids with which *staupus* is paired. This unit is most often recorded as measuring: a) unsurprisingly, the most common liquid ingredients, such as the standard liquefying agents wine, water, and vinegar; b) the final liquid product of a recipe (or a liquid mixture at some stage in the preparation process); and c) notably local liquid ingredients. In BnF lat. 5543, the unit is first used with old

9 BnF lat. 5543, f. 2r: *Item [Cura ad omnes apostomas]. Marrubio ius calices III, apio III, betonica similiter, mel similiter, uinum uetus calices \staupos/ VIIII, coque lento igne in olla rude usque ad staupos XII.* See Appendix 2, entry 2.1.6.

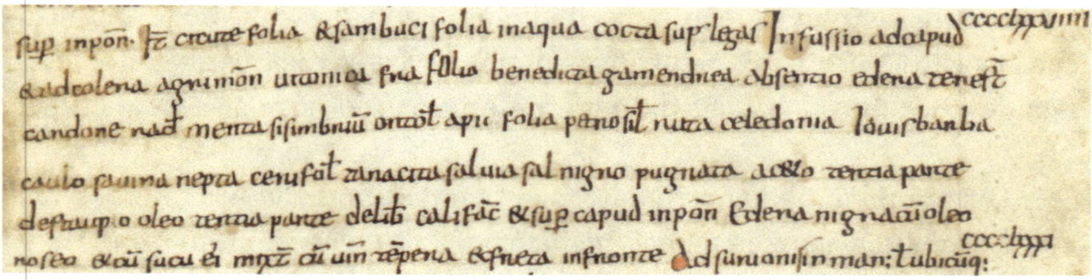

FIGURE 6 *Infussio ad capud et ad colera* in St. Gallen, Stiftsbibliothek, cod. sang. 759 (p. 51), a ninth-century manuscript with a collection of medical texts (https://www.e-codices.unifr.ch/de/csg/0759/51)

wine, one of the most frequently recorded liquid ingredients, and then used as the measurement for the recipe's end result, the volume of the cooked potion.[10] The chapter's opening example, the *Potionem probata ad ilica passio* of BAV reg. lat. 1143, also measures wine by the *staupus*, as does the only other recipe in BnF lat. 5543 that includes the unit. In the latter recipe, a treatment for joint pain, a substantial volume of wine, fifty cups, is required, though it should be noted that this large quantity was intended to last for several weeks: the patient is instructed to drink the potion for fifty days.[11] Turning to examples of other common liquid ingredients, a potion intended to combat paralysis in BnF lat. 11219, for example, includes a full *staupus* of hot water (*plenum staupum de aqua calida*) while an infusion for the head and for jaundice in cod. sang. 759 uses a third of a *staupus* of vinegar (*aceto tertia parte de staupo*; see Figure 6).[12]

In addition to these typical liquefying agents, *staupus* often appears as a liquid measure for a recipe's end product or during the process of preparation, as demonstrated by the second appearance of the unit in the *Cura ad omnes apostomas* of BnF lat. 5543. Similarly, a potion to kill worms in cod. sang. 751 uses *staupus* twice: once to measure an ingredient (three *staupus* of strong vinegar, *tres staupus de aceto uehementi*) and once to measure the potion being prepared.[13] A two-recipe unit found in codd. sang. 397, 752, and 899 contains a striking cluster of ingredients named in the vernacular and explained in Latin.[14] The recipes in cod. sang. 752 were included in the opening example of

10 Cf. Opsomer, *Index de la pharmacopée*.
11 BnF lat. 5543, f. 2v: *Item alia eiusdem* [*Contra artetricos*]. See Appendix 2, entry 2.2.2.
12 BnF lat. 11219, ff. 226va–226vb: *Potio contra paralesin*; cod. sang. 759, p. 51: *Infussio ad capud et ad colera*. See Appendix 2, entries 4.7 and 11.5.
13 Cod. sang. 751, p. 416: *Pocio ad podalo uermo occidere*. See Appendix 2, entry 9.18.
14 The recipes are located in cod. sang. 397, p. 22; cod. sang. 752, p. 158; and cod. sang. 899, p. 131. See Appendix 2, entries 7.1–2, 10.4–5, and 14.1–2.

the previous chapter in relation to their comments on wine, beer, and mead (see Figure 5). Within this recurring two-recipe cluster, the treatment for fevers includes the unit *staupus*, fitting with this unusual, vernacular-heavy context:

> On improving haemorrhoids: take plantain and the sour herb, which by another name is named *gundereba*, and tallow from mutton, this is *unslit*, and these three ingredients should be beaten in a mortar and then roasted in a small pan. And in this way, the fasting [patient] should eat [this] with bread. [They] should drink beer and mead but not water before [they] are healed.
>
> If a tertian or quotidian fever strikes a person: [they] should collect a handful of vervain, which in another way is called *isarnina*, and nine grains of pepper, and mix them together with wine. [They] should drink one *staupus* [of this mixture] before the onset of the fever.[15]

Given the linguistic origins of the term *staupus*, it may, at first, seem surprising that it is not used to measure any of the notably local ingredients, namely, those listed in the vernacular. These ingredients, however, are not liquid products, so the use of *staupus*, should not be expected. Indeed, in the first recipe, no units of measurement are given and, in the second, vervain is measured by the handful, *manipulus*.

Yet, in many of the other recipes in which the unit *staupus* is found, it is paired with liquid substances of a local flavour, the third primary category. A recipe to dry out swellings, *Ad glandolas siccandas*, in cod. sang. 44, for example, ends with six cups of beer, *sex staupos de ceruisa* (see Figure 7).[16] The use of this latinised vernacular unit alongside, as argued in Chapter 4, a locally produced and consumed beverage that was newly introduced into the recorded medical literature is especially noteworthy. Beer is also measured by

---

15 The above translation represents the recipes titled *De fico emendando* and *Si tertiana aut cottidiana febris hominem tangit* in codd. sang. 397 (p. 22), 752 (p. 158), and 899 (p. 131); as an example of the Latin text (which is nearly identical across the three recipes), the following is from cod. sang. 752: *De fico emendando. Accipe plantaginem et herbam acerem, quae alio nomine gundereba nominatur, et seuum de multone, hoc est unslit, et ista tria tundantur in mortario et fricantur in patella et sic ieiunus comedat cum pane. Ceruisam et medum nec aquam bibat antequam sanetur. Si tertiana aut cottidiana febris hominem tangit. Colligat de ueruena manipulum i, quae alio modo isarnina uocatur, et viiii grana de pipero, et cum uino mixtam componat, et ante accessionem inde bibat staupum unum.* See Appendix 2, entries 7.1–2, 10.4–5, and 14.1–2. Note that the order of the two recipes is reversed in cod. sang. 752.

16 Cod. sang. 44, p. 353; *Ad glandolas siccandas*. See Appendix 2, entry 5.23.

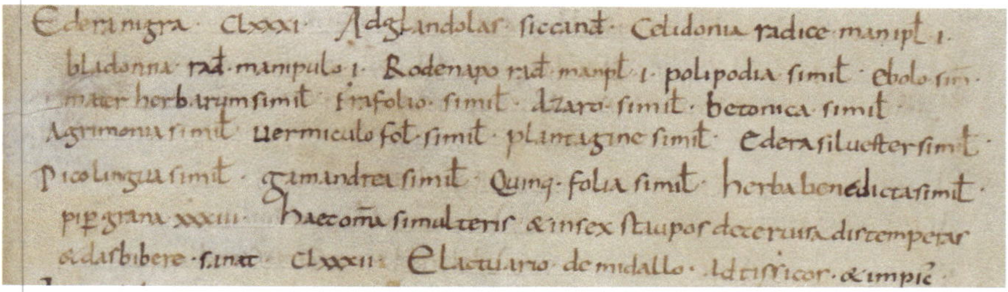

FIGURE 7 *Ad glandolas siccandas* in St. Gallen, Stiftsbibliothek, cod. sang. 44 (p. 353), an early medieval composite manuscript, the second half of which contains medical texts and was written in northern Italy in the ninth century (https://www.e-codices.unifr.ch/de/csg/0044/353)

the *staupus* in recipes in codd. sang. 550, 751, and BnF 11218.[17] In addition to beer, the unit's frequent pairing with local ingredients can be seen in its use to measure the juices of a number of different herbs, vegetables, and weeds that were growing in northern and western Europe, such as plantains, cabbage, savory, betony, fennel, coriander, feverfew, and horehound. Like the additional documentary evidence for beer in the Carolingian world, it is worth highlighting that many of these plants are named in other non-medical texts, including the *Plan of St Gall*'s garden of medicinal plants, Walahfrid Strabo's *Hortulus*, as well as the final chapter of the *Capitulare de villis*, which lists nearly one hundred plants to be cultivated in gardens, reinforcing their particularly local feel.[18] Two treatments for lung problems in cod. sang. 751, for example, call for a full *staupus* of white horehound juice as well as two of vinegar and one of honey.[19]

In this review of the contexts in which the unit *staupus* is used, two further trends have emerged with respect to the recipes in which the term appears. First, in the majority of cases, these recipes rely primarily, if not exclusively, on local ingredients, such as those named in the final category addressed above. The chapter's opening example, the recipe for abdominal problems in BAV reg. lat. 1143, exemplifies this focus on local *materia medica*: all eighteen ingredients

17 Cod. sang. 550, p. 54: *Istam causa facias contra morbum qui dicitur nesse*; cod. sang. 751, p. 447: *Potione ad ebrugine*; and BnF lat. 11218, f. 102r: *Pucione ad ebrugine*. See Appendix 2, entries 8.1, 9.31, and 3.11.

18 See Schedl, *Der Plan von St. Gallen*; Horn and Born, *The Plan of St. Gall*, 181–3; Walahfrid Strabo, *Hortulus*; and *Capitulare de villis*, ed. Boretius, no. 32.

19 Cod. sang. 751, p. 417, *Ad pulmones curandum* (and note that the same recipe is repeated on p. 430). See Appendix 2, entry 9.19.

listed in the recipe could have been grown or found in northern and/or western Europe.[20] Many of the other recipes seen so far also follow this pattern, such as the two recipes from BnF lat. 5543. The first, a treatment for abscesses, combines the juices of horehound, celery, and betony with honey and wine, while the second, a cure for joint pain, lists a wide range of local plants, including wormwood, plantain, ivy, nettles, and sage. Pepper is the sole exception, the only non-local item within the list of nearly twenty different ingredients.

Secondly, 'simple' measurements, as labelled by Jörimann, such as a 'handful' (*manipulus*) or an 'eggshell-ful' (*ouum plenum*), often appear in recipes that use the unit *staupus*.[21] Turning again to BnF lat. 5543, the recipe for joint pain mentioned above begins with a call for handfuls of dittany roots, centaury leaves, and basil.[22] Likewise, the recipe in cod. sang. 44 intended to dry out swellings begins by measuring ingredients by the 'handful', *manipulus*, switching to 'similarly', *similiter*, after the first three ingredients, and ends with the unit *staupus* to measure beer.[23] Like the preceding example, this recipe also relies entirely on local products with the exception of pepper. The infusion for the head and for jaundice in cod. sang. 759 (noted above for its use of a third of a *staupus* of vinegar) uses *pugnata*, 'fistful', as its main measurement for its predominantly local herbal ingredients.[24] Although classical units can also be found in these recipes, such as the use of *calyx* in the first recipe of BnF lat. 5543, the frequent appearance of non-technical language for measuring ingredients alongside the use of *staupus* is striking, revealing a strong tendency within these recipes to communicate information in a straightforward, easily understood manner.

There are, however, some other exceptions to the trends noted above. A treatment in BnF lat. 11219 for those with problems urinating, which includes the unit *staupus* to measure wine, relies on ingredients that cover the full spectrum of 'localness'.[25] Some, such as parsley, celery, and fennel, could have been growing in northern and western Europe, while others were far from local.

---

20 See Appendix 2, entry 18.9 for the full transcription from BAV reg. lat. 1143; the ingredients are: agrimony roots cooked in wine; the roots of butcher's broom, caltrops, asparagus, angelica, celery, parsley, and violets; dried pennyroyal; three heads of garlic; one ounce of marshmallow seeds; four leeks with roots; betony, with its roots either dried or fresh; cress; wild rue or, if necessary, the cultivated variety; coriander; dill; and oil.

21 *Frühmittelalterliche Rezeptarien*, ed. Jörimann, 90.

22 BnF lat. 5543, f. 2v: *Item alia eiusdem* [*Contra artetricos*]. *Diptamnum radices manipulum i, centaurea folia manipulum i, basilisca similiter*… See Appendix 2, entry 2.2.2.

23 Cod. sang. 44, p. 353: *Ad glandolas siccandas*. See Appendix 2, entry 5.23.

24 Cod. sang. 759, p. 51: *Infussio ad capud et ad colera*. See Appendix 2, entry 11.5.

25 BnF lat. 11219, f. 225va, *Ad eos qui urinam facere non possunt*. See Appendix 2, entry 4.6.

Most notably, the recipe incorporates one of the newly recorded ingredients mentioned in Chapter 3, *galinga*, galangal. A recipe for a jaundice treatment in cod. sang. 759, *Ad ycterícus*, offers another example at odds with the general findings presented above.[26] In this case, however, it is one of the two ingredients with which *staupus* has been paired that is exceptional. In the first instance, it is used to measure water—a full *staupus* is to be drunk, fitting with one of the usual uses of *staupus*. The term is then used with *garum*, the famous Roman fish sauce: half a *staupus* should be drunk and then the patient's blood should be let. The use of this term to measure such a conspicuously classical ingredient stands in stark contrast to the largely local, simple, and common liquids with which *staupus* is most frequently paired.[27] The significance of these exceptions will be considered below.

2.3 *The Absence of* Staupus *in Texts on Weights and Measures*

As noted in Chapter 2, brief treatises on weights and measures often circulated alongside (or even within) recipe collections. Augusto Beccaria identified over thirty such texts within the manuscripts included in his catalogue.[28] Of the twenty-four manuscripts under analysis in the present study, seven contain at least one text on weights and measures: codd. sang. 44, 759, BAV pal. lat. 1088, BnF lat. 6882A, and 11218 each include one; BAV reg. lat. 1143 has two; and cod. sang. 751 contains five (see Table 8).[29] Although each text is distinct, they all offer similar information, conveying the volume or weight of each named unit represented and the relationships between these different units. Indeed, in some cases the distinctions between texts are largely in relation to orthographic variation; the two brief texts in BAV reg. lat. 1143, for example, are nearly identical. While they tend to be very short texts, usually taking up less than a full page (and in some cases only a few lines), several, such as the first and fourth examples in cod. sang. 751, extend over multiple folia. The first of

26 Cod. sang. 759, p. 93: *Ad ycterícus*; see Appendix 2, entry 11.23.1.

27 Robert I. Curtis, *Garum and Salsamenta: Production and Commerce in Materia Medica* (Leiden: Brill, 1991).

28 Beccaria, *I codici*, 477.

29 The treatises are as follows: cod. sang. 44, p. 279, *De ponderibus et mensuris*; cod. sang. 751, pp. 35–7, *De ponderibus*, p. 39, *De mensuris uel numeris*, p. 395, *De mensura et ponderibus*, pp. 429–30, *De ponderibus et mensuris*, p. 492, *Incipit de ponderibus et mensuris*; cod. sang. 759, p. 46, *De ponderibus et mensuris medicinalibus*; BAV pal. lat. 1088, ff. 115r–115v, *De ponderibus et mensuris*; BAV reg. lat. 1143, f. 81r, *Incipit pensum obuli*, f. 189v, *Incepit pensum obuli*; BnF lat. 6882A, f. 24r, *De ponderibus et mensuris medicinalis*; BnF lat. 11218, ff. 42r–42v, *Incipit racio ponderum uel mensurarum diuersorum medicinalium*.

TABLE 8 The treatises on weights and measures found within the manuscript sample

Manuscript	Treatise
Cod. sang. 44	*De ponderibus et mensuris*
Cod. sang. 751	*De ponderibus* *De mensuris uel numeris* *De mensura et ponderibus* *De ponderibus et mensuris* *Incipit de ponderibus et mensuris*
Cod. sang. 759	*De ponderibus et mensuris medicinalibus*
BAV pal. lat. 1088	*De ponderibus et mensuris*
BAV reg. lat. 1143	*Incipit pensum obuli* *Incepit pensum obuli*
BnF lat. 6882A	*De ponderibus et mensuris medicinalis*
BnF lat. 11218	*Incipit racio ponderum uel mensurarum diuersorum medicinalium*

these treatises in the manuscript (pp. 35–7) also ends with a list of the many different symbols used to represent these units.

The weights and measures described in these texts are, with few exceptions, those inherited from Antiquity. For measurements of volume, these often include *amphora*, *congius* (an eighth of an *amphora*), *sextarius* (roughly a pint, a sixth of a *congius*), *hemina* and *cotyla* (both equal to half a *sextarius*), *acetabulum* (a quarter of a *hemina*/*cotyla*), and *cyathus* (a twelfth of a *sextarius*). Measurements of weight include *libra* (pound), *uncia* (ounce), and then the many subdivisions of the *uncia*, such as *semuncia* (a half ounce), *sicilicus* (a quarter ounce), *drachma* (a dram, or an eighth of an ounce), *scrupulum* (scruple, or a twenty-fourth of an ounce), *obolus* (a forty-eighth of an ounce), and *siliqua* (carat).[30] Weights based on coins, such as the *denarius* or the *solidus*, are also sometimes listed, and many of the measurements are grounded in

30 As cautioned in the opening 'Note on Weights, Measures, and Their Symbols', the translation of these terms is approximate; that is, a *libra* is not identical to a modern pound, nor is an *uncia* equivalent to an ounce, but they provide a general sense of the amount under consideration. For a review of texts on weights and measures, see also Sigerist, 'Maße und Gewichte', 439–44 and Bischoff, 'Maße und Gewichte', 169–70. Cf. Isidore, *Etymologiae*, 16.15–17.

comparisons to products in the natural world, such as a barley grains (*grana ordei*) or various types of beans. Despite the variety of weights and measures named in these texts, none features the unit *staupus*. While this absence likely reflects the classical origins of these treatises, the preceding chapters have demonstrated that scribes actively updated pharmaceutical writings in relation to their circumstances and with the latest information. This suggests that, if the term *staupus* regularly needed clarification, it, too, would be found in texts defining the various weights and measures that appear in recipes. The lack of *staupus* in these contexts implies that explanations of its volume were seen as unnecessary.

Relatedly, it is also striking that the term *staupus* is often used either multiplied or as a fraction, such as the fifty cups of wine needed for the potion against joint pain or the third of a cup of vinegar recorded in the infusion of cod. sang. 759. In contrast, the classical vocabulary uses a range of different terms to describe such varied amounts. If one *staupus* is understood as roughly equivalent to one *hemina* (this is the classical unit with which it has most recently been associated and, at approximately 300mL, is between the two extremes posited by Guérard and Sigerist), fifty *heminae* would be equivalent to twenty-five *sextarii* or just over four *congii*.[31] Similarly, a third of a *staupus* would be fairly close to one *acetabulum*. Classical units thus present more specialised terminology that covers a full spectrum of sizes. This range, however, creates a rather complicated vocabulary. The adaptation of *staupus* to suit a variety of volumes further supports its user-friendly nature: it offers a single unit that can be increased or decreased by simple multiplication or division as needed rather than exchanged for an entirely new term. Such adaptability suggests that it was in more common parlance—a unit used in everyday life instead of a highly technical term. Moreover, the relatively widespread use of *staupus* and the seemingly accepted, if somewhat vaguely defined, sense of its volume also fits with the other units with which it is often seen alongside, such as 'handful' or 'eggshell-full' (and may help to explain why past attempts to define its precise volume have varied so greatly).

With this understanding of where and how the unit is used, what can now be said about its practicality?

31 *Das Lorscher Arzneibuch*, ed. and trans. Stoll, 40; *Polyptyque de l'abbé Irminon*, ed. Guérard, vol. 1, 188; *Studien und Texte*, ed. Sigerist, 175.

2.4 *The Practicality of the Unit* Staupus

The relative prevalence and widespread distribution of the unit *staupus* as well as its frequent pairing with local ingredients, absence from texts defining weights and measures, and sense of flexible, everyday usage all suggest that the inclusion of this term in recipes was highly practical. Its appearance should not be read as cause for confusion or as evidence of impracticality due to language barriers; rather, as an adaptation made to address a changing linguistic environment, it represents the very opposite. The introduction of the term would have aided in readers' comprehension, which, if the recipes were being formulated, would have been vitally important.

Paradoxically, the exceptions to the general trends highlighted above add further weight to the argument for this unit's practicality. In particular, the *garum* example indicates that the unit *staupus* had become fully integrated into the medical vocabulary circulating in early medieval western Europe. Given the classical origins of this fish sauce, the recipe likely derives from an ancient text. Although I have yet to identify a specific source for this recipe, *garum* is recorded as an ingredient in earlier pharmaceutical writings. It appears in five prescriptions of the *Medicina Plinii*, for example. In the first recipe, a treatment for ears, one *cyathus* of *garum* is used.[32] If the *garum* recipe of cod. sang. 759 is descended, directly or indirectly, from another classical or late antique recipe collection, the original instructions likely used a different term, such as *sextarius*, *hemina*, *cotyla*, *acetabulum*, or, as in the *Medicina Plinii*, *cyathus*, to describe the volume of *garum*. This suggests that the ninth-century recipe has been modified: *staupus* has replaced a classical unit of measurement, rendering the instructions more user-friendly.

Finally, while the individual *garum* example illustrates the adaptation of earlier written sources, the particularly local nature of many of the ingredients with which *staupus* is paired may reflect a different, if related, development. As noted in the previous chapter, the appearance of beer in recipes suggests that medical knowledge was updated to suit local conditions and/or that pharmaceutical information that was previously transmitted orally was now being recorded. The inclusion of a Latinised vernacular unit fits this context of local use and supports the idea that these recipes, though not indicative of the work of a specific *medicus*, do reflect knowledge circulating on the ground. This, in turn, points very strongly to the use of these texts in the context of

32 *Plinii Secundi Iunioris qui feruntur De medicina libri tres*, ed. Önnerfors, 1.6.2: *Gari excellentis cyathus, aceti cyathus unus, mellis cyathus et dimidius: in calice nouo sensim decoquitur, spuma subinde penna tollitur, et cum spuma resederit, remouetur et ex eo tepidum infunditur*. See also *The* Medicina Plinii, trans. Hunt, 1.6.2.

therapy: they capture and transmit the medical knowledge that was in use during this period. The recipes that incorporate the unit *staupus* thus bear witness to scribes' active engagement with a variety of sources, both textual and oral, and their drive to make the texts understandable to their readers. Overall, the inclusion of *staupus* in recipes appears to have been very practical adaptation and is highly suggestive that they were intended for use in medical practice.

3 Wild Versus Cultivated Rue: the Inclusion of an Ingredient Substitution

Near the end of the *Potionem probata ad ilica passio*, this chapter's opening recipe, there is a comment on the type of rue to include: wild rue is preferred but, if not available, cultivated rue would be an acceptable alternative (*ruta siluatica, et si non domestica*). These instructions provide practical advice for what to do if wild rue is not obtainable and recommend a nearly identical plant with which to replace it. Whatever the reason for preferring wild rue (perhaps the wild type was thought to be stronger than the domesticated variety and thus favoured), this note implies that it was not always available. This is a useful reminder that even theoretically local substances were not necessarily accessible; an ingredient's localness might make it *more* likely to be available, but this is no guarantee that the product in question was on hand.

Does the inclusion of information regarding a substitution suggest that this recipe incorporates knowledge gained through experience? Was this recommendation included in reaction to difficulties encountered when attempting to obtain wild rue? Or, like the Terenti(an)us example, might this recipe transmit knowledge from older sources without necessarily addressing Carolingian experiences? In this final case study of Part 1, I examine the presence of information regarding ingredient substitutions within recipes as another possible perspective on the question of practicality: while such notes within prescriptions offer practical solutions if certain ingredients were unavailable, does this information appear to be related to contemporary practices?

3.1 *Instructions for Ingredient Substitutions in the Recipe Sample*

Within the recipe sample, I have identified twenty-six examples of substitutions recorded as part of the recipe's main text (following the model of the opening example) and one instance of a marginal gloss next to the recipe it concerns. Like the *Potionem probata ad ilica passio*, some substitutions suggest replacing wild-type ingredients with their cultivated equivalent, such as the substitution recorded in a recipe to treat spreading ulcers in cod. Sang. 44: 'it is better to use the leaves of wild parsnip than the cultivated type. If you cannot find wild parsnip, use the cultivated one'.[33] In other cases, closely related plant species are listed as substitutes. Two parallel antidotes for stomach problems and various other ailments, the *Antidotum ad stomaco frigido qui dicitur climax* of cod. sang. 751 and *Antidotum ad stomachum frigidum qui dicitur climax* of BnF lat. 11218, for example, recommend using mustard seeds (*senapi semen*) if rocket seeds (*erucae semen*) are unavailable, thereby substituting one member of the Brassicaceae family for another.[34] Alternatively, where multiple parts of the ingredient in question may be used, such as its leaves, seeds, fruits, roots, and/or wood, one part of the plant may be listed as a possible replacement for another. A recipe for expelling various creatures found in codd. Sang. 44, 751, and BAV pal. Lat. 1088, for instance, suggests substituting hemp leaves (*folia de cannabe*) for hemp seeds (*semen de cannabe*) if necessary.[35] The recipes in cod.

33 Cod. sang. 44, pp. 330–1: *Item aliud ad fagidinica…melior enim est pastinace siluestris folia quam domestice, si non inuenis agrestem, domesticam uteris*. See Appendix 2, entry 5.17.2. On the evolving terminology used for certain 'eating diseases', including *phagedaena*, see Luke Demaitre, '"Is It Lupus?"—The Wolf in a Disease, from Metaphor to Medicine', in *Beyond Cadfael: Medieval Medicine and Medical Medievalism*, ed. Lucy Barnhouse and Winston Black (Budapest: Trivent Publishing, 2023), 31–56.

34 Cod. sang. 751, p. 448: *Antidotum ad stomaco frigido qui dicitur climax*; BnF lat. 11218, ff. 98v–99r: *Antidotum ad sthomachum frigidum qui dicitur climax*. See Appendix 2, entries 9.32 and 3.9, respectively.

35 Cod. sang. 44, p. 350: *Ranas et craxantos haec potio expellere solet* [although this title might suggest otherwise, this is part of a group of recipes found under the heading *Item ad ipsum potio bibenda contra ipsos uermes eiciendos aut quacumque maleficio in se habuerit*]. *Et si de hac potione non exierint, bibat alia potione ad occidendos. Ius de mora campestria teris et exprimis et teris folia cannapi manu plena, et si folia non fuerint semen ipsius, dabis ei potione calice pleno, et si ius more non habuerint aut cannapo inuenire non potuerit lacte caprino calido bibat*; cod. sang. 751, p. 423: *Item* [*Ad serpentes uel alios uerme de ominem expellendum potio probata*]. *Ius de mura campestria expremis et teris folia de canepa, miscis simul et dabis bibere calicę pleno, si folia non habes semen mitte, ipsum ualet uel* [note: the instructions appear to end abruptly mid-recipe]; BAV pal. lat. 1088, ff. 37r–37v: *Item* [*Ad serpentes uel aliorum uermes de homine expellendum*]. *Ius de mora campestria exprimis et teris folia de cannabe, miscis simul et dabis bibere calice pleno, et si folia non habes semen mitte, ipsum ualet, si mora non est lacte caprino calidum facit*. For full transcriptions of these recipes, see Appendix 2, entries 5.21.2, 9.23.3, and 16.5.3, respectively. On hemp production, see Marie-Pierre Ruas, 'Productions agricoles en Auvergne carolingienne d'après un dépotoir découvert à Saint-Germain-des-Fossés (Allier)', *Revue archéologique du centre de la France* 39 (2000): 137–60, https://doi.org/10.3406/racf.2000.2849; Corrie C. Bakels, 'Crops produced in the southern Netherlands and northern France during the early medieval period: a comparison', *Vegetation History and Archaeobotany* 14, no. 4 (2005): 394–9, https://doi.org/10.1007/s00334-005-0067-x; and Robert C. Clarke and Mark D. Merlin, *Cannabis: Evolution and Ethnobotany* (Berkeley: University of California Press, 2013).

sang. 44 and BAV pal. lat. 1088 also note that goat's milk can be used as alternative if mulberry juice is unavailable.[36]

Thirteen of the substitutions concern exotic ingredients. In some cases, the recommended replacements are similar products, such as the substitution of cassia (*cassia*) for cinnamon (*cinamomum*) in the *Anthidotus Teodori* of BAV reg. lat. 1143, though the recipe specifies that if cassia is used the amount should be increased from eight scruples to eighteen.[37] Similarly, the *Antidotum qui dicitur acharistus* of BnF lat. 11218 records that if cassia is used in place of cinnamon, it should be doubled: *cinamomum uncia I aut casiae duplum.*[38] Other substitutions concerning *exotica* are not so clearly related, or at least not to a modern reader. Take, for example, the substitution listed in a treatment for incontinence in cod. Sang. 761: if pepper (*piper*) is not available, use natron (*nitri*).[39] Regardless of the efficacy of the substitution in question, the inclusion of instructions for how to proceed when the desired ingredient is not available represents a very practical, problem-solving addition to a recipe. Unlike the appearance of the newly recorded unit *staupus*, however, the degree to which these types of substitution instructions reflect early medieval contexts is less clear. Do they offer advice from early medieval practitioners who attempted to use the recipes or was this information was copied from earlier sources?

3.2 *Ingredient Substitution in Earlier Sources*

Instructions for replacing ingredients must be considered in relation to a late antique pseudo-Galenic text, *Περὶ ἀντεμβαλλομένων*, *On substitute drugs*, that addresses this very topic. The treatise contains a list of 369 ingredient substitutions.[40] Latin versions of the text have circulated under a variety of names; the titles *Antemballomena* or *Antebalumina*, based on a direct transliteration of the Greek title into Latin, are most frequently seen in the surviving early

36 Given the abrupt ending of the recipe in cod. sang. 751 (the next recipe begins immediately after *uel*), it seems that the recipe in its current form is incomplete, and it is thus possible that this second substitution information should have been included.

37 BAV reg. lat. 1143, ff. 81r–82r: *Anthidotus Teodori*. See Appendix 2, entry 18.1.

38 BnF lat. 11218, ff. 57v–58r: *Antidotum qui dicitur acharistus*. See Appendix 2, entry 3.4.

39 Cod. sang. 761, p. 56: *Item [Ad incontinentiam hurinae] … piper ∻ I aut si piper nolueris, nitri ∻ II*. See Appendix 2, entry 12.1.8.

40 Klaus-Dietrich Fischer, 'Drugs to Declare. Two Pharmaceutical Works Attributed to Galen', *Cuadernos de Filología Clásica. Estudios griegos e indoeuropeos* 28 (2018): 225–41, https://doi.org/10.5209/CFCG.59395, at pp. 233–9; Alain Touwaide, 'Quid pro Quo: Revisiting the Practice of Substitution in Ancient Pharmacy', in *Herbs and Healers from the Ancient Mediterranean through the Medieval West: Essays in Honor of John M. Riddle*, ed. Anne Van Arsdall and Timothy Graham (Farnham: Ashgate, 2012), 19–61.

TABLE 9 Copies of *De succedaneis liber* found within the manuscript sample

Manuscript	Treatise
Cod. sang. 759	*Antebalumina Galieni*
BnF lat. 6882A	*Incipit antebalumina Galieni*
BnF lat. 11219	*Incipit prologus antebalumina Galieni medici*

medieval texts, though the manuscripts showcase a high level of orthographic variation.[41] Early printed editions of the text were given the name *De succedaneis liber* and this remains what is most frequently associated with the treatise despite the popularity of *Quid pro quo* in the later Middle Ages.[42] Beccaria identified thirteen copies or fragments of the text in early medieval manuscripts, three of which can be found in codices included in the present study (see Table 9). While the lists of substitutions in BnF lat. 6882A and BnF lat. 11219 cover several folia, only the title of the text survives in an index in cod. sang. 759; the pages containing the substitutions themselves have been lost.[43]

A comparison of the twenty-six substitutions found within this study's recipe sample to those listed in *De succedaneis liber* offers some direct parallels. For example, the replacement of cinnamon with cassia, recorded as *pro cinamum, casia duplu aut bratheos dublo* in a version of *De succedaneis liber* in BnF lat. 6882A, is consistent with the information provided within recipes, even noting that the quantity of cassia should be doubled.[44] Other substitutions in *De succedaneis liber*, though not identical, present similar recommendations. Instead of replacing mustard seeds with rocket seeds as was noted in two recipes, the text suggests similarly peppery watercress seeds as an alternative: *pro sinape, cardamomi semen*.[45]

Some types of substitution, such as the substitution of cultivated plants for their wild-type or *vice versa*, however, seem to be more common in recipes

41 Beccaria, *I codici*, 456.

42 Touwaide, 'Quid pro Quo', 19.

43 Cod. sang. 759, p. 58, *Antebalumina Galieni*; BnF lat. 6882A, ff. 11v–15r, *Incipit antebalumina Galieni*; and BnF lat. 11219, ff. 230ra–233vb, *Incipit prologus antebalumina Galieni medici*.

44 BnF lat. 6882A, f. 12r, *pro cinamum, casia duplu aut bratheos dublo*; BnF lat. 11219, f. 231ra, *pro cinnamomo, casia duplum aut brateu duplum*; Touwaide, 'Quid pro Quo', 37; for Touwaide's tables, see pp. 34–60. The text also offers *bratheos*, savin, as an alternative.

45 BnF lat. 6882A, f. 14v, *pro senape, cardamomum*; BnF lat. 11219, f. 231va, *pro sinape, cardamomi semen*.

than in the pseudo-Galenic text.[46] There are no close parallels, for example, to the suggested substitutions seen in the *Potionem probata ad ilica passio* of BAV reg. lat. 1143 or *Item aliud ad fagidinica ulcera* of cod. sang. 44. The former recommended replacing wild rue with a cultivated variety if the wild type was unavailable and the latter suggested that domesticated parsnips could be swapped for wild parsnips if necessary.[47] That these unparalleled instances of suggested substitutions involve common plant products that could have been grown in Carolingian Francia, whether wild or cultivated, indicates that these recommendations may reflect experience on the ground. Nevertheless, the large amount of overlapping and generally similar information shared between *De succedaneis liber* and individual recipes suggests that this treatise may be the underlying source for many of the substitution instructions seen in the recipe sample.

3.3 *The Practicality of Substitution Instructions in Recipes*

While some of the instructions regarding ingredient substitutions located within recipes, and especially those that replace a wild plant with a domesticated version, might reflect personal experience or local knowledge networks, much of this information appears to descend from classical and late antique traditions. That is not to say that the substitution instructions were not practical, but that their existence within recipes should not be taken as evidence for the use of these recipes in early medieval medical practice. This distinction is key and highlights the importance of a cautious approach to the written record: just as not all signs of a text's use should be interpreted as evidence of its use *in* the practice of medicine, a text's practical features are not automatically indicative of whether it was intended to be used in practice.

Overall, it seems likely that the substitution instructions included within recipes combine earlier traditions with local knowledge and practice. The recording of some potentially new substitutions as well as the substitutions that offer similar but not identical advice (such as mustard being replaced with rocket instead of watercress) points to the incorporation of information outside of the classical canon. The broad similarities between the instructions in these recipes and those presented in *De succedaneis liber*, however, suggests that the information included in early medieval recipes, even in cases where they differ, may be building on these earlier traditions. Ultimately, these substitution

46 For the full texts in the two Paris manuscripts involved in the present study, see BnF lat. 6882A, ff. 11v–15r; BnF lat. 11219, ff. 230ra–233vb.

47 BAV reg. lat. 1143, ff. 185r–185v, *Potionem probata ad ilica passio*; cod. sang. 44, pp. 330–1: *Item aliud ad fagidinica ulcera*; see Appendix 2, entries 18.9 and 5.17.2.

instructions can be said to offer potentially practical information—alternative ideas if certain ingredients were unavailable—but, unlike the other case studies examined in Part 1, they should not be taken as signs that these texts were intended to be consulted in the context of practice.

4 Conclusion

While Chapters 3 and 4 explored practicality by investigating examples of newly recorded *materia medica*, both local and exotic, this chapter reveals that additional features within recipes can also offer valuable insights into this topic.

The inclusion of a vernacular unit and substitution instructions both represent practical features within recipes, yet they have different implications for the question of practicality. First, with respect to *staupus*, the introduction of a Latinised vernacular term in Carolingian medical texts indicates that the recipe literature was an evolving body of knowledge and suggests that scribes actively adapted recipes to make them more accessible to their readers. While earlier studies highlighted singular examples of *staupus* and drew conclusions from these isolated instances, I argue that it is the repeated occurrence of this unit that is even more noteworthy. The analysis of its use, highlighting its connection to local ingredients and adaptability, indicates that the term would have made recipes more understandable—and thus useable—for their potential readers. If these recipes were being consulted in practice, a correct understanding of measurements would have been fundamentally important. Yet the appearance of *staupus* in recipes not only suggests that this material was intended to be used in medical practice, but that it was likely derived from local practice. That is not to say that recipes including *staupus* directly document the activities of a Carolingian *medicus*; rather, such prescriptions may offer a window onto medical knowledge that had traditionally circulated orally. The recording of this unit thus provides strong evidence that these texts were intended to be used in the context of therapy.

In contrast, the inclusion of instructions for ingredient substitutions, though also practical, has significant parallels to the case of Terenti(an)us: these suggestions should not be interpreted as direct evidence for the use of recipes in contemporary medical practice. By offering alternative ingredients if a particular substance was unavailable, they are inherently practical instructions; their similarities with the late antique text *De succedaneis liber*, however, indicate that they may be linked to this tradition. Without further evidence it is impossible to know if such information reflects an individual's personal experiences, a copy of an earlier source, or a combination of the two. I end with this case study not to reduce the weight of the evidence from the preceding studies, but to highlight the complexity of investigating the question of practicality. It is often tempting to interpret all signs of a manuscript's use as indicative of their use in medical practice and, as in this case, all practical elements within recipes as further corroboration of their intention to be used in a therapeutic context. A more cautious and critical approach to the sources, however, must be taken. Ultimately, as analyses of *materia medica* and the unit *staupus* have demonstrated, it is the 'new' elements in the recipe literature, such as the appearance of newly recorded ingredients, that provide the most compelling evidence for the ways in which these recipes offered practical information that was likely intended for, and could have been used in, medical practice.

PART 2

Applicability

CHAPTER 6

Reading Recipes in the Light of Skeletal Remains

An Introduction to the Integration of Osteological Evidence

1 Introduction: Moving From Practicality to Practice, an Investigation Into Applicability

The following chapters, building on the exploration of the practicality of recipes in Part 1, now investigate the question of applicability.[1] While the preceding case studies showcased the practical nature of many of these recipes, including evidence for whether they *could* have been used, the degree to which this information was potentially relevant to the individuals with access to the texts was not considered. Although many recipes appear to have been practical, is there evidence suggesting that they were relevant to populations in this period? A recipe's usability (i.e., its practicality) and utility (i.e., its applicability) should not be conflated. As discussed in Chapter 2, examples of individuals who sought to *apply* medical writings, such as Bishop Cynehard (though he was presumably somewhat unsuccessful in his use of the texts given his complaints about lacking some of the ingredients listed in the recipes), are few and far between.[2] The second part of this book, therefore, asks: were these recipes applicable to individuals in early medieval Europe? Are there signs that they address health concerns that affected people during this period?

As noted in Chapter 1, the question of applicability may seem surprising since it is generally assumed that medical knowledge, due to its very nature, has direct relevance. This assumption must be questioned. The situation is more complex because, as Peregrine Horden has explained, medical knowledge may have been recorded, preserved, studied, and passed on for a multitude of reasons, and its use in the context of therapy represents just one of these reasons.[3] Moreover, modern scholarship has highlighted that a variety of options were available in the 'medical marketplace', but many of these approaches to healing did not necessarily involve medical writings, whether as teaching texts

1 For this study's definitions of practicality and applicability, see Chapter 1.

2 Wallis, *Medieval Medicine*, 110–11; 'Epistula 114', in *Die Briefe des heiligen Bonifatius und Lullus*, ed. Tangl, 247: *sed tamen [p]igmenta ultramarina, quae in eis scripta conperimus, ignota nobis sunt et difficilia adipiscendum*.

3 Horden, 'Prefatory Note', 1–6.

or guides to be consulted in practice.[4] An examination of the applicability of these recipes thus has the potential to cast fresh light on the relationship between recorded medical knowledge and the practice of medicine.

The present chapter introduces this investigation of applicability, first outlining in greater detail why the medical texts' relevance to populations in the Carolingian world deserves a deeper examination. This discussion delineates how the following chapters use the osteological record to re-evaluate the evidence presented by the recipe literature. I then address some of the challenges inherent in bringing together these two bodies of evidence and how they have helped to determine the foci of the case study-based chapters (Chapters 7–9). This introduction ends with an overview of the following chapters' analytical framework, including a review of the archaeological sites considered in the case studies.

2 Establishing the Framework of Part 2

2.1 *Why Question the Relevance of Recipes?*

Although the textual analyses of Part 1 identified the influence of sources beyond the classical canon, the continued significance of classical and late antique medical traditions in the Carolingian period, both as texts themselves and as sources for the recipes analysed in this book, cannot be downplayed.[5] The impact of classical knowledge is important to consider since the 'healthscape' of Mediterranean Antiquity was not the same as that of early medieval Europe. Not only is it likely that diseases would have differed to some degree, but so, too, would individuals' experiences of disease. As Faith Wallis affirms, experiences of health, wellness, and disease are culturally conditioned: 'what human beings—medieval or modern—see in the human body, or in the patterns of disease, is shaped not only by the possibilities and limitations of their experience, but by the structures and meanings that their culture bestows on this experience'.[6]

4 Flint, 'The Early Medieval 'Medicus'', 127–45; Skinner, *Health and Medicine in Early Medieval Southern Italy*, see especially Chapter 5 (pp. 79–107); Clare Pilsworth, 'Could you just sign this for me John? Doctors, charters and occupational identity in early medieval northern and central Italy', *Early Medieval Europe* 17, no. 4 (2009): 363–88, https://doi.org/10.1111/j.1468-0254.2009.00282.x; David Knipp, 'The Chapel of Physicians at Santa Maria Antiqua', *Dumbarton Oaks Papers* 56 (2002): 1–23, https://doi.org/10.2307/1291851.

5 Again, see the discussion of this topic in Chapters 1 and 2.

6 Wallis, *Medieval Medicine*, xxv-xxvii.

The 'possibilities of experience' that every individual encounters are influenced by external forces, including a region's climate and endemic pathogens, as well as internal factors, such as lifestyle, working conditions, hygiene practices, systems of belief, and other socio-cultural features. When addressing crusader medicine, Piers Mitchell considers a similar geographic shift, that of western European crusaders moving to the Middle East, and highlights potential differences in the health experiences of the two regions: 'an individual with a culture and an immune system developed for cooler northern Europe might have been at considerable risk ... He would encounter new diseases to which he might have little immunity, such as the parasites dracunculiasis and schistosomiasis'.[7] While the situation Mitchell describes represents the inverse of this study (Mitchell considers the movement of *people* between different regions rather than the redeployment of *knowledge* in a different time and location), it remains instructive. Most importantly, Mitchell explains that the crusaders' place of origin, northwest Europe (loosely paralleling the territories of the Carolingian world), and their destination, the eastern Mediterranean (corresponding to an area where many classical and late antique medical authors were active), would have had major biological and cultural differences. It is essential to remember that medical knowledge recorded in the classical Mediterranean world had been developed in order to treat the needs of the people living in this region. As a result, some of the medical issues described by classical authors may have been less relevant to Carolingian scribes living in cooler, damper environments.

Despite the potentially stark differences that Mitchell describes, it is also important to recognise that changes to the external forces that shape an individual's healthscape tend to accumulate gradually. Furthermore, this study contains a number of grey areas, such as the Italian peninsula, where the conditions experienced by classical authors may have been similar to those encountered by early medieval individuals. Consider, for example, the climate and living conditions experienced by a monk in St Gall, a courtier at Aachen, or a scribe in San Vincenzo al Volturno. Many of the external forces acting on the latter individual may have been fairly similar to those encountered by Pliny, Dioscorides, and Galen. The health experiences of physicians writing in Antiquity and of early medieval scribes compiling collections of recipes in the eighth and ninth centuries should therefore be viewed along a spectrum.

Finally, it might be expected that there are certain conditions that were as likely to afflict medieval monks as they were classical physicians, such as

7 Mitchell, *Medicine in the Crusades*, 1.

toothache and joint pain. But did they? An individual's health is intrinsically related to social and environmental factors such as diet, lifestyle, and living conditions, so even seemingly universal conditions must be examined without preconceptions. Indeed, the examples of toothache and joint disease will be addressed in Chapters 7 and 8, respectively.

2.2 *Working With the Available Evidence*

My approach to investigating the relationship between medical knowledge and practice has been shaped by the surviving evidence. While Mitchell's work on medicine in the Crusades draws in part on the medical information recorded in surgical texts and chronicles, the early medieval written record is generally lacking such testimony. In later periods, medical treatments are discussed in a wider range of sources. Chroniclers, for example, often document conditions in camps, episodes of disease, and even some specific medical cases, ranging from trauma (such as injuries sustained while fighting, hunting, or horseback-riding) and infectious disease (including the famous case of Baldwin IV's leprosy) to vitamin and mineral deficiencies (such as scurvy).[8] Although these writings were not intended as case reports in the modern sense, medical professionals such as Mitchell can analyse their descriptions and assess the information they record. In some cases, chronicles and histories have provided pathognomonic details or have constructed a sufficiently clear overall picture of a condition for a modern medical diagnosis; this is, however, fairly rare, and the issue of retrospective diagnosis will be discussed below. Evidence from legal texts, such as penalties for malpractice, also provides insights into the types of procedures that were undertaken during this period. Comparable textual sources for the early medieval period, such as annals and law codes, tend to present less medical information, though as Chapter 9 demonstrates, they can still offer important evidence.

Secondly, while early medieval medical texts primarily focused on dietary and pharmaceutical treatments and avoided surgery (with bloodletting representing a significant exception), surgical writings feature prominently within the medical literature of the later Middle Ages. Again, Mitchell's research on medicine in the Crusades offers a useful comparison: he writes that 'sometimes the wording of a medical text uses practical examples that give the impression that it was written primarily to be used to treat the injured and at other

8 Piers D. Mitchell, 'An Evaluation of the Leprosy of King Baldwin IV of Jerusalem in the Context of the Medieval World', in *The Leper King and His Heirs: Baldwin IV and the Crusader Kingdom of Jerusalem*, ed. Bernard Hamilton (Cambridge: Cambridge University Press, 2000), 245–58; Mitchell, *Medicine in the Crusades*, 185–6, 188–90.

times the inclusion of new techniques suggests that they were practised by the author who recommended their use'.[9] Such detailed, first-hand accounts, especially for surgical procedures, are unknown in Carolingian medical writings; instead, the vast majority of references to the use of texts, such as the case of Terenti(an)us, appear to be part of efficacy clauses—stock phrases that should not be used as direct evidence for a text's use in therapy. Although similar phrases continue to be found in later writings, the textual landscape had changed dramatically.

In addition to using the textual record, Mitchell's work on medicine in the Crusades integrates archaeological evidence. His analyses of written sources, skeletal remains, and the results from excavations of hospitals, latrines, and other sites that may produce information regarding health and medicine provide a more comprehensive picture, demonstrating the importance of bringing together complementary types of evidence. Consider, for example, the evidence for surgical interventions. While some surgeries only concern soft tissue, others affect the skeleton and would therefore leave indications of surgical intervention, such as cutmarks, in an individual's remains. Skeletal evidence and surgical tools found in excavations can then be compared to surgical texts to assess whether particular treatments were put into practice. While this combined approach works for the central and later Middle Ages, the relative lack of early medieval Latin surgical writings combined with the absence of medical equipment, such as surgical tools or pharmacy jars, among the material remains found in early medieval excavations makes this type of comparison impossible for the Carolingian period.[10]

Yet, although early medieval written sources and material finds, when compared to both earlier and later periods, provide more limited evidence for

9 Mitchell, *Medicine in the Crusades*, 138.

10 In contrast, excavations at a number of later medieval sites, such as the monastic hospital of Skriðuklaustur, have uncovered a variety of medical tools, including lancets and scalpels: Steinunn Kristjánsdóttir, 'The Tip of the Iceberg: The Material of Skriðuklaustur Monastery and Hospital', *Norwegian Archaeological Review* 43, no. 1 (2010): 44–62, https://doi.org/10.1080/00293651003798796, at p. 52. On surviving surgical texts, see, for example, Klaus-Dietrich Fischer, '*Universorum ferramentorum nomina*. Frühmittelalterliche Listen chirurgischer Instrumente und ihr griechisches Vorbild', *Mittellateinisches Jahrbuch* 22 (1987): 28–44 and Lawrence J. Bliquez, 'Two Lists of Greek Surgical Instruments and the State of Surgery in Byzantine Times', *Dumbarton Oaks Papers* 38 (1984): 187–204, https://doi.org/10.2307/1291505. Cf. the roughly contemporary and much richer tradition of surgical writing in Arabic, e.g., Abū al-Qāsim Khalaf ibn 'Abbās al-Zahrāwī, *Albucasis* On Surgery and Instruments: *A Definitive Edition of the Arabic Text With English Translation and Commentary*, trans. M. S. Spink and G. L. Lewis (Berkeley, CA: University of California Press, 1973).

medical practice, the skeletal record can still be examined. Palaeopathology, the study of disease in the past, thus offers another avenue to explore health and medicine in early medieval Europe.[11] Since many diseases, injuries, and other aspects of health have the potential to leave traces in the skeleton, osteological evidence can provide insights into individuals' lived experiences, and especially their experiences of health, disease, and injury.[12] The following investigation into the question of applicability is therefore grounded in both skeletal remains from early medieval sites in western Europe and the recipe sample at the centre of Part 1: I re-evaluate these recipes in the light of the osteological evidence.

So, what can a skeleton tell us? Bones and teeth react to various stresses and age-related processes, including infection, injury, surgery, and repeated use, and, in some cases, these changes leave indicators on the skeleton. An evaluation of an individual's remains can also reveal information regarding their health and living conditions at various stages of their life: teeth, formed in infancy and childhood, provide information about an individual's early years whereas bones, which continue to remodel throughout life, can shed light on the final decades of an individual's life.[13] Palaeopathological reports from excavations with early medieval remains can therefore offer insights into the applicability of the medical knowledge in circulation: does the osteological record preserve evidence of the conditions described in the texts? Would the recipes under analysis have been sought by individuals in early medieval Europe?

While the osteological evidence provides a wealth of information, there are, as explained below, a number of challenges that must be considered when studying the skeletal record alongside written sources. Many of these challenges, however, are not insurmountable obstacles and instead have helped to shape the parameters of this book's approach. In the following section, I shall address some of the intrinsic issues with archaeological research and theoretical challenges related to the integration of skeletal evidence.

---

11 Charlotte A. Roberts, *Human Remains in Archaeology: A Handbook*, rev. ed. (York: Council for British Archaeology, 2012), 6; Piers D. Mitchell, 'Retrospective Diagnosis and the Use of Historical Texts for Investigating Disease in the Past', *International Journal of Paleopathology* 1, no. 2 (2011): 81–8, https://doi.org/10.1016/j.ijpp.2011.04.002, at p. 81.

12 Mitchell, *Medicine in the Crusades*, 10; Fleming, 'Bones for Historians', 29–48; Fleming, 'Writing Biography', 606–14.

13 Donald J. Ortner, 'What Skeletons Tell Us: The Story of Human Paleopathology', *Virchows Archiv* 459 (2011): 247–54, https://doi.org/10.1007/s00428-011-1122-x, at p. 247.

3 The Challenges of Using Osteological Evidence to Inform Textual Analysis[14]

3.1 *Intrinsic Issues With Archaeological Evidence*

At the most basic level, it is important to recognise that the underlying organisation of archaeological research affects its work in various ways, including influencing (or determining) where an excavation will occur, its scope, and its duration. In academic research archaeology, excavation size and timing may be dictated by funding, resources, and the seasonal limitations of fieldwork scheduled around academic calendars. Emergency or rescue archaeology that occurs as a result of construction and development may be more constrained by the requirements and urgency of the project in question. In recent decades, the number of emergency excavations (especially of cemeteries) has grown, a by-product of roadworks, land development, and the redevelopment of urban spaces.[15] While this has greatly increased the number of excavated cemetery sites, these projects are, necessarily, carried out under major financial and time pressures, limiting their size, duration, and, in terms of analysing skeletal material, level of detail.[16] Although the constraints felt in research archaeology, such as limited funding or fieldwork seasons, may stem from different origins, they often produce similar results. These fundamental restrictions, combined with the potential physical constraints caused by existing structures above ground, often result in only partial excavations of larger sites. This is especially important to bear in mind with excavations of cemeteries, as it makes it difficult to know the extent to which the excavated sample is representative of the site as a whole.[17]

While the inherent nature of rescue archaeology determines where the excavations occur, research archaeology has more latitude in site selection—at least in theory. These types of excavations, however, have often concentrated on elite sites, such as religious institutions, royal settlements, or urban centres, based on the research interests of the investigators, the research interests of

14 This review of challenges focuses on those specific to my use of the osteological evidence, such as the location of excavations. For more information on the physical challenges of studying human remains, such as the impact of disposal and decay on skeletal material or the effect of excavation and conservation on its preservation, see Roberts, *Human Remains in Archaeology*.

15 John Pearce, 'Beyond the Grave: Excavating the Dead in the Late Roman Provinces', in *Field Methods and Post-Excavation Techniques in Late Antique Archaeology*, ed. Luke Lavan and Michael Mulryan (Leiden: Brill, 2015), 441–82, at p. 445.

16 Pearce, 'Beyond the Grave', 445, 461.

17 Ibid, 444.

the project's funding body, or simply because the location of these sites might be better known. While the individuals buried in these contexts may not have been privileged themselves or may have experienced a variety of conditions throughout their life (consider, for example, some of the Carolingian ecclesiastical elite who, despite humble origins, became bishops and courtiers), excavations in these sites are not likely to represent an even cross-section of society and are instead biased towards more privileged individuals. Emergency archaeology often presents a similar picture since many of the excavated cemeteries are in urban contexts.[18] Given the elite environments in which the manuscripts containing medical texts were generally produced and housed, a bias towards elite sites is not a disadvantage. Indeed, excavations of monastic communities, and especially those known to have had medical texts in their libraries, are particularly relevant to this study, as will be detailed below. It must be remembered, however, that some degree of healthcare provision may have been made available to the wider communities attached to these sites, such as the *familia* who worked the lands, as well as visitors passing through, including *missi dominici* and pilgrims.[19] Notably, some of the sites under consideration, such as Lorsch, appear to contain multiple cemeteries, including separate burial areas for the monks, *familia*, and pilgrims.[20]

It must also be remembered that the geographic distribution of excavations is not evenly spread across western Europe, and certain areas are better represented than others. This is particularly noticeable in northern Italy, where large numbers of Lombard necropoli have been excavated due to the regional interest in Lombard migration and settlement.[21] Some of these sites continued to be used in the generations following the Carolingian conquest of Lombard

18 Ibid, 445–8.

19 As noted in Chapter 2, the level of medical practice available within and beyond monastic centres continues to be debated. See, for example, Glaze, 'The Perforated Wall', 13–14, 69–79; Horden, 'What's Wrong with Early Medieval Medicine?', 8, 10–13, and 16; Nutton, 'Early Medieval Medicine and Natural Science', 326; Park, 'Medicine and Society', 65–6.

20 Claus Kropp, Anne-Karin Kirsch, Wilfried Rosendahl, Jörg Orschiedt, and Lukas Fischer, *Begraben und Vergessen? Knochen erzählen Geschichte: Anthropologische Ausstellung im Schaudepot Zehntscheune des UNESCO Welterbe Kloster Lorsch* (Bad Homburg v. d. Höhe: Verwaltung der Staatlichen Schlösser und Gärten, 2017). My thanks, too, to members of the scientific board of Lorsch, including Claus Kropp and Hermann Schefers, for sharing their insights into the cemeteries and discussing unpublished data from the excavations.

21 Alexandra Chavarría and Maurizio Marinato, 'Frammentazione e complessità nelle pratiche funerarie altomedievali in Italia settentrionale', in *VII Congresso Nazionale di Archeologia Medievale. Palazzo Turrisi. Lecce, 9–12 settembre 2015*, ed. Paul Arthur and Marco Leo Imperiale, vol. 2 (Florence: All'Insegna del Giglio, 2015), 61–8.

Italy and are therefore considered in the case studies of Part 2. While I shall return to the representativity of this concentration of sites below, significantly, as mentioned in Chapter 2, the inclusion of a northern Italian cluster aligns well with the surviving manuscript evidence since a number of the codices involved in the present study appear to have been produced in this region, moving north soon after their composition.

Moreover, many of the recent, well-documented northern Italian excavations under consideration have published analyses of skeletal remains, something essential to this investigation and that is often lacking in older archaeological reports due to funerary archaeology's traditional focus on the study of burial contexts and grave goods rather than the osteological material itself.[22] While it is important to recognise that skeletal remains are not always available to study (perhaps a result of cremation—a practice that continued in the Rhineland into the eighth and, in some cases, even the ninth centuries—or later disturbances of the burial site),[23] there has been a significant increase in research on osteological evidence in recent decades, coinciding with the development of new techniques and methodologies, such as stable isotope analysis, that are producing alternative approaches to studying the skeletal record.[24] The growing number of publications from excavations across the Carolingian world that not only examine burials but also address their skeletal remains has made this study's dual approach possible.

22 Roberts, *Human Remains in Archaeology*, 11, 40.

23 Willem A. van Es and Willem J. H. Verwers, *Excavations at Dorestad 4: The Settlement on the River Bank Area* (Amersfoort: Cultural Heritage Agency of the Netherlands, 2015), 227: 'in Groningen and further eastwards [cremation] continues until after 800'. For more on early Frankish burial practices, see the work of Guy Halsall, such as Guy Halsall, *Cemeteries and Society in Merovingian Gaul: Selected Studies in History and Archaeology, 1992–2009* (Leiden: Brill, 2010) and Guy Halsall, *Settlement and Social Organization: The Merovingian Region of Metz* (Cambridge: Cambridge University Press, 1995).

24 Fleming, 'Writing Biography', 611–13. On stable isotope analysis, see, for example, Susanne Hakenbeck, 'Potentials and Limitations of Isotope Analysis in Early Medieval Archaeology', *European Journal of Post-Classical Archaeologies* 3 (2013): 95–111. On the relevance of stable isotope analysis to specific questions of past population health, such as dietary practices or age of weaning, see Sam Leggett and Tom Lambert, 'Food and Power in Early Medieval England: A Lack of (Isotopic) Enrichment', *Anglo-Saxon England* 49 (2020): 155–96, https://doi.org/10.1017/S0263675122000072; Takumi Tsutaya and Minoru Yoneda, 'Reconstruction of breastfeeding and weaning practices using stable isotope and trace element analyses: A review', *American Journal of Biological Anthropology* 156, supplement 59 (2015): 2–21, https://doi.org/10.1002/ajpa.22657.

3.2 *Theoretical Challenges Related to the Integration of Skeletal Evidence*

3.2.1 Retrospective Diagnosis

Retrospective diagnosis, the identification of 'an individual case of illness or a disease in history by a modern name or diagnostic category', can be highly problematic for a wide variety of reasons.[25] In particular, there are extensive debates regarding the potential utility of retrospective diagnosis (what is gained from applying a modern medical diagnosis to a past disease experience?), its accuracy (if modern medicine sometimes makes errors in diagnosis, what is the likelihood of correctly diagnosing individuals in the past?), appropriateness from an intellectual standpoint (*can* a modern diagnosis be applied given the cultural and environmental differences between the diagnosing physician and diagnosed individual?), and potential ethical problems (have the individuals in question given consent?). The following section will review the debates involving retrospective diagnosis, the responses to these issues, and how this study fits into the discussion.

In many cases, retrospective diagnoses have been pursued by physicians interested in the health of a famous individual. Studies of this kind, sometimes labelled 'anachronistic diagnoses', are often criticised for their modern medical approach to a historical question combined with their less rigorous study of the appropriate historical evidence.[26] Axel Karenberg, a physician-turned-historian, explains that retrospective diagnosis 'runs the risk of restricting the understanding of history to a biologic process'; this is particularly true if the cases are not adequately contextualised within their historical period.[27] Osamu Muramoto expands on these concerns, noting that retrospective diagnoses rarely address 'the possibility that different diseases might have existed in historical time, or [that] the same disease might have been described through different illness experiences that are bound by a particular historical time and place'.[28] This raises the question, is retrospective diagnosis useful? And does applying a modern medical label on a past disease experience make sense? Andrew Cunningham takes a hard-line against retrospective diagnosis, arguing that it is neither legitimate nor possible to diagnose diseases from

25 Axel Karenberg, 'Retrospective Diagnosis: Use and Abuse in Medical Historiography', *Prague Medical Report* 110, no. 2 (2009): 140–5, at p. 140.

26 Osamu Muramoto, 'Retrospective Diagnosis of a Famous Historical Figure: Ontological, Epistemic, and Ethical Considerations', *Philosophy, Ethics, and Humanities in Medicine* 9 (2014), https://doi.org/10.1186/1747-5341-9-10.

27 Karenberg, 'Retrospective Diagnosis', 144–5.

28 Muramoto, 'Retrospective Diagnosis of a Famous Historical Figure'.

historical evidence given the differences between past experiences and understandings of disease and our own.[29] Instead, he suggests that past disease, as experienced and identified by the people who were affected by it, should be understood in the past as exclusively historical studies without the introduction of modern medical concepts.[30] Mitchell and Muramoto, despite agreeing with aspects of Cunningham's argument, have shown how retrospective diagnosis can provide valuable insights into understanding past populations. More specifically, Muramoto has advanced an effective counter argument from a theoretical perspective while Mitchell has shared constructive guidance on the best practices for incorporating textual evidence in the study of past disease.[31]

In addressing the ontological challenge presented by making a diagnosis in the past, Muramoto uses the example of tuberculosis, or rather a *Mycobacterium tuberculosis* infection. Many retrospective diagnoses are interested in asking 'whether Disease X which we recognise as tuberculosis today is the same and identical disease as "phthisis", "consumption", or whatever they called [it] in historical time'.[32] This, he argues, is not an appropriate way to investigate a past disease because it does not account for changing environmental, biological, and cultural differences. Instead, he suggests framing the investigation by questioning the ontology of a disease, its persistence and existence through time: 'consider modern tuberculosis representing Disease X, while historical tuberculosis Disease X^1. Diseases X and X^1 may be related to each other, but they are not identical, or may be clinically similar but may be different entities with different aetiology and pathophysiology'.[33] Accepting both the difference *and* similarity or relatability between Diseases X and X^1 is crucial to the present study. Continuing with the tuberculosis example, although in a modern medical setting tuberculosis is understood to be caused by *Mycobacterium tuberculosis*, historical tuberculosis ('consumption', 'phthisis', etc.) may have been caused by other pathogens (such as *Mycobacterium bovis*) that produced a similar result.

Given the underlying questions of this book, thinking about a range of related or similar diseases is more fitting: when considering the potential applicability of medical remedies, I am interested in the symptoms that diseases

29 Andrew Cunningham, 'Identifying Disease in the Past: Cutting the Gordian Knot', *Asclepio* 54, no. 1 (2002): 13–34, https://doi.org/10.3989/asclepio.2002.v54.i1.133.

30 Cunningham, 'Identifying Disease in the Past', 16.

31 Muramoto, 'Retrospective Diagnosis of a Famous Historical Figure'; Mitchell, 'Improving the Use of Historical Written Sources', 88–95.

32 Muramoto, 'Retrospective Diagnosis of a Famous Historical Figure'.

33 Ibid.

produced rather than a specific disease label. Although tuberculosis is not one of the selected conditions addressed in the following chapters, it provides a useful example. It would be inappropriate to take the medieval Latin medical term *phthisis*, which is commonly translated as 'consumption' or 'tuberculosis', to mean an infection of *Mycobacterium tuberculosis* and to look for skeletal indicators of this particular disease exclusively. Instead, it would be more appropriate to read *phthisis* as a collection of symptoms that loosely correspond to diseases like tuberculosis, such as coughing and weight loss. With a group of symptoms in mind, it is then possible to consider whether skeletal indicators might be present.

Although retrospective diagnosis continues to be debated, this type of non-specific, conservative approach is generally accepted by many historians of medicine. Faith Wallis, for example, writes, 'it can sometimes be useful for the purposes of historical analysis to try to determine what modern disease category might match a medieval description; indeed, it can actually enhance our understanding of what the medieval writer is attempting to convey'.[34] This fits with what the following chapters aim to do: by thinking about the 'disease categories' suggested by the texts with respect to the osteological evidence, it is possible to re-evaluate whether the texts might have been applicable—that is, whether they record treatments for conditions (or rather the symptoms of conditions) that, based on skeletal remains, individuals experienced in this period.

Returning to Muramoto's in-depth examination of retrospective diagnosis, he also takes issue with one of the standard approaches to the question 'how do we know what disease a person had?' Many opponents of retrospective diagnosis point out that modern researchers can never know the full medical 'reality' of an individual in the past since historical evidence, whether textual, art historical, or archaeological, does not represent medical data, or at least not the type of medical data recorded today for the purpose of diagnosis. Yet, fundamentally, 'medical diagnosis is a process of hypothesis-making and hypothesis-adjustment' as well as 'a probabilistic judgment under uncertainty rather than an apodictic judgement under certainty'.[35] If modern diagnoses are not given with complete certainty, then retrospective diagnoses should not be held to a higher, impossible standard. Additionally, Muramoto explains that 'a clinician is not a natural scientist whose task is to uncover a hidden state of affairs of nature; she is only applying natural sciences to more pragmatic

34 Wallis, *Medieval Medicine*, xxvii.

35 Muramoto, 'Retrospective Diagnosis of a Famous Historical Figure'.

tasks of caring and treating a sick patient, explaining the condition, and prognosticating the future course of his suffering'.[36] Understanding diagnosis as an explanatory device is critical: it is less about defining a patient's exact, certain, and total disease reality, and instead concerned with determining the next course of action and possible long term expectations. This can be easy to forget since modern medical diagnoses involving advanced laboratory tests and imaging are often seen as the definition of an individual's condition rather than as an explanatory device based on probability and subject to revision. Recognising that diagnosis, whether modern or medieval, is intended to provide a framework for treatment and care is essential for understanding the textual evidence under consideration.[37]

Muramoto tackles one further epistemological point: the methodologies involved in diagnosis. Modern medicine can diagnose conditions from a number of different approaches: 'by clinical signs and symptoms (clinical diagnosis); by laboratory tests (laboratory diagnosis); by genetic tests (genetic diagnosis); by identifying aetiology (aetiological diagnosis); [and] by pathological examination (pathological diagnosis)'.[38] Although the study of skeletal remains makes possible the examination of pathologies and even some medical tests, many of the above methods are not available when making diagnoses in the past, adding a further degree of uncertainty. An assessment of the evidence should therefore take these methodological limitations into account, framing the possible diagnosis cautiously, such as 'X and Y symptoms or markers are consistent with Z disease'.[39] Mitchell similarly advocates a cautious approach to the identification of past disease and suggests using phrases such as 'possible example of', 'is compatible with', 'a probable example of', or 'very likely to represent' Disease X.[40]

Finally, with this theoretical framework in mind, the question of medical ethics must be addressed. Since this book examines general trends and patterns in the palaeopathological data regarding a selection of conditions, many of the ethical concerns related to retrospective diagnosis pose less of an issue. First, the selected conditions, such as joint disease and oral pathologies, are not diseases that could damage someone's reputation posthumously (i.e., reveal information that someone would want to conceal), and secondly, given

36 Ibid.

37 This take on diagnosis also aligns more closely to the early medieval focus on prognostication. See Wallis, 'Signs and Senses', 265–78.

38 Muramoto, 'Retrospective Diagnosis of a Famous Historical Figure'.

39 Ibid.

40 Mitchell, 'Improving the Use of Historical Written Sources', 89.

the nature of the sample, the individuals are nearly always anonymous (the discovery of Abbot Talaricus' grave representing a rare exception) and not linked to any living people.[41]

3.2.2 The Osteological Paradox

In 1992, James Wood, George Milner, Henry Harpending, and Kenneth Weiss presented the osteological paradox, a series of conceptual challenges that have had a significant impact on the study of palaeopathology.[42] While elements of their landmark report have been debated and revised, the points they originally outlined remain essential to consider when analysing the skeletal record in relation to health and disease in the past.[43] They identified three major problems: demographic nonstationarity (populations are not stationary but in a constant state of flux), selective mortality (a skeletal sample is inherently biased because it only represents the dead *and* only represents them at their age of death), and hidden heterogeneity in risks (an individual's 'underlying frailty or susceptibility to disease and death' is unknown).[44] The combination of these problems results in the paradox that skeletal remains with evidence of pathologies may actually represent the healthier individuals of the population. To clarify, those individuals with signs of 'disease X' lived long enough with disease X for signs of its presence to be recorded in their bones. Individuals from the same burial group without indicators of disease X may have also suffered from disease X but died before it could be recorded in their skeleton. Consequently, individuals who appear healthy based on an assessment of their skeletal remains may actually have been frailer than those with evidence of disease.

While the osteological paradox remains an important collection of concepts with which to engage given the integration of skeletal evidence in the

41 Richard Hodges, John Mitchell, and Lucy Watson, 'The discovery of Abbot Talaricus' (817–3 October 823) tomb at San Vincenzo al Volturno', *Antiquity* 71 (1997): 453–6, https://doi.org/10.1017/S0003598X00085082.

42 James W. Wood, George R. Milner, Henry C. Harpending, and Kenneth M. Weiss, 'The Osteological Paradox: Problems of Inferring Prehistoric Health from Skeletal Samples', *Current Anthropology* 33, no. 4 (1992), 343–70.

43 Consider, for example, the twelve pages of responses to the original article (Wood, Milner, Harpending, and Weiss, 'The Osteological Paradox', 358–70) and later responses such as Mark Nathan Cohen, James W. Wood, and George R. Milner, 'The Osteological Paradox Reconsidered', *Current Anthropology* 35, no. 5 (1994): 629–37; Sharon N. DeWitte and Christopher M. Stojanowski, 'The Osteological Paradox 20 Years Later: Past Perspectives, Future Directions', *Journal of Archaeological Research* 23 (2015): 397–450, https://doi.org/10.1007/s10814-015-9084-1.

44 Wood, Milner, Harpending, and Weiss, 'The Osteological Paradox', 344–5.

following chapters, the aspects of health and disease under investigation in Part 2—dental health, joint disease, and surgery and trauma (elaborated below)—are comparatively less affected by the problems raised by the paradox than many other areas of death and disease. Consider, for example, a traumatic injury sustained from falling off a horse: whether a person was more or less susceptible to disease would likely have had a relatively low impact on their exposure to the traumatic incident. That is, although their underlying level of health and living conditions could have affected their recovery from such an injury, the skeletal evidence bearing witness to the initial traumatic injury would be unchanged. The other groups of conditions analysed in the following chapters, oral pathologies and joint diseases, tend to increase in severity and/or extent over time. The skeletal changes under consideration in these cases are mostly the result of gradual processes rather than fast-acting pathogens that could have killed an individual without leaving a trace in their remains. The osteological paradox thus presents less of a conceptual challenge in the case studies addressed in Chapters 7–9.

3.2.3 Selection of Conditions

Palaeopathological evidence for disease, injury, and treatment is grounded in what can be seen on an individual's remains. That not all medical conditions leave marks on the skeleton restricts the comparison of textual and skeletal evidence to conditions that have the potential to be recorded in teeth and bones. As a result, there are many medical issues that, though they are mentioned by medical texts, cannot be investigated with this approach, including conditions affecting soft tissues (such as stomachaches, liver and spleen pain, and eye problems), external areas (such as hair loss and skin diseases), and mental health. There are, of course, some exceptions. A limited number of conditions affecting soft tissues may be revealed through palaeopathological analysis, but they are often challenging to identify and can go unnoticed fairly easily.[45] In the case of cardiovascular disease, for example, abnormal, enlarged blood vessels may leave an impression of their expansion in certain areas of the skeleton, especially around the heart.[46] Mummified remains present another exception because soft tissues may be preserved and analysed; the archaeological material under consideration, however, does not contain remains preserved in this

45 Tony Waldron, *Palaeopathology* (Cambridge: Cambridge University Press, 2009), 224–35.
46 Waldron, *Palaeopathology*, 224.

manner.[47] Given the challenges of identifying soft tissue conditions in skeletal assemblages and lack of suitable remains, soft tissue diseases have not been included in the present study.

Similarly, some conditions that may at first appear to be unable to leave any skeletal indicators, such as head pain or vision changes, could, in fact, be related to pathologies observable in skeletal remains. For example, an osteoma, a type of benign tumour that can be found in the skull and frontal sinus, could explain these two symptoms, head pain and vision changes.[48] A criterion in selecting the conditions to investigate in Part 2 has therefore been the likelihood of a probable correspondence between, on the one hand, a pain or problem described in the texts and, on the other hand, evidence that can be seen on skeletal remains. In the case of an osteoma, it would be impossible to compare these two bodies of evidence given all the possible causes of head pain and vision changes. In contrast, an issue such as tooth pain, loose teeth, and related descriptions can be more meaningfully compared to dental remains from early medieval individuals.

Despite the various limitations outlined above, many conditions can be studied through palaeopathological analyses of human remains. Primary research areas include joint diseases, infectious diseases, metabolic diseases, trauma, disorders of growth and development, dental diseases, and certain cancers.[49] Taking the methodological challenges into account and using my knowledge of the recipe literature, the following chapters focus on three of these categories: dental diseases (Chapter 7), joint diseases (Chapter 8), and surgery and trauma (Chapter 9).

3.2.4 Absence of Evidence as Evidence of Absence?

One additional theoretical challenge to consider is the potential absence of osteological evidence for conditions recorded in the texts. If symptoms relating to 'Disease X' are described in the recipes but unidentified in skeletal remains, does this indicate that the texts were, at least with respect to this disease, irrelevant to early medieval populations? While such a case could suggest that the

47 Michael R. Zimmerman, 'The Analysis and Interpretation of Mummified Remains', in *A Companion to Paleopathology*, ed. Anne L. Grauer (Chichester: Wiley-Blackwell, 2012), 152–69; Waldron, *Palaeopathology*, 221–3.

48 Waldron, *Palaeopathology*, 170–2.

49 Arthur C. Aufderheide and Conrado Rodríguez-Martín, *The Cambridge Encyclopedia of Human Paleopathology* (Cambridge: Cambridge University Press, 1998); Anne L. Grauer, ed., *A Companion to Paleopathology* (Chichester: Wiley-Blackwell, 2012); Waldron, *Palaeopathology*.

recorded treatments preserved information that was not applicable to communities in Carolingian Europe, the absence of osteological evidence must not be interpreted as simply the evidence of absence. There are many reasons why a condition that *could* be preserved in skeletal material has not been identified (or recorded), including a number of the challenges highlighted above, such as the potentially incomplete nature of excavations, the skeletal material's state of preservation, and the variation in the degree to which skeletal remains are analysed and recorded. This book, therefore, is most concerned with the positive evidence, that is, the cases where the osteological evidence parallels the treatments recorded in the texts, as this correlation indicates that the medical knowledge in question could have been used in the practice of medicine.

4 Outlining the Analytical Approach to Chapters 7–9

4.1 *Overview of Sites*

The osteological evidence consulted in the following chapters comes from excavations of early medieval sites found across the Carolingian world, and, like the manuscript evidence, represents communities from both the Frankish heartlands as well as more peripheral areas. In total, Chapters 7–9 have considered reports on skeletal material from twenty-one different sites located within the Carolingian Empire and one on the very southern edge, San Vincenzo al Volturno (see the map). The selected sites are located in present-day Germany, the Netherlands, France, Switzerland, and Italy and include excavations from Acqui Terme, Biel, Bolgare, Cairate, Campione d'Italia, Caravate, Cherbourg, Cremona, Desenzano, Kirchheim am Ries, Lorsch, Maastricht, Neresheim, Nusplingen, Ovaro, Quingentole, Rivoli, San Cassiano, Schretzheim, Seckenheim, and Tolmezzo. References are also made to skeletal evidence from contemporary sites in the British Isles (Chapters 8 and 9) as well as to excavations of early Frankish burials (Chapter 9) for comparative purposes. Paralleling the manuscript review of Chapter 2, it is important to comment on the representativity of these sites, especially in relation to their chronological range and geographical distribution.

In many cases, the dates of a site's occupation and/or the use of a burial area are only known with relative precision based on stratigraphic evidence or material remains. Occasionally, more exact dating methods, such as radiocarbon dating, are used on osteological remains, providing a date typically within the range of two to three generations. Many of the dates for early medieval skeletal assemblages must therefore be interpreted as approximate rather than absolute. Rarely, however, the existence of complementary documentary evidence can provide a more precise date for site occupation or burial; the excavation of Abbot Talaricus' tomb at San Vincenzo al Volturno presents one such example.[50]

The duration with which a site was used also deserves mention since many sites were active over a relatively long period of time, often spanning several centuries, and may have been used for multiple purposes over this period (settlement, cemetery, quarry, disposal area, etc.), complicating the establishment of a firm chronology.[51] As a result, although the sites involved in this study were in use during the Carolingian period, many pre- and/or post-date it, too. This chronological breadth means that some of the skeletal material consulted in the following case studies does not align perfectly with the chronologically narrower textual record. Yet, as noted above, the external and internal factors affecting health and disease, such as the environment and culture, tend to change gradually, thereby allowing for some flexibility with respect to dating. Cemeteries that contain remains pre- or post-dating the Carolingian period by a few generations should, in the majority of cases, still be comparable and relevant to this study. Consider, for example, the cemetery areas of the Abbey of Lorsch. Although they may contain burials spanning the entire period in which the monastery was active (i.e., up to the sixteenth century), radiocarbon dating has provided definite evidence of Carolingian burials within the so-called *Mönchsfriedhof*, the cemetery that is thought to have contained the monks.[52] Additional archaeological evidence, including the cemetery area's size and uniformity, suggests that many of the un-dated individuals also lived during the Carolingian period (or at least within a few generations of it) rather than the later Middle Ages. The Lorsch skeletal material, moreover, represents a particularly interesting reference point given its connections with medical texts in the late eighth and ninth centuries: surviving library catalogues indicate that its library housed several medical manuscripts during this period and its scriptorium produced the *Lorscher Arzneibuch* in *c.* 800.[53] As this codex

50 Hodges, Mitchell, and Watson, 'The discovery of Abbot Talaricus', 453–6.

51 Pearce, 'Beyond the Grave', 467.

52 Kropp, Kirsch, Rosendahl, Orschiedt, and Fischer, *Begraben und Vergessen?*, 38–9 and personal communications with members of the scientific board of Lorsch, including Claus Kropp and Hermann Schefers. See Figures 8–14 for a selection of images of skeletal remains from the *Mönchsfriedhof*.

53 Bamberg, Staatsbibliothek, Msc. Med. 1; *Das Lorscher Arzneibuch*, ed. and trans. Stoll; Bernhard Bischoff, *Die Abtei Lorsch im Spiegel ihrer Handschriften*, 2nd ed. (Lorsch: Laurissa, 1989); Keil and Schnitzer, eds., *Das Lorscher Arzneibuch und die frühmittelalterliche Medizin*; Adelheid Platte and Karlheinz Platte, eds., *Das Lorscher Arzneibuch: Klostermedizin in der Karolingerzeit* (Lorsch: Laurissa, 1990); Klaus-Dietrich

contains recipe collections comparable to many of those involved in the present study, it is especially important to consider osteological evidence from Lorsch in relation to the treatments recorded in the texts.[54]

Lorsch, situated in the Rhineland, represents a site at the heart of the Frankish Empire. Likewise, excavations from sites in the Netherlands, southern Germany, and Switzerland come from core territories within the Carolingian world. On the other hand, some of the skeletal material considered in Part 2 was excavated on the fringes of Carolingian Francia, such as the burials from Cherbourg. As discussed above, there is also a strong focus on sites from northern Italy. Given Charlemagne's conquest of the Lombard Kingdom in 774, I have consulted palaeopathological reports from sites in northern Italy which have evidence of continued use during this period. Crucially, these sites not only overlap with the period of Carolingian control of northern Italy but, like Lorsch, they present a particularly relevant sample to study since several of the core manuscripts involved in this study were produced in northern Italian writing centres. The movement of many codices to communities in the Alps and beyond, such as St Gall, Reichenau, and Fulda, speaks to the interconnectedness of these sites and a shared intellectual culture, thus indicating the importance of considering skeletal remains from both sides of the Alps. Finally, I have also included evidence from San Vincenzo al Volturno, a site just on the edge of the Carolingian Empire at its greatest extent, given the known links between this important ecclesiastical centre and others further north.

4.2 *The Spectrum of Specificity*

Returning to the texts, it is essential to outline a central feature of my assessment of the recipes in the light of the osteological record. As mentioned in Chapter 2, recipes vary enormously in their specificity: an antidote may claim to treat over fifty different conditions, while a simple may intend to heal a single ailment. This variety is important to bear in mind when considering the question of applicability as there is a difference between, on the one hand, a reference to tooth pain in a very general antidote and, on the other hand, a highly targeted remedy for toothache. In the former, tooth pain is one of many conditions that the antidote intends to treat, whereas it is the primary focus of the latter. These examples represent the two ends of the spectrum of

Fischer, 'Das Lorscher Arzneibuch im Widerstreit der Meinungen', *Medizinhistorisches Journal* 45, no. 2 (2010): 165–88.

54 Note: the recipe books of the *Lorscher Arzneibuch* do not form part of the present study's textual sample since they have received extensive scholarly attention in recent decades. On the *Lorscher Arzneibuch*, see the references in the preceding note.

specificity: the first is a catch-all panacea while the second is a highly specific treatment. I have used this variable, i.e., the specificity of a recipe's approach to treatment, in the following analyses to differentiate recipes, identify patterns in the information they present, and assess how the textual evidence compares to the osteological record. It has been especially useful to combine an analysis of specificity with other features, such as target area(s) of treatment.

In the following chapters, I shall classify recipes as belonging to one of three levels of specificity: a) non-specific, b) semi-specific, and c) highly specific.[55] Generally, antidotes and other recipes that claim to treat a large variety of seemingly unrelated conditions, ranging from snake bites to fevers to stomach pains to gout, fall into the non-specific group; recipes that target a range of similar conditions are considered semi-specific; and recipes that intend to treat a single condition have been classified as highly specific. While the difference between these levels of specificity is subjective, their divisions become easier to see when mapped onto the recipe literature. Consider, for example, recipes that target joint pain: when joint pain is listed as one of a host of different conditions, the recipe is classified as non-specific, but when it is found alongside a more limited number of other symptoms, such as dislocations and fractures, the recipe is considered semi-specific (all of the conditions the recipe intends to treat involve pain management). In contrast, a remedy that only targets joint pain, whether general arthritic pains or a named joint area, falls under the highly specific category. Given the particularly focused nature of highly specific treatments, the following case studies tend to concentrate on this category of recipes in relation to the skeletal evidence.

Having reviewed the significance of the question of applicability and outlined my approach to re-evaluating the recipe literature, it is now possible to turn to the first case study, an investigation into the applicability of early medieval treatments for dental problems.

---

55 In the tables of Chapters 7–9, these categories are generally abbreviated as: NSp, SSp, and HSp, respectively.

CHAPTER 7

Dental Disease

From Caries to Cosmetics

1 Introduction: a Monk From Lorsch

When considering human health in the past, few sights are more compelling than a skeleton that shows clear signs of disease. Figure 8 offers one such encounter, presenting a skull with evidence of a variety of dental problems, including caries, deposits of dental calculus, and periodontal disease. Figures 9 and 10 provide a closer look at the state of this individual's dentition, highlighting carious lesions (pointed out by arrows in Figure 9), deposits of calculus (seen as the deposits on the surface of the teeth in Figure 10), and dental enamel hypoplasia, DEH (evidenced by the horizontal bands across the teeth in Figure 10). This individual, a male aged thirty-five to forty years old at the time of his death, was uncovered in excavations at Lorsch in 1999.[1] His burial was part of the so-called *Mönchsfriedhof*, a cemetery within the Abbey complex that is thought to have been used primarily by the monastic community. Radiocarbon dating indicates that he lived during the late Carolingian period.[2] What can be learnt about early medieval dental health by studying this monk and other individuals from this period? And how do their teeth compare to the descriptions of dental problems recorded in recipes?

Teeth provide a wealth of information. The oral pathologies recorded in the Lorsch monk's dentition, for example, do not present a straightforward case of disease but can offer a much more nuanced picture of the state of his health, both at the time of his death and in earlier phases of his life. Unlike bones, which remodel throughout an individual's life, teeth can provide a snapshot of the period in which their growth occurred, generally infancy or childhood, while simultaneously recording later dietary and disease experiences. Thus, the presence of carious lesions and calculus point to poor dental hygiene as an adult and illustrate the state of his oral health at the time of his death. The existence of DEH, on the other hand, reveals that he may have suffered from malnutrition or serious, growth-interrupting disease(s) at a young age.

1 Kropp, Kirsch, Rosendahl, Orschiedt, and Fischer, *Begraben und Vergessen?*, 38–9.

2 The date range given by radiocarbon dating is 888–966. Kropp, Kirsch, Rosendahl, Orschiedt, and Fischer, *Begraben und Vergessen?*, 38–9.

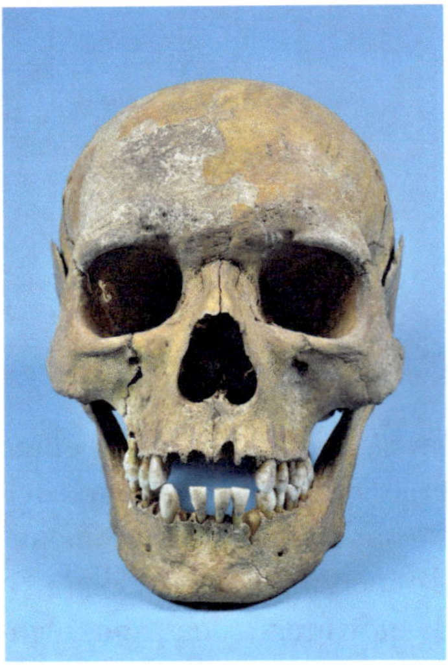

FIGURE 8
A skull from an individual buried in the monastic burial area at Lorsch

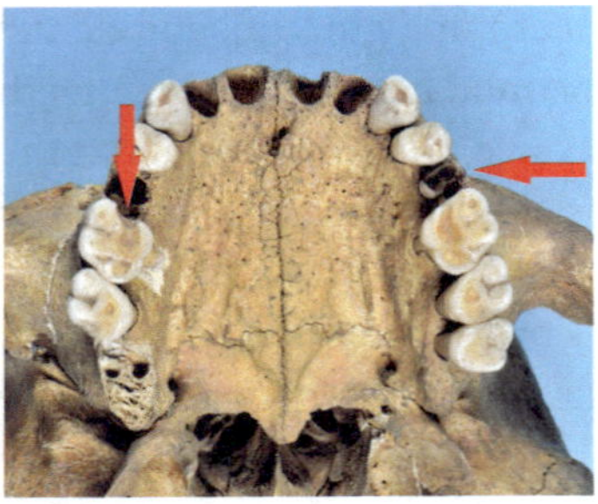

FIGURE 9
Carious lesions visible on skeletal remains excavated at Lorsch

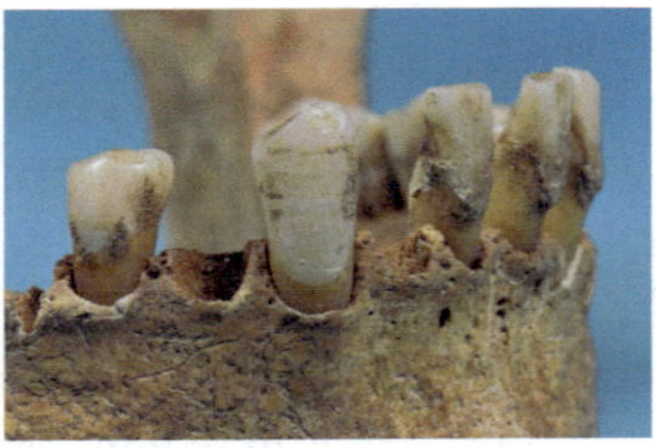

FIGURE 10
Dental calculus and DEH visible on skeletal remains excavated at Lorsch

In this chapter, I shall concentrate on dental disease, first reviewing evidence from early medieval skeletal remains and then analysing recipes that concern treatments for toothaches, lost teeth, mouth sores, and other aspects of oral health. With both bodies of evidence in mind, I then consider the question of applicability. Overall, many of the symptoms listed in the texts appear to have a high degree of overlap with conditions seen in the osteological record: treatments for toothache, mouth sores, lost/loose teeth, putridity, and gum problems fit with the pathologies observed in the skeletal remains in essentially all of the sites consulted. I argue, therefore, that the treatments for dental problems recorded in the texts would have been highly applicable to many individuals in early medieval Europe. A consideration of several categories of recipes, such as treatments that target specific types of teeth, adds further weight to this argument.

2 Oral Health in the Skeletal Evidence

Dental remains represent one of the best materials to study when investigating health and disease in the past, and not simply because of the range of information they can provide as noted above. Crucially, teeth tend to 'resist destruction and taphonomic conditions better than any other body tissue' due to their protective layer of enamel.[3] Before examining the state of dental health as seen in early medieval skeletal assemblages, I shall provide a brief review of dental anatomy and common conditions and address several tooth-specific methodological challenges.

2.1 *Dental Disease in the Archaeological Record: an Overview*

All mammals have two sets of teeth: a set of primary, deciduous teeth that are lost after weaning and a set of secondary, permanent teeth; in humans, the primary dentition contains twenty teeth while the secondary has thirty-two.[4] The permanent dentition is made up of four types of teeth (incisors, canines, pre-molars, and molars), each with a different function related to processing food.[5] Teeth consist of four primary tissues: enamel, dentine, cementum, and

3 Luis Pezo Lanfranco and Sabine Eggers, 'Caries Through Time: An Anthropological Overview', in *Contemporary Approach to Dental Caries*, ed. Ming-Yu Li (Rijeka: IntechOpen, 2012), 3–34, https://doi.org/10.5772/38059; Odin M. Langsjoen, 'Diseases of the Dentition', in *The Cambridge Encyclopedia of Human Paleopathology*, ed. Arthur C. Aufderheide and Conrado Rodríguez-Martín (Cambridge: Cambridge University Press, 1998), 393–412, at p. 393; Waldron, *Palaeopathology*, 236–48.

4 Langsjoen, 'Diseases of the Dentition', 394.

5 Langsjoen, 'Diseases of the Dentition', 395. As this chapter focuses on the state of dental health generally, I shall not detail the nomenclature and annotation used to describe each tooth and tooth area, but it is important to note that there are several systems used to record the state of teeth uncovered in excavations, including the International Coding System (recommended by the Fédération dentaire internationale) and the Standards System (similar to the ICS but with a visual format); differences in recording and analysing teeth and associated pathologies may account for some of the variation observed when comparing results from multiple sites. For more information on tooth anatomy, see Simon Hillson, *Dental Anthropology* (Cambridge: Cambridge University Press, 1996), 6–105.

dental pulp. Enamel, the outer-most protective layer, is almost entirely made up of mineral content (96%), making it among the hardest substances in the body.[6] The second layer, dentine, also called the root of the tooth, forms another layer of protection for the pulp, though it is less hard than enamel. Cementum, a bony connective tissue, links the root of the tooth to the periodontal ligament.[7] Finally, the pulp, the inner-most part of the tooth, contains the soft tissue. Collectively, the tissues supporting and affixing a tooth to the alveolar bone are called the periodontium.[8] While this study concentrates on teeth, an analysis of dental health cannot ignore the surrounding tissues, such as the gingiva (gums) and alveolar bone.

Turning to the types of pathologies recorded in the skeletal remains, caries, a term derived from the Latin *caries*, meaning decay or rottenness, is 'the most common cause of oral pain and tooth loss' and 'one of the few conditions which has been recorded unfailingly in almost all reports on human remains from archaeological sites'.[9] As seen in Figure 9, the Carolingian monk from Lorsch was suffering from multiple carious lesions when he died. The disease is a progressive bacterial condition that affects the calcified dental tissues, demineralising the inorganic material and destroying the organic components.[10] Caries tend to occur at two different locations on the tooth surface, either at the crown or the root, resulting in several types of lesions with differing aetiologies.[11] Coronal caries begin with the destruction of the enamel, then the dentine, and eventually penetrate the pulp chamber; molars and pre-molars tend to be the most affected by this type of lesion due to their complex network of fissures, fossae and groves.[12] Root caries occur more frequently in later life due to the effects of periodontal disease (addressed below), whereby the recession of the gingivae and underlying supporting tissues exposes a tooth's cementum and roots, making them susceptible to infection.[13]

In their review of evidence for caries from prehistory to the present day, Luis Pezo Lanfranco and Sabine Eggers reported that the disease reached a

6 Langsjoen, 'Diseases of the Dentition', 396.

7 Ibid.

8 Ibid.

9 First quotation from Waldron, *Palaeopathology*, 236; second quotation from Simon Hillson, 'Recording Dental Caries in Archaeological Human Remains', *International Journal of Osteoarchaeology* 11, no. 4 (2001): 249–89, https://doi.org/10.1002/oa.538, at p. 249. Note that the term 'caries' remains the same whether singular or plural.

10 Langsjoen, 'Diseases of the Dentition', 402.

11 Hillson, 'Recording Dental Caries', 250.

12 Ibid.

13 Ibid.

peak in the early Middle Ages, having increased steadily from *c.* 1200 BC.[14] This peak was followed by a period of relative stability for several centuries, before rising dramatically with the largescale introduction of sugar in the early modern period.[15] Although skeletal evidence indicates that both sexes were heavily affected by carious lesions, males tend to exhibit a lower prevalence of caries than females. While the cause of this difference continues to be debated, females may be predisposed to the development of caries due to earlier tooth eruptions and hormonal fluctuations as well as 'culturally regulated' differences, such as gendered access to certain foods in some populations.[16] The recording and analysis of caries in the archaeological record is complicated other pathologies, such as the effects of abrasion or the accumulation of dental calculus.

The aging process has been linked to a number of degenerative changes in the dentition, including attrition (wear), erosion, and abrasion.[17] Paradoxically, the rate of attrition and abrasiveness of an individual's diet have been tied to both the development *and* inhibition of caries.[18] On the one hand, abrasive foods and extensive wear may increase the risk of chipping teeth, creating spaces in which dental plaque can collect while simultaneously exposing lines of weakness and/or areas of dentine.[19] On the other hand, a high level of dental wear and abrasion can erode the carious tissue and dislodge plaque, protecting the teeth from the accumulation of bacteria.[20] The degree to which these processes support or inhibit the initiation of caries remains a contentious issue in the field.

Dental calculus also presents a complex relationship with caries. Deposits of calculus are formed over time as plaque, a biofilm made up of bacteria and fragments of food particles, accumulates on the surface of a tooth and eventually mineralises.[21] In theory, there is an inverse relationship between the development of caries and the build-up of calculus since the latter requires an alkaline environment (resulting in net mineralisation) while the former requires an acidic environment (resulting in net demineralisation).[22] Both

14 Pezo Lanfranco and Eggers, 'Caries through Time', 8.
15 Ibid, 8–9.
16 Ibid, 17.
17 Langsjoen, 'Diseases of the Dentition', 398.
18 Hillson, 'Recording Dental Caries', 263–5.
19 Ibid, 263.
20 Ibid.
21 Waldron, *Palaeopathology*, 240–1.
22 Ibid.

pathologies, however, are often found together, indicating that other factors play a role in the development of both caries and calculus.[23]

Periodontal disease, or periodontitis, is a chronic, destructive inflammatory process that affects the tissues of the periodontium over time.[24] This occurs as plaque accumulates at the gum margin and is one of the main causes of antemortem tooth loss (AMTL), a topic addressed in more detail below.[25] In the archaeological record, the condition is identified by a receded alveolar margin and the bone often exhibits signs of inflammation and remodelling.[26]

Cysts, abscesses, and granulomas are three different types of lesions found at the apex of the tooth that are caused by an infection of the dental pulp.[27] If the infected tooth is not removed, the infection induces an immune response in the periapical tissue, a cavity.[28] While acute abscesses and granulomas tend to be less than 3 mm, cysts and chronic abscesses can be much larger, making them easily recognisable in the archaeological record (as seen in Figures 12 and 13 below).[29]

Tooth loss, though not necessarily pathological, must also be mentioned since many teeth may be missing from excavated skeletal remains. It is often possible to determine whether teeth were lost before or after death based on the appearance of the tooth's socket. Post-mortem tooth loss (PMTL), which can occur as a result of taphonomic processes or during excavation and conservation, leaves a 'pristine' tooth socket with no signs of remodelling.[30] In the case of AMTL, the alveolar bone will 'show some degree of remodelling' and the socket will eventually smooth over (an example of a jaw with extensive AMTL can be seen below in Figure 14a).[31] AMTL is a useful measure of dental health since teeth tend to be lost as a result of carious lesions, periodontal disease, and/or intentional extraction due to these causes, though it must be remembered that they can also be lost due to trauma, non-medical extraction (e.g., ritual or cosmetic extractions), and other diseases (such as scurvy).[32] Although

23 Hillson, 'Recording Dental Caries', 265; Waldron, *Palaeopathology*, 241.
24 Langsjoen, 'Diseases of the Dentition', 398–9.
25 John R. Lukacs, 'Oral Health in Past Populations: Context, Concepts and Controversies', in *A Companion to Paleopathology*, ed. Anne L. Grauer (Chichester: Wiley-Blackwell, 2012), 553–81, at p. 560.
26 Waldron, *Palaeopathology*, 240.
27 Waldron, *Palaeopathology*, 241–3; Lukacs, 'Oral Health in Past Populations', 560.
28 Waldron, *Palaeopathology*, 241–3; Langsjoen, 'Diseases of the Dentition', 408.
29 Waldron, *Palaeopathology*, 241–3.
30 Ibid, 238–9.
31 Ibid.
32 Ibid.

it is often possible to differentiate AMTL from PMTL, it remains largely impossible to determine the cause of AMTL. That being said, since some cases of AMTL were almost certainly caused by caries, it is important to remember that the reported incidence of carious lesions in archaeological contexts most probably under-reports their actual incidence. In terms of recording caries, the biases created by attrition and dental calculus must also be mentioned: heavy attrition and calculus build-up may erase or obscure the existence of carious lesions.[33]

Finally, temporomandibular joint disease and DEH will not be discussed in this chapter. Temporomandibular joint disease, or osteoarthritis of the jaw, is less concerned with oral health, though it occurs in the same area of the body, and more reflective of osteoarthritic changes over time.[34] DEH, mentioned in relation to the Lorsch monk pictured above (see especially Figure 10), documents periods of stunted growth that coincided with the time at which the tooth was developing. The disruption of growth in infancy and childhood is generally due to poor nutrition, starvation, or disease at a 'life-threatening magnitude of severity'.[35] As such, DEH is understood as a non-specific indicator of stress and is studied in relation to diet, nutrition, and overall disease load. Although the striations caused by enamel hypoplasia create areas that are more prone to developing caries, the condition is not otherwise linked to dental disease and will therefore be omitted from the following analysis.[36]

2.2 *Skeletal Evidence for Oral Pathologies in Early Medieval Europe*

Stereotypes of medieval dentition are often extremely negative. Caricatures of medieval people have ensured that the popular image of pre-modern teeth is one of decay, disease, and poor hygiene. Is this picture an accurate portrayal of the situation or a gross exaggeration? The review of caries over time conducted by Pezo Lanfranco and Eggers noted that carious lesions, as recorded by archaeological evidence, increased throughout Antiquity and then peaked in roughly 750 AD.[37] Their findings suggest that common assumptions about the state of medieval oral health may not be far from the truth.

33 Hillson, 'Recording Dental Caries', 264.

34 Langsjoen, 'Diseases of the Dentition', 399–400; Lukacs, 'Oral Health in Past Populations', 560.

35 Langsjoen, 'Diseases of the Dentition', 405–7.

36 Hillson, 'Recording Dental Caries', 265; Waldron, *Palaeopathology*, 265–7.

37 Pezo Lanfranco and Eggers, 'Caries through Time', 8–9.

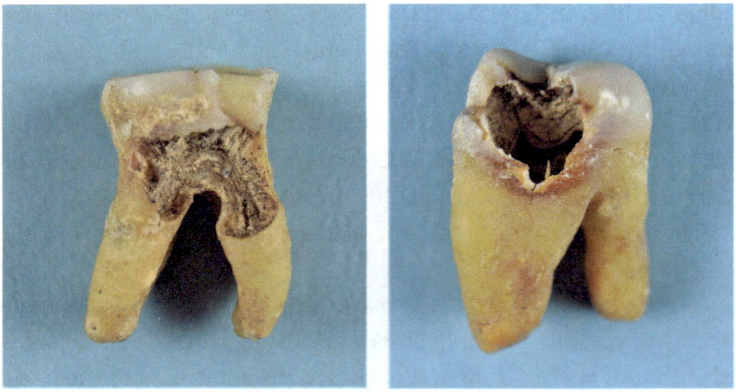

FIGURE 11 A close-up of carious lesions from skeletal remains excavated at Lorsch

The dental health of the individual from Lorsch highlighted above, however, might not have been *as* bad as popular stereotypes suggest. Although he clearly suffered from carious lesions, was missing teeth, and exhibited deposits of calculus, these features must be examined in more detail. The missing teeth, for example, appear to have been lost post-mortem (see Figure 9) and the build-up of calculus is relatively light (see Figure 10). While it cannot be said that his dental health was *good*, it was also not extremely poor. How does his dental record fit with the rest of the sample from Lorsch?

Overall, the dental remains excavated at Lorsch contain a relatively high percentage of teeth affected by caries.[38] Figure 11, for example, illustrates two teeth excavated at Lorsch that have been severely damaged by carious lesions. Many teeth also exhibit calculus deposits, and often of a higher degree than that seen in the opening example. Compare the relatively light presence of calculus seen in Figure 10 with the much heavier accumulation seen in Figure 12. The deposits of calculus are clearly visible in the three remaining molars of the maxilla. A large cyst in the mandible is also observable in Figure 12. It is likely that this stemmed from a carious lesion in the molar, now missing, under which it is located. Similarly, Figure 13 provides evidence of both extensive calculus deposits (best seen on the left-most tooth) and a deep abscess in the

38 Kropp, Kirsch, Rosendahl, Orschiedt, and Fischer, *Begraben und Vergessen?*, and supplemented by personal communications with members of the scientific board of Lorsch, including Claus Kropp and Hermann Schefers.

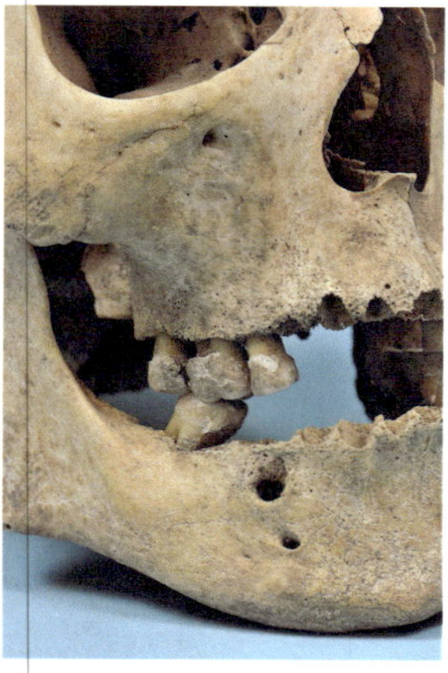

FIGURE 12
Evidence of calculus build-up and a cyst seen on skeletal remains excavated at Lorsch

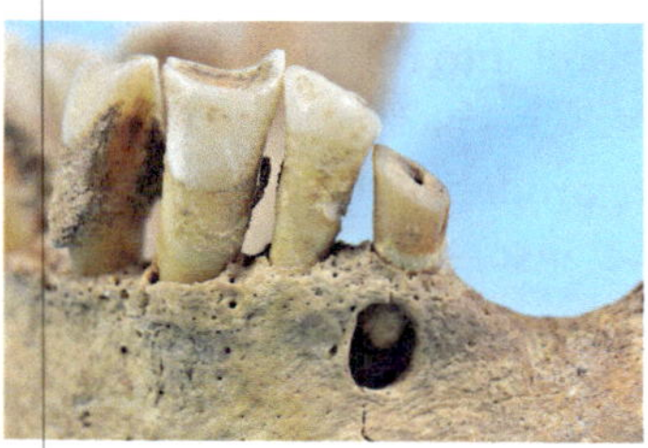

FIGURE 13
Evidence of calculus deposits and an abscess on skeletal remains excavated at Lorsch

mandible. In this case, the abscess has exposed the root of a tooth affected by a carious lesion. These images, combined with the general assessments made by the researchers at Lorsch, illustrate the overall poor state of dental health in medieval Lorsch.

Despite these general signs of dental disease, it must be stressed that the sample from Lorsch displays a high degree of variability. Consider, for example, the two jaws pictured in Figure 14. The image on the left shows clear signs of extensive AMTL: not a single tooth remains in this mandible and nearly all sockets appear to have been fully remodelled, suggesting that the vast majority of teeth were lost at least several years before the individual died. This example fits with the evidence highlighted above, adding further weight to the picture of poor dental health. The image on the right, however, provides a stark contrast. In this case, all of the teeth are present and intact; none exhibits signs of caries, major calculus build-up, or periodontal disease; and there is little evidence of attrition. This serves as a valuable reminder, demonstrating that, even

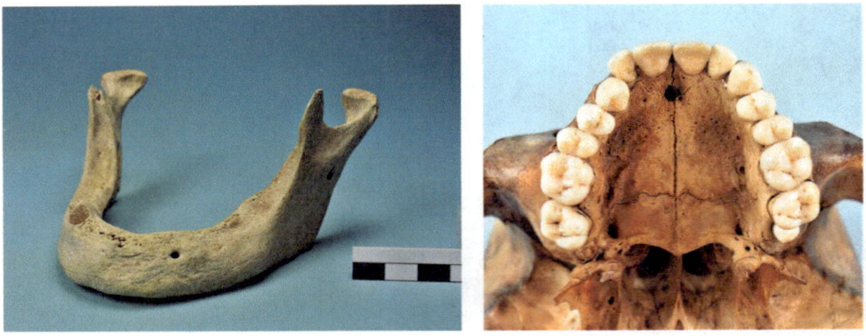

FIGURE 14 Contrasting dental health visible in the skeletal remains excavated at Lorsch

at sites with many examples of dental pathologies, there is often a spectrum of oral health.

The Lorsch assemblage offers a visual entry point into this overview of evidence for early medieval dental disease, and one that is particularly significant given that the monastic centre is known to have produced medical texts containing recipe collections during this period. Yet, just as the skeletal remains excavated at a single site can vary immensely, so, too, can there be major differences between sites. While, in some cases, this may be due to differing excavation and recording systems, on the other hand, variation may arise due to differences in diet and other health factors. So, how do the findings at Lorsch compare to other sites in early medieval Europe?

To illustrate the potential for variation between sites, consider the disparities between the results of the excavations of Biel-Mett and San Lorenzo di Desenzano. The report from Biel-Mett, a cemetery in the present-day Canton of Bern used from the late sixth or early seventh centuries to the late eighth or early ninth centuries, included an assessment of the dentitions from forty-three skulls. The authors noted that 'most of the individuals had suffered from periodontal disease' and that the population exhibited a high degree of abrasion as well as a relatively high frequency of caries (30% of recovered teeth were affected) and AMTL (23%).[39] In contrast, archaeologists working at San Lorenzo di Desenzano, a northern Italian site whose second phase of use has been dated to the Carolingian period, recorded significantly fewer incidences

39 Jean-François Roulet and Susi Ulrich-Bochsler, 'Zahnärztliche Untersuchung frühmittelalterlicher Schädel aus Biel-Mett', *Schweizerische Monatsschrift für Zahnheilkunde* 89, no. 6 (1979): 526–40, at p. 526.

of oral pathologies. Caries were noted in only 6.1% of teeth, AMTL accounted for just 10.8% of teeth, and very few abscesses were observed.[40] While the significant differences between these two sites could be due, at least in part, to differences in the excavation and data recording methods employed by the research teams responsible for this work, it is likely that these populations experienced different living conditions and/or variations in diet. Regardless, even though individuals buried at San Lorenzo di Desenzano appear to have enjoyed relatively good dental health overall, some people still suffered from caries, AMTL, and abscesses.

Age is another factor that sometimes helps to explain the high level of variation between sites. Excavations at a Merovingian-Carolingian cemetery in Cherbourg, for example, uncovered 111 subadult individuals dating from the seventh to eleventh centuries.[41] Within this sample, there was no evidence of carious lesions on permanent teeth, while only 1.3% of deciduous teeth were affected by the disease.[42] This is a strikingly low incidence of caries and unlike any other site involved in the present study: barely any carious lesions were reported despite the relatively large sample size. The results appear less unusual, however, when the age of the individuals is considered. This study focused on a sample of subadults, meaning that, at the time of their death, their teeth had been exposed to cariogenic environments for only a short period of time. Since caries is an age-linked disease that progresses over time, this very low frequency would be expected.

Excepting cases such as Cherbourg, the evidence from most sites looks more like that from Lorsch or Biel-Mett, exhibiting some intra-site variation but, on the whole, moderate to high levels of caries and AMTL. The excavation report of the cemetery at Santa Maria Assunta di Cairate, a rural monastic site used from the late sixth to ninth centuries, provides a detailed assessment of the

40 Alessandro Canci, Alexandra Chavarría Arnau, and Maurizio Marinato, 'Il cimitero della chiesa altomedievale di San Lorenzo di Desenzano (BS): note di bioarcheologia', in *VI Congresso Nazionale di Archeologia Medievale. Sala Conferenze "E. Sericchi", Centro Direzionale CARISPAQ "Strinella 88". L'Aquila, 12–15 settembre 2012*, ed. Fabio Redi and Alfonso Forgione (Florence: All'Insegna del Giglio, 2012), 452–5.

41 V. Garcin, P. Velemínsky, P. Trefny, A. Alduc-Le Bagousse, A. Lefebvre, and J. Bruzek, 'Dental Health and Lifestyle in Four Early Mediaeval Juvenile Populations: Comparisons between Urban and Rural Individuals, and between Coastal and Inland Settlements', *HOMO—Journal of Comparative Human Biology* 61, no. 6 (2010): 421–39, https://doi.org/10.1016/j.jchb.2010.06.004, at pp. 423–4.

42 Garcin, Velemínsky, Trefny, Alduc-Le Bagousse, Lefebvre, and Bruzek, 'Dental Health and Lifestyle', 430.

dental remains recovered from three distinct burial areas.[43] The dental material from Group A, which included sixteen individuals, nearly all of whom were female, were relatively poorly preserved: only fifty-two teeth (out of a possible 512) were identified and all maxillae and mandibles were fragmentary.[44] Given this state of preservation, it is not surprising that only three individuals exhibited signs of caries. However, the carious lesions of one of these individuals were very severe and, despite the fragmentary nature of the jaw bones, extensive AMTL was also noted.[45] Group B, which appears to have been used as the burial area for an elite family, included eight individuals.[46] Although only one individual exhibited evidence of caries, this was another particularly severe case: thirteen teeth, mostly pre-molars and molars, were affected.[47] Finally, the dental remains of Group C, representing the population of the surrounding area, also experienced relatively poor preservation, and only fifteen of the sixty-eight individuals uncovered were analysed.[48] Yet within this sample, eight individuals exhibited carious lesions (five of whom were female), representing a higher frequency of caries than what was reported in Groups A and B. Again, pre-molars and molars were the most affected teeth.[49]

In the excavation reports of early medieval cemeteries in Acqui Terme and Rivoli, the former in use between the seventh and ninth centuries and the latter between the sixth and eighth centuries, it was noted that individuals exhibited high levels of AMTL and caries.[50] Indeed, at least one carious lesion was recorded on all of the female individuals studied and nearly two-thirds of the males.[51] Likewise, a higher incidence of caries was noted among females excavated at the Saint Servatius complex in Maastricht, a site from which eighty-three individuals have been dated to the so-called 'Basilica Phase' of its use,

43 Anny Mattucci, Cristina Ravedoni, and Elena Rettore, 'Analisi antropologica e paleopatologica della popolazione rinvenuta nel monastero dell'Assunta di Cairate', in *Un monastero nei secoli. Santa Maria Assunta di Cairate: scavi e ricerche*, ed. Valeria Mariotti (Mantua: SAP, 2014), 519–32.

44 Mattucci, Ravedoni, and Rettore, 'Analisi antropologica e paleopatologica', 520, 524–5.

45 Ibid, 524–5.

46 Ibid, 520–1.

47 Ibid, 524–5.

48 Ibid, 521–3, 525.

49 Ibid, 525.

50 Francesco Mallegni, Elena Bedini, Angelica Vitiello, Laura Paglialunga, and Fulvio Bartoli, 'Su alcuni gruppi umani del territorio piemontese dal IV al XVIII secolo: aspetti di paleobiologia', in *Archeologia in Piemonte*, ed. Liliana Mercando, Marica Venturino Gambari, and Egle Micheletto, vol. 3 (Turin: Allemandi, 1998), 233–61.

51 Mallegni, Bedini, Vitiello, Paglialunga, and Bartoli, 'Su alcuni gruppi umani', 233–61.

which roughly overlaps with the Carolingian period.[52] Overall, of the thirty-two adults with sufficiently preserved dental remains, over half exhibited evidence of caries and AMTL.[53]

Other sites present a similar picture. Caries were reported for approximately two-thirds of the fifty-eight adults excavated at San Lorenzo di Quingentole, a cemetery used from the late sixth or early seventh to eighth centuries.[54] At Bolgare, a late Lombard necropolis containing the remains of over 400 individuals, the widespread presence of carious lesions was also noted.[55] However, in contrast to these particularly high frequencies, only two out of eleven individuals (18.2%) uncovered at the Church of San Zeno, Campione d'Italia, a site thought to have been used by the descendants of the Lombard merchant Totone, exhibited signs of caries.[56] One of these individuals, however, a male aged roughly fifty years old at the time of his death, presented numerous carious lesions, reflecting the progressive nature of the disease.[57]

While caries are typically the dental pathology most thoroughly addressed in archaeological reports, other aspects of dental health, such as patterns of attrition, evidence of periodontal disease, and the presence of calculus and abscesses are often noted, as well. The dental remains of the single burial found in the church of San Vito di Illegio in Tolmezzo, Udine, for example, were

52 Panhuysen, 'Demography and Health in Early Medieval Maastricht', 206. In total, the excavations of the Saint Servatius site identified 244 individuals buried in and around the church complex dated between *c.* 350 and *c.* 950; the 'Basilica Phase' covers the third and final period of use within this date range (pp. 120–1).

53 Ibid, 206–8.

54 Marco Dal Poz, Francesca Ricci, Bruno Reale, Maddalena Malvone, Loretana Salvadei, and Giorgio Manzi, 'Paleobiologia della popolazione altomedievale di San Lorenzo di Quingentole, Mantova', in *San Lorenzo di Quingentole: archeologia, storia ed antropologia*, ed. Alberto Manicardi (Mantua: SAP, 2001), 151–98.

55 Cristina Cattaneo and Andrea Mazzucchi, 'Popolazioni tardo antiche e dell'alto medioevo narrate dai resti ossei: il progetto di una banca dati lombarda', in *La via Carolingia: uomini e idee sulle strade d'Europa. Dal sistema viario al sistema informativo*, ed. Paola Marina De Marchi and Stefano Pilato (Mantua: SAP, 2013), 87–98.

56 Note: this site contains many more individuals when all phases of use are considered; Phase 2, with eleven individuals, was the most relevant period of use to include in this study. Paul Blockley, Roberto Caimi, Donatella Caporusso, Cristina Cattaneo, Paola Marina De Marchi, Lucia Miazzo, Davide Porta, and Cristina Ravedoni, 'Campione d'Italia. Scavi archeologici nella ex chiesa di San Zeno', in *Carte di famiglia. Strategie, rappresentazione e memoria del gruppo familiare di Totone di Campione (721–877)*, ed. Stefano Gasparri and Cristina La Rocca (Rome: Viella, 2005), 29–80.

57 Blockley, Caimi, Caporusso, Cattaneo, De Marchi, Miazzo, Porta, and Ravedoni, 'Campione d'Italia', 56–8.

described in detail.[58] Dated to the Carolingian period, this individual, another male aged approximately fifty, exhibited evidence of mild periodontitis and deposits of dental calculus. Notably, his teeth were very worn, and this high degree of attrition may explain the relatively low levels of caries reported.[59] Returning to the Saint Servatius complex, periapical abscesses were observed in over half of the assessed individuals (seventeen of thirty-two), while dental calculus was seen in nearly all cases (twenty-eight of thirty-two).[60]

The three groups at Santa Maria Assunta di Cairate display some differences in the degree to which they were affected by the long-term processes of wear as well as their level of calculus accumulation. It was recorded that individuals from Group A, despite their relatively poor preservation, exhibited evidence of periodontitis and a significant build-up of calculus, especially on the canines and pre-molars.[61] Moderate levels of attrition and two cases of abscesses were also recorded. In Group B, all recovered teeth exhibited evidence of wear, though it was fairly light, and, in one case, a large amount of calculus had accumulated.[62] Attrition was greater in Group C, with most individuals exhibiting a moderate level of wear; four individuals, however, showed signs of exceptionally intense wear, resulting in the erosion of the dental crown to the dentine in some teeth.[63] Calculus was noted on the teeth of many individuals, with a particularly large amount reported on two males. Four severe abscesses were recorded, three of which affected females.

An extraordinary case from Seckenheim, a cemetery used from the sixth to eighth centuries, deserves special mention.[64] The individual buried in grave 595 exhibited dental calculus on seven of nine recovered teeth, with two teeth displaying an extremely large build-up of calculus, 'almost dwarfing the teeth

58 Valeria Amoretti, Aurora Cagnana, Paola Greppi, and Andrea Saccocci, 'Lo scavo della chiesa di San Vito di Illegio (Tolmezzo, UD). Una "Eigenkirche" carolingia nelle Alpi Carniche', in *v Congresso Nazionale di Archeologia Medievale. Palazzo della Dogana, Salone del Tribunale (Foggia); Palazzo dei Celestini, Auditorium (Manfredonia); 30 settembre-3 ottobre 2009*, ed. Giuliano Volpe and Pasquale Favia (Florence: All'Insegna del Giglio, 2009), 487–91.

59 Amoretti, Cagnana, Greppi, and Saccocci, 'Lo scavo della chiesa di San Vito di Illegio', 487–91.

60 Panhuysen, 'Demography and Health in Early Medieval Maastricht', 210.

61 Mattucci, Ravedoni, and Rettore, 'Analisi antropologica e paleopatologica', 524–5.

62 Ibid.

63 Ibid, 525.

64 J. L. Hansen and K. W. Alt, 'An Exceptional Case of Dental Calculus in a Merovingian Skeleton from Mannheim-Seckenheim', *Bulletin of the International Association for Paleodontology* 6, no. 2 (2012): 70–6.

themselves'.[65] Five periapical lesions were also noted in the sockets of teeth that were lost ante-mortem and caries were present on one of the remaining teeth, revealing that this individual suffered from very poor dental health.[66] Yet it is the size of the calculus deposits that are the most striking feature: their dimensions 'indicate that the teeth were not used for mastication for some time before death', suggesting that this individual must have consumed a particularly liquid diet in the final years of their life.[67]

The findings reviewed above indicate that many early medieval individuals suffered from a number of different oral health problems. Although there are large variations between sites, it is evident that dental disease would have been a serious concern for all populations: carious lesions were recorded at all sites involved in the present study and are a common cause of AMTL. The loss of teeth in life was probably not only a very painful process, but also potentially debilitating, affecting an individual's ability to eat as well as their appearance. Although most reports did not comment on sex-based differences, at several sites, such as Saint Servatius, Acqui Terme, and Rivoli, it appears that females were more frequently affected by caries, a result that fits with studies from other periods.[68] Molars and pre-molars were often noted as being particularly affected by carious lesions in several reports (and illustrated by Figures 9 and 11), findings that also correspond with the scientific literature on the disease.[69] Although many excavation reports focus more on caries, there is still an extensive record of periodontal disease, abscesses, and calculus build-up within the literature. Overall, the generally high frequency of caries and AMTL, combined with the presence of a number of other pathologies reported at some sites, suggests that dental disease took a significant toll on many individuals during this period.

3 Recipes to Treat Dental Disease

As might be expected based on the osteological record, early medieval medical texts preserve many examples of treatments for dental problems. An in-depth

65 Hansen and Alt, 'An Exceptional Case of Dental Calculus', 72.

66 Ibid.

67 Ibid.

68 Pezo Lanfranco and Eggers, 'Caries through Time', 17. See also Belén López Martínez, Antonio Fernández Pardiñas, Eva García Vázquez, and Eduardo Dopico Rodríguez, 'Socio-Cultural Factors in Dental Diseases in the Medieval and Early Modern Age of Northern Spain', *HOMO—Journal of Comparative Human Biology* 63, no. 1 (2012): 21–42, https://doi.org/10.1016/j.jchb.2011.12.001.

69 Hillson, 'Recording Dental Caries', 250.

review of the recipe literature may provide deeper insights into the nature of this overlap: do treatments comment on particular symptoms or describe the specific problems they target? To what extent does the evidence presented by the osteological remains align with or reshape how the texts have been understood?

Within the recipe sample, 248 recipes are presented as treatments for conditions of the teeth and mouth, such as tooth pain, cavities, and ulcers. In other words, approximately five percent of all recipes analysed in this study address dental disease and related concerns. While many other recipes concern conditions *near* the mouth, such as those intended to treat sore throats, inflamed tonsils, and cracked lips, only recipes that clearly indicate that they were intended to treat symptoms that can be linked to dental conditions have been selected for analysis (this includes recipes in which dental conditions are the only treatment target named as well as recipes in which dental conditions are one of multiple possible targets). A number of prescriptions with ambiguous phrasing that could potentially treat problems of the teeth and mouth have been excluded given their uncertainty.

As seen in Table 10, the recipes can be divided into six general categories according to the information they record. That is, if an early medieval reader came across this text, what would the recipe seem to be intended to treat? Or if an individual were seeking a treatment for a particular condition, such as toothache or putrid breath, what key words would they look for in a recipe collection? As a result, this categorisation is often based on the titles of recipes, though, where applicable, any additional information provided within recipes is also taken into account. The categories are: 1) toothache, 2) ulcers, sores, wounds, and burns, 3) cavities and tooth loss, 4) putridity and cosmetics, 5) general, unspecified mouth complaints, and 6) gum problems.

TABLE 10 Categories of dental pathologies

Categories	# of recipes	% of total (248)
Toothache	121	48.8%
Ulcers, sores, etc.	33	13.4%
Cavities and tooth loss	31	12.5%
Putridity and cosmetics	26	10.5%
Mouth complaints (unspecified)	20	8.1%
Gum problems	17	6.9%

TABLE 11 Specificity of dental pathologies

Specificity	# of recipes	% of total (248)
NSp	22	8.9%
SSp	34	13.7%
HSp	192	77.4%

Naturally, there is some overlap between these categories—ulcers or sores of the mouth, *ulcera oris*, could be due to an underlying cavity, for example, and putrid breath was surely a result of generally poor dental hygiene and related to other oral health problems. Some recipes also mention multiple conditions and could therefore be classified in more than one of the categories. In many of these cases, the recipe's title may present a single (primary) condition/symptom it is intended to treat with additional (secondary) conditions/symptoms listed at the end of the recipe. A recipe to treat bloody gums, *Ad gengiuas plenas sanguinem*, in cod. sang. 751, for instance, ends with a note stating that it is not only a useful treatment for the gums but also for the teeth, throat, and uvula.[70] Similarly, where a series of recipes is listed under a single heading with a primary treatment aim, individual recipes within the series may present extra conditions and symptoms for which these recipes can also be used. Consider a group of nine recipes in BnF lat. 11218 listed under the title *Ad oris uicia*.[71] While this heading indicates that the following recipes are intended to treat unspecified mouth problems, several also record more targeted applications. For example, the sixth recipe in this series, titled *Item ad gingiuas qui reumatizant*, is aimed at treating the gums in addition to more general mouth complaints.[72] When applicable, I have grouped recipes according to their primary treatment target (generally the condition/symptom named in the title), though it is important to remember that some recipes were recorded as treatments for multiple aspects of dental health.

Before considering each category, the specificity of these recipes must be mentioned (see Table 11). As discussed in Chapter 6, it can be helpful to sort recipes into non-specific, semi-specific, and highly specific categories. Non-specific recipes represent very broad, cure-all treatments (typically antidotes) whereas

70 Cod. sang. 751, p. 473: *Ad gengiuas plenas sanguinem ... non solum gengiuas cumtetiris utile est, sed a dentes et faucis et uuam oportum est.* See Appendix 2, entry 9.37.1.

71 BnF lat. 11218, ff. 89r–89v, *Ad oris uicia*. See Appendix 2, entry 3.5.

72 BnF lat. 11218, f. 89v, *Item ad gingiuas qui reumatizant*. See Appendix 2, entry 3.5.6.

TABLE 12 Categories of dental pathologies with breakdown of specificity

Categories	Total	NSp	SSp	HSp
	# of recipes % of 248	# of recipes % of 22	# of recipes % of 34	# of recipes % of 192
Toothache	121 49.1%	11 50.0%	27 79.4%	83 43.2%
Ulcers, sores, etc.	33 13.3%	1 4.5%	2 5.9%	30 15.6%
Cavities and tooth loss	31 12.5%	5 22.7%	1 2.9%	25 13.0%
Putridity and cosmetics	26 10.5%	2 9.1%	2 5.9%	22 11.5%
Mouth complaints (unspecified)	20 8.1%	2 9.1%	2 5.9%	16 8.3%
Gum problems	17 6.9%	1 4.5%	0	16 8.3%

semi-specific recipes treat multiple, potentially related issues, such as general head pain *and* toothache (i.e., a narrowed range of conditions rather a complete panacea). All recipes that target oral pathologies exclusively have been classified as highly specific, including those listing several oral pathologies. Overall, there are very few non- and semi-specific recipes: out of the 248 dental recipes, only twenty-two (8.9%) and thirty-four (13.7%) can be categorised as non- and semi-specific, respectively. The vast majority, 192 (77.4%), are highly specific treatments. Tables 12 and 13 provide a more detailed breakdown, visualising how the specificity of the recipes maps onto the six primary areas of dental health as recorded in recipe titles and descriptions. In the following sections, I consider each of these six categories in more detail before exploring the collective implications of this analysis with respect to the question of applicability.

3.1 *Category 1: Toothache*

As seen in Table 10, 121 recipes mention toothache, *dentium dolorem*. That is, roughly half (48.8%) of all of the recipes within the sample that claim to treat dental conditions fall into this category. Eleven non-specific recipes include

TABLE 13 Specificity of dental pathologies with breakdown of categories

Specificity	Toothache	Ulcers, sores, etc.	Cavities and tooth loss	Putridity and cosmetics	Mouth complaints (unspecified)	Gum problems
	# of recipes % of 121	# of recipes % of 33	# of recipes % of 31	# of recipes % of 26	# of recipes % of 20	# of recipes % of 17
NSp	11 9.1%	1 3.0%	5 16.1%	2 7.7%	2 10.0%	1 5.9%
SSp	27 22.3%	2 6.1%	1 3.2%	2 7.7%	2 10.0%	0
HSp	83 68.6%	30 90.9%	25 80.7%	22 84.6%	16 80.0%	16 94.1%

toothache as one of many, unrelated conditions they are intended to treat, such as the *Antidotus Atrianus* of cod. sang. 217, where *dentium dolorem* is listed alongside over a dozen other ailments, from epilepsy to stomach problems to fevers.[73] Ten of the eleven recipes are explicitly named antidotes.[74] Like the *Antidotus Atrianus*, they each list tooth pain as one of many ailments they claim to cure; these include the *Antidotum sotira* of cod. sang. 44, the *Antidotum Theodosion* also of cod. sang. 217, four antidotes in BAV pal. lat. 1088 (the *Antidotum panchristum* and *Antidotum gera Galieni fortissimo* as well as the *Antidotum Adrianum* and *Antidotum sotira*, variants of two of those already mentioned), the *Antidotum Sancti Paulini* of BAV reg. lat. 598, the *Antidotus polichristus* of BAV reg. lat. 1143, and another version of the *Antidotum sotira* in BnF lat. 11218 (here, titled *Antidotum sotirie*).[75] A preparation for rose oil in cod. sang. 44 represents the only other non-specific recipe that mentions toothache in the sample; although it is not an antidote, it opens with a similarly wide-ranging list of its possible uses and should therefore be grouped with the other catch-all recipes.[76] While these eleven recipes represent a small proportion of the treatments that name toothache (9.1%), they make up half (50.0%) of all non-specific dental recipes within the sample.

Twenty-seven toothache recipes can be considered semi-specific, all of which are intended for a more general condition (or range of conditions) relating to the head and include toothache as part of this broader treatment package. On pp. 257a–258b of cod. sang. 217, for example, a cluster of ten recipes can be found under the heading *Ad capitis*, though the first recipe immediately clarifies that it is intended to treat not only head pain but also problems of the ears, nose, mouth, and, more specifically, long-standing tooth pain, *dentem diutius dolentibus*.[77] Additional examples of recipes aimed at treating head problems and tooth pain jointly can also be found in cod. sang. 217 as well as cod. sang.

73 Cod. sang. 217, p. 262: *Antidotus Atrianus*; see Appendix 2, entry 6.2.

74 On the genre of complex, composite recipes known as antidotes, see Chapter 2.

75 Cod. sang. 44, pp. 234–6: *Antidotum sotira*; cod. sang. 217, pp. 263b–264b: *Antidotum Theodosion*; BAV pal. lat. 1088, ff. 52v–53r: *Antidotum Adrianum*; ff. 53r–53v: *Antidotum panchristum*; ff. 55v–56r: *Antidotum gera Galieni fortissima*, and ff. 59r–59v: *Antidotum sotira*; BAV reg. lat. 598, f. 124r: *Antidotum sancti Paulini*; BAV reg. lat. 1143, ff. 161v–162v: *Antidotus polichristus*; and BnF lat. 11218, ff. 113v–114v: *Antidotum sotirie*. For transcriptions of each of these recipes, see Appendix 2, entries 5.1, 6.3, 16.19–22, 17.1, 18.6, and 3.12, respectively. As seen in the entries of Appendix 2, even when multiple prescriptions share a title and may be related, their ingredients, aims, and overall presentation can vary enormously.

76 Cod. sang. 44, pp. 256–7: *Oleo roseo*. See Appendix 2, entry 5.11.

77 Cod. sang. 217, pp. 257a–258b: *Ad capitis*. See Appendix 2, entry 6.1.

751, BAV reg. lat. 1143, and BnF lat. 11218.[78] Although these twenty-seven recipes represent less than a quarter of those concerning toothache, they make up approximately eighty percent of all semi-specific recipes.

With the aforementioned non- and semi-specific toothache recipes collectively comprising less than a third of the total toothache recipes identified in the sample, the majority of this category of recipes (68.6%) are highly specific. Of these eighty-three recipes, essentially all are titled *Ad dentium dolorem* or present very similar variants. Consider, for example, three different two-recipe clusters in cod. sang. 759: *Ad dentes dolorem trociscus* ('A pill for pain of the teeth', p. 48), *Ad dentes ut numquam doleant* ('So that the teeth never hurt', p. 73), and *Ad dentium dolorem* ('For pain of the teeth', pp. 75–6).[79] A recipe titled *De dentes dolores* in BnF lat. 2849A provides a simple treatment using ivy juice and 'the roots [of a plant] called *spana*' (*de illa radice que dicitur spana*).[80] In addition to these individual recipes or small groupings, toothache treatments can be found in larger clusters. In cod. sang. 217, for example, a group of fourteen recipes for tooth pain is listed under the heading *Item ad dentium dolorem*.[81]

Paradoxically, although there are many more highly specific toothache recipes than non- or semi-specific recipes (eighty-three compared to eleven and twenty-seven, respectively), they comprise a smaller percentage of their specificity category (43.2% as opposed to 50.0% and 79.4%, respectively). The remaining five categories, making up just over half of the dental disease-related treatments in the sample (51.2%), present a somewhat different picture, and I shall return to the significance of these different trends after reviewing the findings from Categories 2–6.

3.2 *Categories 2–6: the Other Half of the Recipes Concerning Oral Health*

Categories 2–6 share a number of features. First, in contrast to the very large number of treatments that fall under Category 1, each of the remaining five

78 Cod. sang. 217, p. 267: *Item ad emigranium seu ad dentium dolorem*; and lower on the same folio, the fourth entry under the heading *Ad dolorem auricule uel aque ingressu*; cod. sang. 751, p. 457: *Purgaturium capitis*; BAV reg. lat. 1143, f. 99r: *Ad emigranium siue dentium dolorem*; and BnF lat. 11218, ff. 50r–50v: *De capite dicit*. See Appendix 2, entries 6.4.11, 6.5.4, 9.34, 18.2, and 3.3, respectively.

79 Cod. sang. 759, p. 48: *Ad dentes dolorem trociscus*; p. 73: *Ad dentes ut numquam doleant*; pp. 75–6: *Ad dentium dolorem*. See Appendix 2, entries 11.4, 16, and 18.

80 BnF lat. 2849A, f. 19r: *De dentes dolores*. See Appendix 2, entry 1.1.

81 Cod. sang. 217, p. 335: *Item ad dentium dolorem*. See Appendix 2, entry 6.9.

categories includes a much smaller number of recipes (see Table 10), since, taken together, they represent approximately half of the recipes relating to dental conditions within the sample (127 recipes). They also have a relatively even distribution of recipes, ranging from thirty-three to seventeen recipes (13.4% to 6.9%) each.

Furthermore, while the majority of the recipes in Category 1 can be classified as highly specific (68.6%), the percentages of highly specific recipes in Categories 2–6 is—without exception—even higher. Collectively, nearly ninety percent of these recipes are highly specific (109 out of 127 recipes), while non- and semi-specific recipes (with eleven and seven recipes, respectively) comprise less than ten percent each. To put it another way, although the toothache recipes of Category 1 are predominantly highly specific, non- and semi-specific recipes still represent a sizeable minority. In contrast, nearly all recipes in Categories 2–6 are highly specific, with only eighteen recipes categorised as either non- or semi-specific. These trends will be reconsidered below.

3.2.1 Category 2: Ulcers, Sores, Wounds, and Burns

In contrast to the consistent Latin phrase seen in Category 1, *dentium dolorem*, several different terms are frequently paired with the standard word for 'mouth', *os* (genitive *oris*), such as *ulcus* (ulcer, sore), *uulnus* (wound, injury), and *ustio* (burn), that suggest various types of mouth sores. The words *ulcus* and *uulnus* have a wide range of meanings, so I have tended to take a broad and flexible approach to interpreting their use in recipes and translate accordingly. Ulcers or sores, *ulcera*, occur most frequently, appearing in nineteen of the thirty-three recipes. Examples include *Ad ulcera oris*, 'For sores of the mouth', in BAV pal. lat. 1088; *Ad ulcera quae in ore nascuntur*, 'For sores that grow in the mouth', in cod. sang. 751; and *Ad ulcera oris uel quicquid in labia fuerint*, 'For sores of the mouth or that are in the lips', in cod. sang. 44.[82] Treatments that mention wounds appear in codd. sang. 217 and 759, such as *Ad uulnera in ore*, 'For wounds in the mouth', in the latter manuscript.[83] All but three of the thirty-three recipes that mention these different types of mouth sores (90.9%) are highly specific treatments. Two treatments found in BnF lat. 11219, including the *Puluis ad uuam leuandam uel oris ulcera*, a powder intended to lift the uvula and treat ulcers of the mouth, align with the semi-specific category,

82 BAV pal. lat. 1088, f. 35v: *Ad ulcera oris uel quidquid intra labiis fuerit*; cod. sang. 751, p. 435: *Ad ulcera quae in ore nascuntur*; cod. sang. 44, p. 361: *Ad ulcera oris uel quicquid in labia fuerint*. See Appendix 2, entries 16.4, 9.26, and 5.26, respectively.

83 Cod. sang. 217, p. 273: *Ad uulnera oris siue tumores gingiuarum*; cod. sang. 759, p. 5: *Ad uulnera in ore*. See Appendix 2, entries 6.7 and 11.2, respectively.

while a panacea-type plaster in BnF lat. 11218 provides the sole example of a non-specific treatment.[84]

3.2.2 Category 3: Cavities and Tooth Loss

The thirty-one recipes making up Category 3 all concern various aspects of tooth loss, including cavities, lost teeth, and loose teeth. Like the varied vocabulary seen in Category 2, an assortment of terms is used to describe to these related issues, associated symptoms, and approaches to treatment. As examples in codd. sang. 44, 751, and BAV pal. lat. 1088 demonstrate, some recipes bear the title *Ad dentem cauum*, offering treatments for cavities.[85] In other cases, teeth are described as moving. Cod. sang. 751, for example, contains a recipe for teeth that move labelled *Item ad dentes qui mouentur*, while BAV pal. lat. 1088 includes a 'Powder for movement of the teeth' titled *Puluis ad dentium commotionem*.[86] Loose teeth are also described, as seen in treatments in cod. sang. 759 and BAV reg. lat. 1143 titled *Ad dentes laxos*.[87] While many of these recipes mention putridity, confirming that there is often overlap between categories, it appears that for all recipes grouped in Category 3, the primary concerns are cavities, tooth loss, and/or tooth mobility whereas putridity is secondary to, or dependent on, the cavities and lost/loose teeth. Consider, for example, the recipe titled *Ad dentes stringendos uel si dolent uel putriscunt aut sanguinant*: keeping or stabilising the teeth is the first stated aim of the treatment, while it also addresses tooth pain and putrid or bleeding teeth.[88]

Twenty-five of the thirty recipes, including all those highlighted so far, represent highly specific treatments; of the remaining six, five are non-specific panaceas while one is a semi-specific recipe. Three of the non-specific recipes are found together in BnF lat. 11218: the first in this group is a plaster titled *Inplastrum Afrodites* and the following two recipes, both beginning with *Item*,

84 BnF lat. 11219, f. 225rb: *Puluis ad uuam leuandam uel oris ulcera*. See Appendix 2, entry 4.5.

85 Cod. sang. 44, p. 360: *Ad dentem cauum*; cod. sang. 751, p. 472: *Item ad dentem cauam*; and BAV pal. lat. 1088, f. 35v: *Item ad dentem cauum*. See Appendix 2, entries 5.24, 9.36.3, and 16.2.7, respectively.

86 Cod. sang. 751, p. 472: *Item ad dentes qui mouentur*; BAV pal. lat. 1088, f. 50r: *Puluis ad dentium commotionem*. See Appendix 2, entries 9.36.6 and 16.14, respectively.

87 Cod. sang. 759, p. 5: *Ad dentis laxos*; BAV reg. lat. 1143, f. 148v: *Ad dentes laxos*. See Appendix 2, entries 11.3 and 18.5, respectively.

88 Cod. sang. 759, p. 92: *Ad dentes stringendos uel si dolent uel putriscunt aut sanguinant*. For similar examples, see also cod. sang. 751, p. 472: *Ad dentes ne cadent neque putriscant*; cod. sang. 899, p. 141: *Ne cadant dentes neque putrescant*; BnF lat. 11218, f. 122r: *Ad dentes stringendas uel si dolent uel putrescunt*. See Appendix 2, entries 11.22, 9.36, 14.6, and 3.14, respectively.

'likewise', are thus linked to it.[89] The plaster names over thirty different conditions it is intended to help, ranging from stomach problems to the bites of various animals (rabid dogs, snakes, and even humans), thereby fitting the model of an antidote despite not being named as such.[90] Within this list, it is noted that the plaster is effective in treating various types of wounds and injuries, including those of the dentition. Since it seems that teeth are mentioned here in relation to being lost (or at least needing to be 'corrected' or 'straightened') as a result of a head injury, I have classified the recipe as fitting with Category 2.[91] The one example of a semi-specific treatment comes from cod. sang. 217. Within a five-recipe cluster intended to treat 'throat constraint', *Ad synances*, the fourth entry notes that this recipe is also intended to help teeth remain in place (*ad dentes constringit*).[92]

3.2.3 Category 4: Putridity and Cosmetics

As seen in Category 3, putridity is noted with some frequency as a secondary or linked dental issue. In other recipes, however, it is named as the primary concern, as illustrated by a cluster of recipes titled *Ad fetorem oris* ('For foul smells of the mouth') in cod. sang. 217.[93] Also included in this category are recipes that seem to put a more positive spin on the attempts to mask rotten teeth and bad breath, such as dentifrices intended to whiten the teeth and/or improve the breath. BAV pal. lat. 1088, for example, includes a 'Dentifrice for brightness of the teeth', *Dentifricium ad dentium splendorem*, followed by one to counteract bad smells emerging from the mouth, *Dentifricium odoris fetorem*.[94]

While the vast majority (84.6%) of these treatments are highly specific, this category also includes two semi-specific and two non-specific recipes. The aforemetioned *Dentifricium odoris fetorem speculare* as well as another dentifrice in cod. sang. 44, *Dentisfritium bonum et salubrem*, can both be considered semi-specific since, in addition to treating bad breath, the recipes address a wider range of issues; although these conditions are largely in the same area

89 BnF lat. 11218, ff. 45v–46r, *Inplastrum Afrodites*, f. 46r, *Item de Afroditis*, ff. 46r–46v, *Item catapodias Eufimie*. See Appendix 2, entries 3.1.1–2 and 3.2, respectively.

90 BnF lat. 11218, ff. 45v–46r, *Inplastrum Afrodites*. See Appendix 2, entry 3.1.1.

91 BnF lat. 11218, ff. 45v–46r, *Inplastrum Afrodites*. E.g., *statim curat et recte dentis capitis plagas*. For the full transcription, see Appendix 2, entry 3.1.1.

92 Cod. sang. 217, p. 338: for the fourth entry of *Ad synances*. See Appendix 2, entry 6.12.4.

93 Cod. sang. 217, p. 274: *Ad fetorem oris*. See Appendix 2, entry 6.8.

94 BAV pal. lat. 1088, f. 50r: *Dentifricium ad dentium splendorem*; f. 50r: *Dentifricium odoris fetorem*. See Appendix 2, entries 16.15–16.

of the body (e.g., in the mouth, throat, and uvula), there are a few exceptions, such as *frigorem*, chills.[95] Although neither of the two remaining recipes, such as the *Sales ieraticas* of cod. sang. 751, are named antidotes, they are both classified as non-specific given the wide array of different conditions they claim to treat, ranging from eye problems to breathing difficulties, alongside rotten teeth.[96]

3.2.4 Category 5: General, Unspecified Mouth Complaints

While the types of tooth and mouth problems listed in some of the preceding categories, such as 'wound' or 'ulcer', usually do not provide much, if any, detail regarding the nature of these ailments, other recipes are even broader in their approach. Category 5 includes all recipes that list *oris uitia*, 'complaints of the mouth', as their intended target. Nineteen such recipes appear in the sample, as does a single recipe for unspecified tooth complaints, *Ad dentium uitiae*.[97] Like the cluster of recipes in BnF lat. 11218 listed under the title *Ad oris uicia* noted above, codd. sang. 217 and 751 also contain small groups of treatments under the headings *Ad uitium oris* and *Ad uitia oris*, respectively.[98] Despite their broad remit, eighty percent (sixteen of the twenty recipes) are classified as highly specific treatments because their only named purpose relates to healing these general afflictions of the mouth.

In addition to these sixteen highly specific recipes, four recipes represent non- and semi-specific treatments. Two recipes, the *Oleo lentisscinum* of cod. sang. 44 and *Emplastrum somato filax* of cod. sang. 761, are catch-all panaceas. Like the aforementioned rose oil preparation, the *Oleo lentisscinum* (mastic oil) is said to be applicable for a wide-ranging list of different ailments, including uterine pain, hardness of the stomach, dysentery, and mouth problems.[99] The *Emplastrum somato filax* claims to treat an even more detailed and diverse list of conditions, opening with dog bites—rabid or otherwise—and also including problems of the eyes, ears, and parotid glands; kidney stones; coughs; gout; etc. The phrase *oris uitia curat*, 'it cures complaints of the mouth', is found near

95 BAV pal. lat. 1088, f. 50r: *Dentifricium odoris fetorem*; cod. sang. 44, p. 248: *Dentisfritium bonum et salubrem*. See Appendix 2, entries 16.16 and 5.8.

96 Cod. sang. 751, p. 418: *Sales ieraticas qui faciunt ad acies oculorum usque senectutę et flegma impetum deducit et suspirium relaxat et dentes putresce non sinit*. See Appendix 2, entry 9.20.

97 Cod. sang. 751, p. 409: *Ad dentium uitiae*. See Appendix 2, entry 9.15.

98 BnF lat. 11218, ff. 89r–89v: *Ad oris uicia*; cod. sang. 217, p. 273: *Ad uitium oris*; cod. sang. 751, p. 435: *Ad uitia oris*. See Appendix 2, entries 3.5, 6.6, and 9.27, respectively.

99 Cod. sang. 44, p. 258: *Oleo lentisscinum*. See Appendix 2, entry 5.12.

the end of this extensive list.[100] A recipe in BnF lat. 11219 with a narrower treatment focus falls into the semi-specific category. Like the *Puluis ad uuam leuandam uel oris ulcera* mentioned in Category 2 (and, in fact, located on the same folio in BnF lat. 11219), the *Puluis uera ad faucium tumorem et omnis oris uitia siue sordicia,* a powder for throat swellings as well as all mouth complaints and unpleasantness, targets a range of problems in the same general area of the body.[101] Another dentifrice found in BAV pal. lat. 1088, the *Dentifritium qui omnem humorem exsiccat,* is similarly semi-specific: its title mentions drying out the humours, and it then opens by claiming to treat all diseases of the mouth before listing more specific applications that extend to the throat.[102]

3.2.5 Category 6: Gum Problems

Seventeen recipes present gum problems as their primary target, such as the several recipes titled *Ad gengiuas*, treatments for the gums, in cod. sang. 751 or those under the heading *Ad exasperationem gingiuarum*, treatments for irritation of the gums, in cod. sang. 44 and BAV pal. lat. 1088.[103] A dentifrice in cod. sang. 44, *Dentisfritium ad gingiuas confortandas et dissicandas,* is more specifically intended to heal and dry out the gums, while a treatment in cod. sang. 217 tackles swollen gums.[104] All but one of the recipes (94.1%) are highly specific; the one exception, the non-specific *Trociscus Eraclio,* is presented as a cure for a diverse assortment of conditions, from ear complaints to various wounds and sores, and problems of the gums are included in this mix.[105]

3.3 *Summary*

With treatments for dental disease and related conditions appearing in nearly five percent of all recipes analysed in this study, oral health represents a significant area of interest within the sampled recipe literature. Treatments intended to combat toothache represent about half of these recipes, while treatments

---

100 Cod. sang. 761, pp. 62–3: *Emplastrum somato filax*. See Appendix 2, entry 12.3.

101 BnF lat. 11219, f. 225ra: *Puluis uera ad faucium tumorem et omnis oris uitia siue sordicia*. See Appendix 2, entry 4.4.

102 BAV pal. lat. 1088, ff. 50r–50v: *Dentifritium qui omnem humorem exsiccat*. See Appendix 2, entry 16.17.

103 Cod. sang. 751, p. 473: *Ad gengiuas plenas sanguinem*; cod. sang. 44, p. 361: *Ad exasperatione gingiuarum*; BAV pal. lat. 1088, f. 35v: *Ad experatione gingiuarum*. See Appendix 2, entries 9.37, 5.25, and 16.3, respectively.

104 Cod. sang. 44, p. 248: *Dentisfritium ad gingiuas confortandas et dissicandas*; cod. sang. 217, p. 337: *Item ad uuam reprimendum et gingiuas tumentes*. See Appendix 2, entries 5.9 and 6.11.3, respectively.

105 Cod. sang. 751, p. 364, *Item trociscus Eraclio*; see Appendix 2, entry 9.4.

for tooth loss and cavities, gum problems and sores affecting the soft tissues, as well as rottenness and putridity (in terms of both odour and appearance) also occur. The vast majority of these treatments are restricted to the oral cavity: in total, 77.4% of the dental health-related recipes can be considered highly specific. In some of these highly specific recipes, multiple dental issues are named, such as cavities and foul smells or tooth loss and gum problems. The thirty-four semi-specific treatments (representing 13.7% of the recipes) target a limited range of additional conditions, and generally those in the vicinity of the mouth, such as problems with the throat. Less than ten percent of the recipes (8.9%) represent cure-all panaceas, revealing that, when a recipe names an aspect (or aspects) of dental health as its intended use, this is consistently—nearly four times out of five—its *only* intended use. In other words, treatments for dental problems often list dental problems exclusively, offering a very targeted approach. Having now reviewed the recipes, it is possible to consider their applicability in the light of the osteological evidence presented above.

4 The Applicability of the Recipe Sample to Early Medieval People

The evidence analysed in this chapter indicates that there is a significant degree of overlap between the skeletal remains and the textual record: the conditions and symptoms that dental remedies claim to treat largely fit with what is observed in the osteological evidence. The early medieval dental remains show clear evidence of dental disease, and this was most often manifested by carious lesions and AMTL, though signs of periodontal disease, calculus build-up, and abscesses were also noted. The recipes, meanwhile, target standard issues that would have arisen from poor dental hygiene, such as toothache, mouth sores, loose or lost teeth, gum problems, and foul-smelling breath. Some of these treatment targets, such as those for cavities and lost or loose teeth, mirror the skeletal remains. Others, including the many recipes for toothache or the dentifrices intended to improve bad breath, treat symptoms that are impossible to see in the osteological record *directly*. However, the surviving skeletal evidence makes clear that such symptoms would have been pressing concerns for many individuals. Indeed, the regular occurrence of dental disease and its ensuing symptoms may help to explain why the vast majority of the recipes offer fairly simple and relatively focused treatments. Ultimately, the parallels between the textual and archaeological evidence indicate that many of the recipes would have been relevant to the individuals who had access to these texts and suggest that these treatments could have been written with the intention of being used in the context of therapy.

While the general picture created by the evidence is thus one of applicability, a closer look at several trends and types of recipes can push this analysis further.

4.1 *Specific Types of Teeth*

As noted above, molars and pre-molars, due to their fissured surfaces and less accessible location at the back of the mouth, are the teeth most susceptible to the development of carious lesions. This fact is not only illustrated by Figures 9 and 11 but was also emphasised in a number of reports; at Santa Maria Assunta di Cairate, for example, molars and pre-molars were recorded as being particularly affected in the second and third burial groups. If, then, these teeth were typically the ones most frequently and severely affected by caries, it is particularly notable that several recipes within Category 1, toothache, mention the molars explicitly. A total of six recipes, such as *Ad dentes molares* of codd. sang. 217 and 1396, are named as molar-specific treatments.[106] Intriguingly, these are the only recipes to target an individual type of tooth. Overall, the osteological evidence suggests that treatments intended for the molars would have been highly relevant, adding further weight the argument that many of the dental recipes would have been applicable to individuals in early medieval Europe.

4.2 *Specific Types of People*

The skeletal evidence at some sites, such as Acqui Terme, Rivoli, and the Saint Servatius complex in Maastricht, suggests that females were more prone to developing carious lesions. These results fit with known, though not fully understood, sex-linked differences regarding the experience and severity of dental disease: certain biological and cultural factors may predispose females to developing caries. Given the direct parallel seen above in the case of molars, it might have been expected that the textual evidence would reflect this difference, as well. However, no treatments are presented as being intended to treat women specifically, and there is no apparent gender-based division of recipes. While the listing of uterine issues in a number of non-specific recipes could be seen as a possible exception to this general finding, gynaecological problems are often included in panaceas, and I would therefore suggest that a gendered reading of these recipes is inappropriate.

While treatments for women are not recorded, a different person-based category did emerge: age. Four recipes targeted teething infants, such as the

---

106 Cod. sang. 217, p. 336: *Ad dentes molares*; cod. sang. 1396, p. 19: *Ad dentes molares*. See Appendix 2, entries 6.10 and 15.1.

treatment titled *Ut infantibus dentes sine dolore exeant* in cod. sang. 44.[107] With this age-based differentiation, it is perhaps surprising that there were no recipes intended for the aging population given that, as confirmed by the osteological evidence, the frequency and severity of dental disease increases with age. It could be argued, however, that most treatments would have simply become *more* applicable with age, thereby making separate recipes that target the tooth conditions of older adults unnecessary. In other words, once an individual's teeth had developed, recipes for toothache, mouth sores, and tooth loss would have been relevant regardless of their age, and senility would not have resulted in new types of oral health problems but rather in higher frequencies of their occurrence and/or increasing severity. In contrast, the teething process is a distinct issue and requires a different treatment. The inclusion of such recipes thus fits with the overall picture of applicability presented by the evidence.

When considering whether different types of patients are recorded in the recipes, it is also important to reflect on another group of people: the potential practitioners (if, of course, these treatments were being consulted in the context of practice). Given that the treatment of dental conditions is found alongside all other types of health concerns rather than separated into distinct treatises focused exclusively on dentistry, there is no sign of specialisation in this respect. Such a finding fits with the general observation that the terminology used to distinguish between different types of medical practitioners expanded in later centuries and was less specialised during the early Middle Ages.[108] It remains possible, however, that the medical marketplace included more specialised practitioners whose activities were not recorded in the surviving written record.

4.3 *Cosmetics*

Given the evidence for severe dental disease, it may seem that dentifrices and tooth whitening treatments are somewhat frivolous: why worry about the whiteness of teeth if they have already been lost or are on their way out? A consideration of the contexts in which these recipes were produced, however, suggests the opposite. As discussed in Chapter 2, the locations in which medical texts were written and housed, whether monastic centres or courtly libraries, were generally elite sites that involved the upper-most strata of society. The privileged circles of the court, aristocratic households, and the ecclesiastical elite represent groups of individuals who may have been especially

107 Cod. sang. 44, p. 304, *Ut infantibus dentes sine dolore exeant*. See Appendix 2, entry 5.16.
108 Park, 'Medicine and Society', 70.

interested in whitening their teeth and avoiding putrid breath. Monica Green has highlighted the 'continuity between "medical" and "cosmetic" concerns' in the context of women's medicine, and I suggest that an interest in cosmetic recipes, such as these dental treatments, should also be read in this light, and with the potential to appeal to men and women alike.[109] Furthermore, Patricia Skinner has argued that the emphasis on injuries (and their penalties) seen in many early medieval law codes reflects not only the practicality of maintaining law and order, but also the significance of an 'unblemished personal appearance' in relation to an individual's honour.[110] While physical injuries, including, notably, dental trauma, are often listed in the law codes, more superficial damage, such as the cutting of hair, can also be found. This focus on appearance and presentation helps to explain the inclusion of cosmetic preparations alongside seemingly more serious issues, from chronic pain to open sores, in early medieval recipe collections. Accordingly, the inclusion of recipes for cosmetic purposes should not be seen to counter their potential applicability.

4.4 *Possible Sources for Dental Recipes*

As mentioned above, it has been suggested that dental health declined between *c.* 1200 BC and *c.* 750 AD.[111] With this in mind, it is important to think about how these recipes compare to classical texts and to reflect on the origins of these treatments. Do many recipes derive from classical and late antique medical writings? Or does a wave of new material appear to have been introduced, coinciding with increasing demands for dental care? As the case studies of Part 1 have shown, both of these patterns, that of preservation and that of addition, have been identified in the recipes under analysis. Within newly compiled recipe collections, some entire clusters of recipes can be traced to known sources while, in other cases, single recipes appear to have been selected from earlier texts individually. A recipe titled *Ad dentium uitiae* noted in Category 5, for example, is located in a short section of recipes derived from Pseudo-Antonius Musa's *De herba vettonica liber* in cod. sang. 751.[112] Here, in the middle of an enormous recipe collection, two groups of recipes on pp. 408–9 present

109 Green, 'Bodies, Gender, Health, Disease', 4.

110 Patricia Skinner, 'Visible Prowess?: Reading Men's Head and Face Wounds in Early Medieval Europe to 1000 CE', in *Wounds and Wound Repair in Medieval Culture*, ed. Larissa Tracy and Kelly DeVries (Leiden: Brill, 2015), 81–101, at pp. 85–9.

111 Pezo Lanfranco and Eggers, 'Caries through Time', 8.

112 Cod. sang. 751, p. 409: *Ad dentium uitiae*. See Appendix 2, entry 9.15.

a selection of material from this late antique herbal. The recipe in question parallels the seventh entry in *De herba vettonica liber*, *Ad dentium uitia*.[113]

For many recipes, however, a direct link a classical or late antique treatise has yet to be identified and their origins remain unknown. In fact, in a handful of cases, some of the new developments in pharmaceutical literature discussed in Part 1 can be seen: the second recipe within a cluster titled *Ad dentium dolorem*, 'for tooth pain', in cod. sang. 759, for example, includes beer in its ingredients.[114] The overall range of recipes relating to dental health—i.e., that many have a basis in classical and late antique traditions, while others reflect new influences—documents an active process of selection. Carolingian scribes engaged with a variety of sources and brought together this assortment of information in new and different ways. As demonstrated in Part 1, the hybrid nature of recipe collections further supports the idea that they were intended to be used in practice.

5 Conclusion

The early medieval skeletal evidence reveals that treatments for tooth problems would have been necessary in the Carolingian world: poor dental health, while not universal, was frequent. All sites reviewed in this chapter provided evidence of dental disease. The recipe literature displays many examples of overlap with the skeletal remains, such as treatments for toothache, tooth loss, and/or mouth sores. Based on the undeniable parallels between the textual and osteological evidence, I argue that the medical knowledge in circulation would have been highly applicable to contemporary populations. Furthermore, certain types of recipes, such as those concerning appearance, suggest that these recipes may have been particularly relevant to the individuals with access to these manuscripts, such as members of royal, aristocratic, or ecclesiastical communities.

This opening case study of Part 2 thus offers a fairly straightforward example of overlap between the two bodies of evidence under analysis: by reading the recipes in the light of the osteological record, it reinforces the idea that these treatments were intended to be put into practice. While this conclusion may not come as a surprise, the process of reaching it has involved a non-traditional

113 Pseudo-Antonius Musa, *De herba vettonica liber*, in *Antonii Musae De herba vettonica liber. Pseudoapulei Herbarius. Anonymi De taxone liber. Sextii Placiti Liber medicinae ex animalibus etc.*, ed. Ernst Howald and Henry E. Sigerist, CML 4 (Leipzig; Teubner, 1927), 3–11, no. 7.

114 Cod. sang. 759, pp. 75–6: *Ad dentium dolorem*; see Appendix 2, entry 11.18.

approach that avoids circular arguments regarding the relationship between medical knowledge and practice. This approach, therefore, enhances our understanding of whether the recipes could have been applied in practice. In the next chapter, I shall employ the same approach to investigate the topic of joint diseases.

CHAPTER 8

Joint Disease

Problematising Podagra

1 Introduction: the Pains of Gout—and the Problems of Translation

Gout, an erosive arthropathy most commonly manifested by excruciating pain in the big toe caused by a build-up of uric acid crystals, is a disease with baggage. Historically, gout has been linked to elites, people with access to rich food and alcohol; today, it is on the rise, affecting between one and four percent of the population in the west.[1] As early as the fifth century BC, there was thought to be a connection between gout and wealth, with Hippocrates describing the condition as the 'arthritis of the rich'.[2] The link between wealth—often interpreted more specifically as dissolute overindulgence—and gout stems from the realisation that those with a meat- and alcohol-heavy diet, i.e., the elite, were more susceptible to developing the disease. Galen agreed with his predecessor, but also posited that there was a hereditary aspect to the condition.[3] Modern medical studies have since confirmed that diet, sex, age, and genetics all play a role in the onset of the disease: males are more prone to developing gout, and risk factors include obesity and weight gain, increasing age, a genetic predisposition, and a diet involving foods and drinks rich in purines, such as meat, seafood, and alcohol.[4] The stereotype that it tends to be seen in older, elite males is not without reason.[5]

How does this stereotype fit with the experience of individuals in early medieval Europe? Do the textual and osteological records provide evidence for the occurrence of gout during this period? And, if so, do they suggest any variation in the prevalence of gout between different populations? A diet rich in meat and alcohol and a more sedentary lifestyle could have been available

1 Gaafar Ragab, Mohsen Elshahaly, and Thomas Bardin, 'Gout: An old disease in new perspective—A review', *Journal of Advanced Research* 8, no. 5 (2017): 495–511, https://doi.org/10.1016/j.jare.2017.04.008, at p. 496.

2 George Nuki and Peter A. Simkin, 'A concise history of gout and hyperuricemia and their treatment', *Arthritis Research and Therapy* 8 (2006), https://doi.org/10.1186/ar1906.

3 Ibid.

4 Ragab, Elshahaly, and Bardin, 'Gout: An old disease in new perspective', 496.

5 Nuki and Simkin, 'A concise history of gout'.

to males in the most privileged strata of society, such as members of royal and aristocratic households and, depending on the strictness with which dietary rules were enforced, ecclesiastical communities, or at least certain members within them.[6] On the other hand, fasting has also been linked to the onset of acute gout attacks, suggesting that members of male ecclesiastical communities may have been particularly susceptible to developing the disease.[7] This subset of the population, as discussed in Chapter 2, overlaps with those individuals who would have been among the most likely to have had access to the medical texts. With these factors in mind, an investigation into gout that brings together written sources and the osteological record is much needed. Moreover, although female religious houses cannot be discounted as centres of manuscript production, the majority of the individuals in royal, aristocratic, and ecclesiastical settings with access to medical texts were probably male, adding further weight to the idea that treatments for gout may have been highly relevant to individuals in these communities.[8]

The evidence for gout is strong in the recipe literature. The Latin term *podagra* (from the Greek *ποδάγρα*) is typically understood to refer to gout in the big toe. I identified *podagra*, related terms (e.g., *podagricum*, as in the *Antidotum podagricum*), and their orthographic variants in nearly 150 recipes within the sample, examples of which will be reviewed below. Indeed, recipes intended to help those suffering from gout have already been seen in several chapters, including the two treatments with which this book opened, the *Potio ad podagra* of cod. sang. 759 and *Antidotum podagricum* of cod. sang. 751. Both provide instructions for a potion involving birthwort, myrrh, laurel berries, and centaury (the treatment in cod. sang. 759 also includes cardamom and parsley) and claim that drinking this mixture for a year will cure the patient of gout.[9] The prevalence of *podagra* in the written sources fits with the idea that the

6 Dietary rules were relaxed, for example, for the ill and elderly; see, for example, *RB 1980*, ed. and trans. Fry, especially Chapters 36–41; *Saint Columban: His Life, Rule, and Legacy*, trans. Terrence G. Kardong (Collegeville, MN: Liturgical Press, 2017), especially Chapters 10 and 15.

7 Leo A. B. Joosten, Mihai G. Netea, Eleni Mylona, Marije I. Koenders, R. K. Subbarao Malireddi, Marije Oosting, Rinke Stienstra, et al., 'Engagement of Fatty Acids with Toll-like Receptor 2 Drives Interleukin-1β Production via the ASC/Caspase 1 Pathway in Monosodium Urate Monohydrate Crystal-Induced Gouty Arthritis', *Arthritis & Rheumatism* 62, no. 11 (2010): 3237–48, https://doi.org/10.1002/art.27667, at p. 3246.

8 See Chapter 2 for more on the environments in which manuscripts were produced. On gynaecological texts in medieval medical writings, see Horden, 'What's Wrong with Early Medieval Medicine?', 11–13; and on female medical practitioners within monastic contexts, see Green, 'Bodies, Gender, Health, Disease', 13–14.

9 Cod. sang. 759, p. 60: *Potio ad podagra*; cod. sang. 751, pp. 489–90: *Antidotum podagricum*. See Appendix 2, entries 11.8 and 9.38, respectively.

individuals most likely to have engaged with the manuscripts in which these recipes are recorded may have been at a higher risk of developing gout. Does the osteological evidence support this idea? Given the underlying assumptions about the potential users of these texts and their possible elevated risk factors for the disease, it is crucial to look beyond the written sources in order to avoid a circular argument.

The evidence for gout in early medieval skeletal remains, addressed below, provides a stark contrast to the rich textual record of *podagra*: osteological evidence for gout is almost entirely lacking in this period. A simple comparison of these two bodies of evidence suggests that the large number of *podagra*-related recipes would have been irrelevant to early medieval populations—can this disconnect be explained? I return to this question after analysing the skeletal and textual evidence for joint disease in other areas of the body. A more general study of joint disease provides a fuller picture of the arthropathies observed in early medieval skeletal remains as well as the treatments for joint pains and related problems recorded in the recipes. Informed by the wider context, it is then possible to revisit the gout-*podagra* paradox. I argue that the apparent incongruence between the textual and osteological evidence can be resolved by recalibrating our interpretation of the term *podagra*. Reading *podagra* as equivalent to a modern medical definition of gout inappropriately restricts our analysis of the Carolingian texts to a contemporary understanding of this disease and its effects. A broader interpretation of *podagra*, however, fits with the textual and osteological evidence. I therefore suggest that the term should often be understood as referring to a collection of symptoms relating to toe and foot joint pain. Such an interpretation could include true gout but is not restricted to this meaning alone. This re-evaluation of *podagra* highlights the danger of understanding a medieval Latin medical term as aligning with a single, clinically defined *modern* medical condition and contributes to current discussions in the field concerning medieval medical terminology and lexicography. Secondly, the new interpretation of *podagra* has major implications for the question of applicability, indicating that, despite the initially conflicting evidence, many of the treatments recorded in the recipe collections would have been highly relevant to individuals in early medieval Europe.

2 The Appearance of *Podagra* in Medical Recipes

The textual evidence from eighth- and ninth-century recipe collections appears to support the idea that gout was a fairly common condition and a pressing concern among those who compiled and had access to the texts: 140 recipes within the sample of recipes involved in this study (roughly 2.5%) claim to cure *podagra* and/or to alleviate the pain linked to the disease.[10] This relative frequency seems to fit with the aforementioned idea that those individuals, whether writing in monastic centres or active at the royal court, were most probably members of the elite and enjoyed a more privileged lifestyle associated with a number of the risk factors for gout.

As with the other case studies in Part 2, the following review of recipes takes into account their specificity. With respect to *podagra*, recipes that list *podagra* as one of many unrelated conditions, such as antidotes, are considered non-specific; recipes that treat a small number of conditions presenting potentially similar or related symptoms, such as those that treat both *podagra* and *artriticus* ('afflictions of the joints', discussed below), are classified as semi-specific; and those that only refer to *podagra* are considered highly specific. The distribution of recipe specificity will be important to keep in mind when comparing *podagra*-related treatments to those of other joint diseases later in this chapter.

Nearly fifty percent of the recipes that mention *podagra* (sixty-seven of the 140 recipes) are non-specific treatments (see Table 14). Unlike the dental conditions considered in the previous chapter, *podagra* and related terms are frequently named as one of the many ailments targeted by antidotes. The *Antidotum gera Galieni fortissimo* of BAV pal. lat. 1088, for example, presents a list of just under fifty different conditions it is intended to treat, including epilepsy, paralysis, eye problems, gynaecological conditions, fevers, breathing problems, and skin conditions; in the middle of the list, it is noted that the antidote provides relief to those suffering from *podagra*.[11] Other examples of non-specific treatments include the *Antidotum gira deacoloquintidis* (noted in Chapter 3 for its use of camphor, *cafora*), which is also found in BAV pal. lat. 1088. This antidote claims to help individuals suffering from approximately twenty-five different ailments, ranging from vertigo to liver pain, and, like the *Antidotum gera Galieni fortissimo*, includes those afflicted with *podagra*.[12] As mentioned in Chapter 3, the list ends with the particularly bold claim that, in addition to curing present infirmities, this potion will also defend against future ills (*non solum presentes infirmitates curat, sed futuras egritudines defendit*). The *Anteditum Teodoritum* of cod. sang. 759, offers another cure-all treatment; the term *podagricis* can be found near the end of a long list of maladies. In line with the *Antidotum gira deacoloquintidis*, this antidote not only claims

10 As noted above, I include recipes using the terms *podagra*, *podagricis*, etc. as well as their orthographic variants.

11 BAV pal. lat. 1088, ff. 55v–56r: *Antidotum gera Galieni fortissima*. See Appendix 2, entry 16.21.

12 BAV pal. lat. 1088, f. 90r: *Antidotum gira deacoloquintidis*. See Appendix 2, entry 16.26.

TABLE 14 Overview of the specificity of recipes that mention *podagra*

Specificity	NSp	SSp	HSp	Total
# of Recipes	67	31	42	140
% of total	47.9%	22.1%	30.0%	100%

to take care of a host of different diseases in the present, but also to repel the onset of future infirmities.[13]

Not all non-specific antidotes, however, aim to treat scores of different conditions: the *Antidotum pigra Gallieni optimum* and *Antidotum filantropum*, both of cod. sang. 44, for example, only list about a dozen different afflictions.[14] While these antidotes may appear to be more specific due to the reduced number of diseases they are intended to treat, they continue to list a wide range of unrelated ailments, from stomach pain to epilepsy, and both, importantly, include *podagra*, within this mix.[15] These 'simplified' antidotes, therefore, represent abridged versions of comprehensive cures rather than more specialised treatments.

In contrast to the frequent appearance of *podagra* within the antidotes seen above, only thirty-one recipes, or 22.1% of the recipes that target *podagra*, represent semi-specific treatments. These preparations continue to treat multiple conditions, but they do not cover the full range of health problems seen in the non-specific reicpes. The *Oxira podagricis* of cod. sang. 751, for example, is presented as a treatment for sufferers of gout as well as *omnem dolorem*, all pain.[16] While the inclusion of *omnem dolorem* makes the scope of this treatment very broad, it relates entirely to pain management. As such, the *Oxira podagricis* is intended for one type of medical issue—admittedly, one very wide-ranging

13 Cod. sang. 759, p. 2: *Anteditum Teodoritum*. Not unlike the *Antidotum gera Galieni fortissima* (above), this antidote includes the phrase: *non solum presentibus curat egritudines sunt et futuris aduenientis infirmitates repellit*. See Appendix 2, entry 11.1.

14 Cod. sang. 44, p. 238: *Antidotum pigra Gallieni optimum* and *Antidotum filantropum*. See Appendix 2, entries 5.2–3.

15 The *Antidotum pigra Gallieni optimum* begins by listing the following conditions: *Qui facit stomaicis, epilenticis, melancolicis, freneticis, epaticis, spleneticis, podacricis, uertigines, caligines, typus subito, metus saltus, membrorum neruorum contractiones, perfrictiones, et quod liber stupor, uel mulieris uitia, et ad omnes causas quę subito ueniunt emendant.* The *Antidotum filantropum* lists the following conditions: *Facit tissicis, dipnoicis, cefalargicis, stomaticis, ad toraces, limosotis dissolutis, epaticis, spleneticis, colicis, aliis doloribus, nefreticis, podacricis*. For full transcriptions, see Appendix 2, entries 5.2–3.

16 Cod. sang. 751, p. 419: *Oxira podagricis*. See Appendix 2, entry 9.22.

issue—and not the full spectrum of conditions and concerns listed in the panaceas.

Some semi-specific recipes, however, are narrower in their focus. An earlier recipe in cod. sang. 751, the *Unguentum acupo galastico*, is intended to cure gouty or arthritic pains and swellings, for example.[17] In this case, although the treatment targets more than *podagra* alone, the range of conditions it claims to cover is limited to a cluster of potentially related issues. Similarly, the *Malagma aduersus dolores fracturas et podagra ad luxum* of cod. sang. 759 treats pain from fractures, gout, and dislocations.[18] BAV pal. lat. 1088 offers a comparable treatment on f. 65v, the *Potio contra artreticam siue nesciam uel podagram*, which combats gout, hip pain, and arthritis.[19] While none of these recipes targets gout exclusively, each one is intended to treat a range of ailments that would have had somewhat similar symptoms, especially with respect to pain.

Finally, out of the 140 remedies that mention gout, forty-two (30.0%) offer treatments highly specific to *podagra* (again, see Table 14). Cod. sang. 44, for example, records the following recipe:

> For gout: take equal measures of birthwort, centaury, and acacia powder and mix with cyclamen juice; apply this on [the toe].[20]

The *Potio ad podagra* of cod. sang. 759 and *Antidotum podagricum* of cod. sang. 751, the two Terenti(an)us recipes noted above, also fall into the specific category as they target *podagra* exclusively. Intriguingly, their recipes contain some parallels to the previous example, *Ad podacra* of cod. sang. 44, with all three prescriptions listing birthwort and centaury among their ingredients.[21] Cod. sang. 751 presents another treatment titled *Antidotum podacricum* forty-five pages earlier; this *Antidotum podacricum*, however, offers an unrelated recipe involving pepper, cumin, and ginger.[22] This entry also specifies that the treatment helps to reduce foot pain (*ad pedis dolorem sedatur*).

---

17 Cod. sang. 751, p. 319: *Unguentum acupo galastico ad omnem dolorem uel tumorem tam podagricis quam artetricis*. See Appendix 2, entry 9.2.

18 Cod. sang. 759, p. 63: *Malagma aduersus dolores uel fracturas et podagra ad luxum*. See Appendix 2, entry 11.11.

19 BAV pal. lat. 1088, f. 65v: *Potio contra artreticam siue nesciam uel podagram*. See Appendix 2, entry 16.25.

20 Cod. sang. 44, p. 260: *Ad podacra. Aristologia rotunda, centauria, agatia puluis ęquali pondere, cum succu ciclaminis distemperas et superpone proficit*. See Appendix 2, entry 5.13.

21 Cod. sang. 759, p. 60: *Potio ad podagra*; cod. sang. 751, pp. 489–90: *Antidotum podagricum*. See Appendix 2, entries 11.8 and 9.38, respectively.

22 Cod. sang. 751, p. 444: *Antidotum podacricum ad pedis dolorem sedatur*. See Appendix 2, entry 9.30.

Having now reviewed recipes in which *podagra* is mentioned, the evidence for gout in the skeletal remains must be considered.

3 The Absence of Gout in Archaeological Contexts

In contrast to the prevalence with which *podagra* is named in textual sources, osteological evidence for gout is extremely limited in this period. Analyses of early medieval skeletal remains have produced very few examples of probable cases of gout, though it is important to recognise that preservation biases may have contributed to the lack of evidence for this erosive arthropathy. Since the metatarsal-phalangeal joint at the base of the big toe is the most common and well-known site of an acute inflammatory gout attack, this is the most useful skeletal element to assess, but small bones, such as the phalanges, are more fragile and susceptible to decay. Male skeletal remains, however, tend to be found more often and in a better state of preservation due to both excavation biases and biological factors.[23] Since males are more predisposed to developing gout, these particular excavation and preservation biases work in this study's favour, offering a greater chance of recovering sufficiently preserved skeletal material from the individuals who would have been more likely to suffer from this condition. With this in mind, the relative absence of gout is even more striking.

It must also be noted that a number of other conditions can present similar destructive arthropathies on the bones of the feet, including leprosy, rheumatoid arthritis (RA), and osteomyelitis, but each one has distinguishing features which, if there is sufficient preservation of skeletal material, would allow for a differential diagnosis.[24] RA and leprosy, for example, would typically present pathologies in other parts of the skeleton: RA tends to affect multiple joints in addition to the feet and toes (most notably the hands), while leprosy results in necrosis of the face and hands alongside the feet and toes. It is therefore possible that the actual incidence of gout is higher than reported, but, due to the state of preservation, such a specific diagnosis has not been given.

23 For biases of preservation, see Roberts, *Human Remains in Archaeology* (see especially Chapter 3, 'Resting Places for the Dead, and Factors Affecting Preservation of Bodies').

24 Gaspare Baggieri and Francesco Mallegni, 'A Probable Case of Gout', *Medicina Historica* 1, no. 1 (2017): 23–8, at pp. 25–7; Jenna M. Dittmar, Piers D. Mitchell, Peter M. Jones, Bram Mulder, Sarah A. Inskip, Craig Cessford, and John E. Robb, 'Gout and 'Podagra' in medieval Cambridge, England', *International Journal of Paleopathology* 33 (2021): 170–81, https://doi.org/10.1016/j.ijpp.2021.04.007.

At present, probable cases of gout have only been identified among individuals buried at two early medieval sites within the Carolingian Empire (both in northern Italy), though additional cases have been recorded in both earlier and later periods as well as in other geographic areas, such as the British Isles.[25] The urban cemetery of Piazza Marconi in Cremona, in use from the seventh to the tenth centuries, contained 141 individuals, while the burial area in Bolgare, with over 400 individuals, was used in the seventh and eighth centuries.[26] The sheer size of these cemeteries may help to explain why gout was observed: given that the disease only affects one to four percent of the population today (a population with a diet relatively high in purines), a higher frequency of gout should not be expected in the past.[27]

A number of the other excavations considered in this study, however, uncovered large cemeteries comparable to Cremona and Bolgare and yet yielded no skeletons with evidence suggestive of probable cases of gout. The burial area excavated at Santa Maria Assunta di Cairate, for example, produced ninety-two individuals, and the excavations at Seckenheim, a site in use from the sixth to the late eighth centuries, analysed 112 skeletons; evidence of gout was reported from neither excavation.[28] It is worth remarking that the skeletal remains at Seckenheim have been noted for their exceptionally good preservation. Furthermore, many of the sites under consideration are thought to have contained elite burials, such as Lorsch, where separate burial areas for the monks, *familia* of the monastery, and possibly pilgrims have been uncovered, and Campione d'Italia, which appears to have contained the remains of a privileged merchant family, the descendants of a certain Totone.[29] Overall, the lack of evidence for gout at many different sites around the Carolingian

25 Baggieri and Mallegni, 'A Probable Case of Gout', 23–8; Juliet Rogers, Iain Watt, and Paul Dieppe, 'Arthritis in Saxon and Mediaeval Skeletons', *British Medical Journal* 283 (1981): 1668–70, https://doi.org/10.1136/bmj.283.6307.1668; Dittmar, Mitchell, Jones, Mulder, Inskip, Cessford, and Robb, 'Gout and 'Podagra''.

26 Cattaneo and Mazzucchi, 'Popolazioni tardo antiche e dell'alto medioevo', 87–98.

27 Ragab, Elshahaly, and Bardin, 'Gout: An old disease in new perspective', 496.

28 Valeria Mariotti, ed., *Un monastero nei secoli. Santa Maria Assunta di Cairate: scavi e ricerche* (Mantua: SAP, 2014); Denise Navitainuck, Christian Meyer, and Kurt W. Alt, 'Degenerative Alterations of the Spine in an Early Mediaeval Population from Mannheim-Seckenheim, Germany', *HOMO—Journal of Comparative Human Biology* 64, no. 3 (2013): 179–89, https://doi.org/10.1016/j.jchb.2013.03.007; and Hansen and Alt, 'An Exceptional Case of Dental Calculus', 70–1.

29 Kropp, Kirsch, Rosendahl, Orschiedt, and Fischer, *Begraben und Vergessen?*, and personal communications with members of the scientific board of Lorsch, including Claus Kropp and Hermann Schefers; Blockley, Caimi, Caporusso, Cattaneo, De Marchi, Miazzo, Porta, and Ravedoni, 'Campione d'Italia', 29–80.

world, combined with its low frequency in large burial complexes, suggests that this disease was not a significant medical problem for many people during this period.

The absence of gout in the skeletal remains may seem puzzling given the relatively high frequency with which *podagra* is mentioned in medical recipes. Can the gap between the written sources and osteological record be reconciled? Or does the lack of overlap between these two bodies of evidence suggest that some of the medical knowledge circulating in the eighth and ninth centuries did not, in fact, relate to the needs of contemporary individuals? To answer these questions, it is necessary to assess the textual and osteological evidence for other joint diseases to build a more complete picture of arthropathic conditions in the Carolingian world. The gout-*podagra* paradox can then be re-evaluated against this background.

4 Moving Beyond Gout: Evidence for Other Arthropathies in the Osteological Record

Although gout has been recorded very rarely, many other forms of arthritis have been consistently noted in skeletal assemblages from early medieval sites. Fundamentally, joint diseases tend to be separated into two categories, proliferative and erosive, based on their pathology. Osteoarthritis (OA), the bony reaction to the degeneration of articular cartilage, is the 'archetypical proliferative joint disease' and the most commonly seen pathology overall, often affecting the vertebrae, shoulders, hips, knees, ankles, and feet.[30] Gout represents a classic erosive arthropathy: well-defined round or oval erosions of the bone are caused by 'the precipitation of uric acid crystals in structures either in or around a joint', most frequently the metatarsal-phalangeal joint of the big toe.[31] Other erosive joint diseases include RA, psoriatic arthritis, and ankylosing spondylitis. Like gout, these conditions only affect a small percentage of the total population and would therefore be expected to be found in archaeological contexts only relatively rarely. Unlike gout, however, descriptions of these diseases are fairly recent (no earlier than the seventeenth century), and

30 Tony Waldron, 'Joint Disease', in *A Companion to Paleopathology*, ed. Anne L. Grauer (Chichester: Wiley-Blackwell, 2012), 513–30, at p. 513; Waldron, *Palaeopathology*, 24–71; Adelaide Tosi, Paola Badino, Barbara Pezzoni, 'Medical Conditions Observed in Osteoarchaeological Remains: Arthropathies, Traumatic Lesions, Tumours, Metabolic Diseases and Dental Pathologies', *Medicina Historica* 1, no. 1 (2017): 29–34, at p. 30.

31 Waldron, *Palaeopathology*, 68.

their diagnostic features are not recorded in pre-modern texts.[32] With this in mind, I shall concentrate primarily on osteological evidence for OA.

Changes that occur on the surface of a bone as a result of OA include the formation of new bone, often seen as bone spurs; pitting on the surface of the joint; alterations of the joint contour, such as widening or flattening; and the development of an eburnated, highly polished area on the surface of the joint.[33] According to Tony Waldron, OA can only be said to be present if eburnation is apparent or if at least two of the other changes noted above exist.[34] It is necessary to take a conservative approach to the diagnosis of OA since there can be a 'difference between skeletal appearances and clinical experiences', and palaeopathological analyses will lack information about pain as reported by a patient.[35] Similarly, when considering joint disease in the vertebrae, the development of Schmorl's nodes (protrusions formed as a result of damage to the vertebral endplate) does not necessarily cause back pain.[36] Schmorl's nodes are, however, often linked to other spondyloarthropathies (joint diseases of the spine) and seen in association with bio-mechanical stress on the lower back.[37] Therefore, if evidence of these nodes is found alongside other spinal pathologies, it can be assumed that the populations under consideration would have experienced back pain to some degree.

The development of OA is primarily linked to the aging process and the long-term wear on joints through daily activity, though metabolic and genetic factors as well as injuries, obesity, and sex also have an impact on the prevalence and severity of this pathology.[38] The natural effects of aging and physical activity, especially among populations involved in heavy labour, such as agricultural work, help to explain the pervasiveness of these conditions. I shall elaborate on the evidence for OA and joint stress in the following categories: 1)

32 Waldron, *Palaeopathology*, 46–74; Waldron, 'Joint Disease', 521–9.

33 Waldron, *Palaeopathology*, 27–8.

34 Ibid, 33.

35 Ibid, 31.

36 Waldron, *Palaeopathology*, 45; Tosi, Badino, Pezzoni, 'Medical Conditions Observed in Osteoarchaeological Remains', 30. See, too, the discussion on 'clinical correlation' in Robert D. Jurmain and Lynn Kilgore, 'Skeletal Evidence of Osteoarthritis: A Palaeopathological Perspective', *Annals of the Rheumatic Diseases* 54 (1995): 443–50, https://doi.org/10.1136/ard.54.6.443, at p. 446.

37 Ibid.

38 Waldron, *Palaeopathology*, 28; Tosi, Badino, Pezzoni, 'Medical Conditions Observed in Osteoarchaeological Remains', 29–30; Mattucci, Ravedoni, and Rettore, 'Analisi antropologica e paleopatologica', 523–4.

the spine, 2) large joints and limbs: shoulders, elbows, hips, and knees, and 3) small joints: hands and feet.

4.1 *The Spine*

In the palaeopathological reports consulted in this study, the spine tends to be recorded as the area most frequently and severely affected by arthropathies.[39] At the site of Seckenheim, 112 adults with largely complete and well-preserved spines were analysed. This sample yielded 2599 vertebrae and 106 sacral bones, allowing for a particularly detailed analysis.[40] Evidence of stress and arthritis of the spinal column was present in 111 individuals (99.1%), and the frequency and severity with which individuals were affected by arthritic changes increased with age.[41] Furthermore, nearly three-quarters (73.2%) of these individuals presented at least one vertebra with evidence of Schmorl's nodes.[42] While this site has recorded exceptionally high frequencies of OA and signs of associated pathologies, it must be noted that, in many cases, these arthropathic changes were not very severe. The high prevalence of spondyloarthritis within the Seckenheim sample may therefore be explained by their unusually good state of preservation. Indeed, the authors of this report suggest that the lower frequencies of OA recorded at other sites are due to their less-well preserved skeletal remains.[43] This interpretation fits with the contrasting results from the excavation of the La Perosa site in Rivoli, a rural cemetery used from the sixth to eighth centuries.[44] Here, just under ten percent of the sample of thirty-four adults presented evidence of joint diseases. As a corollary to the Seckenheim report, this study's authors acknowledge that such a low incidence of joint disease is probably due to the poor state of preservation of the skeletal remains.[45]

Most sites report evidence of joint disease, and especially OA of the vertebrae, at frequencies between the two extremes of Seckenheim and La Perosa, often affecting between thirty and forty percent of individuals. This intermediate level of joint disease reporting is probably due in large part to the more moderate degree of preservation seen at many of the sites under consideration. While the extremely good preservation seen at Seckenheim is uncommon,

39 Mallegni, Bedini, Vitiello, Paglialunga, and Bartoli, 'Su alcuni gruppi umani', 233–61.
40 Navitainuck, Meyer, and Alt, 'Degenerative Alterations of the Spine', 179–83.
41 Ibid.
42 Ibid, 183.
43 Ibid, 185.
44 Mallegni, Bedini, Vitiello, Paglialunga, and Bartoli, 'Su alcuni gruppi umani', 233–61.
45 Ibid.

in-depth palaeopathological studies are rarely pursued when preservation is very poor. At the rural cemetery excavated at Corso Roma in Acqui Terme, in use from the seventh to ninth centuries, roughly thirty percent of the sample of twenty-nine adults presented evidence of joint disease, with spondyloarthritis the most commonly recorded condition.[46] Similarly, of the ninety individuals uncovered at San Lorenzo di Quingentole, a rural church with a surrounding burial area dated to the eighth century, 38.4% exhibited signs of stress in their vertebrae.[47]

Although the vertebral column is almost universally the most severely affected area of the skeleton (an exception to this will be discussed below), particular areas of the back exhibit varying levels of severity at different sites. For instance, all adult males from Campione d'Italia (three individuals out of a group of eleven skeletons) present evidence of spinal arthritis, with the lumbar vertebrae the most affected area.[48] Similarly, among the individuals dated to the 'Basilica Phase' of the Saint Servatius site, the lower back tended to exhibit more signs of degenetive disc disease than the cervical and upper thoracic vertebrae.[49] These findings contrast with the rural cemetery excavated at San Martino di Ovaro. This cemetery was in use from the sixth to early eleventh centuries and included thirty-one individuals, thirteen of whom can be more precisely dated between the seventh and ninth centuries. The individuals dated to this period exhibited a greater degree of degeneration in their thoracic vertebrae.[50] Not unlike the population buried at Seckenheim, spondyloarthropathies were seen in nearly all individuals. Certain patterns of wear are often related to particular activities, working conditions, and walking surfaces, and therefore suggest that individuals at the sites under examination experienced different lifestyles and/or engaged in a variety of different activities, some of which stressed specific parts of the back more than others. Overall, however, it is evident that joint diseases of the spine were very prevalent in these populations. Given the diversity of sites under analysis, the relatively high frequencies with which these conditions are seen reflect the great extent with which individuals in early medieval Europe were affected by spondyloarthritis.

---

46 Ibid.

47 Dal Poz, Ricci, Reale, Malvone, Salvadei, and Manzi, 'Paleobiologia della popolazione altomedievale di San Lorenzo di Quingentole', 171–6.

48 Blockley, Caimi, Caporusso, Cattaneo, De Marchi, Miazzo, Porta, and Ravedoni, 'Campione d'Italia', 56–8.

49 Panhuysen, 'Demography and Health in Early Medieval Maastricht', pp. 191–3.

50 Valeria Amoretti, 'Analisi paleobiologiche dei resti scheletrici', in *Lo scavo di San Martino di Ovaro (sec. V–XII). Archeologia della cristianizzazione nel territorio di Aquileia*, ed. Aurora Cagnana (Mantua: SAP, 2011), 481–536.

4.2 *Large Joints and Limbs: Shoulders, Elbows, Hips, and Knees*

While the spine often appears to be the most frequently and severely affected area of the skeleton, there is extensive evidence for arthropathies in other joints. Regular physical activity engages the large joints of the shoulders, hips, knees, and elbows, leading to wear and tear over time. The intense physical labour associated with agricultural work, blacksmithing, horseback-riding, carrying heavy objects, etc., would put these joints under even more significant bio-mechanical stress, and the skeletal remains from early medieval cemeteries confirm the active living and working conditions experienced by most people during this period. For many individuals who lived long enough, this intense physical activity has been documented by their skeletal remains.

Although the excavation of San Lorenzo di Quingentole recorded typical levels of spinal arthropathies (with approximately forty percent of the population exhibiting signs of stress on their vertebrae), it is exceptional in that the spine was not the *most* severely affected part of the body. Unlike all other sites considered in this study, the skeletal remains from San Lorenzo di Quingentole display more evidence of arthropathies affecting the shoulder.[51] Signs of stress were also recorded in the elbows and extremities, though the severity of stress decreased along the upper limbs.[52] That is, while the shoulder was the most acutely affected area of the body, evidence of joint disease in the elbows was not as severe and the hands even less so. In-depth analyses of the pathologies of several individuals at this site were highlighted as case studies in the excavation report. The skeleton buried in Tomb 33, for example, a male aged between forty and fifty years old, presented evidence of OA in the shoulders, hips, and knees based on eburnation and signs of bone formation.[53] Although the shoulders exhibited more signs of OA than the spine at this site, the authors of the report do not interpret this atypical finding as suggestive of particularly unusual or distinctive labour, such as mining, but regard it as evidence of fairly standard activities, such as agricultural work, wood chopping, and fishing. It is, however, noted that the heavy, clay-rich soil may have played a role in the accumulation of shoulder-stress in relation to agricultural activities and land reclamation.[54]

The excavation of the large, rural monastic cemetery at Santa Maria Assunta di Cairate produced over two hundred skeletons, and the third phase of its

51 Dal Poz, Ricci, Reale, Malvone, Salvadei, and Manzi, 'Paleobiologia della popolazione altomedievale di San Lorenzo di Quingentole', 171–6.

52 Ibid.

53 Ibid.

54 Ibid.

use, dated between the sixth and ninth centuries, included ninety-two individuals. While the spine was the area most affected by OA, signs of arthritic changes were present on the bones of the shoulders, hips, and knees of many individuals.[55] Similarly, at Acqui Terme, three of the twenty-nine adults, over ten percent, had markers of OA in their hips; the sacroiliac joints of two individuals and coxofemoral joint of the third were particularly affected.[56] Looking to comparative sites beyond the Carolingian world, cemeteries from the British Isles paint a similar picture. Juliet Rogers, Iain Watt, and Paul Dieppe's study of arthritis in medieval English skeletons, for example, noted that 'hip and shoulder osteoarthritis were both common' in the seven cemeteries analysed.[57] Of the fifty skeletons dated to the early medieval period involved in their study, roughly a quarter presented evidence of advanced osteoarthritic changes in the shoulders and nearly thirty percent in the hips.[58] Overall, the skeletal evidence indicates that OA was a common condition during this period, affecting not only the spine but also the large joints, and especially the shoulders and hips.

4.3 *Small Joints: Hands and Feet*

Although evidence for gout was very limited at the sites involved in this study, signs of OA in the small joints of the extremities have been noted in many reports. At Bolgare, for example, arthritis and other foot problems were frequent: roughly thirty percent of the population exhibited small fractures in their feet and toes due to repeated microtraumata that resulted from the accumulation of bio-mechanical stress and injuries.[59] Two males from Acqui Terme showed signs of OA in their feet: the left calcaneus and talus of one individual was particularly affected, while the phalanges of the right foot of the other individual recorded bony changes associated with the condition.[60] At Lorsch, an individual buried in the cemetery area associated with pilgrims and dated to the ninth or tenth centuries presented similar pathologies in his right ankle, including osteophytic growth around the calcaneus.[61] One of the three males from Campione d'Italia with spondyloarthritis also exhibited severe OA in his

55 Mattucci, Ravedoni, and Rettore, 'Analisi antropologica e paleopatologica', 523–4.

56 Mallegni, Bedini, Vitiello, Paglialunga, and Bartoli, 'Su alcuni gruppi umani', 233–61.

57 Rogers, Watt, and Dieppe, 'Arthritis in Saxon and Mediaeval Skeletons', 1669.

58 Ibid.

59 Cattaneo and Mazzucchi, 'Popolazioni tardo antiche e dell'alto medioevo', 88–90.

60 Mallegni, Bedini, Vitiello, Paglialunga, and Bartoli, 'Su alcuni gruppi umani', 233–61.

61 Personal communications with Claus Kropp and unpublished notes from the 1990 excavation season at Lorsch.

feet; this individual died at a relatively advanced age (fifty to sixty years old), fitting the severity of his arthritis.[62] As noted above, the excavation report of San Lorenzo di Quingentole concentrated on a handful of skeletons (out of the ninety-two excavated), providing detailed analyses of their pathologies.[63] One of these individuals, a male aged between forty and fifty, exhibited major signs of stress in a variety of joints: in addition to evidence of OA in the vertebrae, shoulder, elbow, hips, and knees, extensive osteophytic growth was observed in the ankles as well as roughness around the surfaces of these joints.[64] These types of developments suggest that the affected individuals either experienced prolonged periods of walking or running and/or carried substantial weight that resulted in significant stress on the ankles and feet.[65]

Arthropathies of the hands were less frequently recorded, though still noted at a number of sites. Individuals at Santa Maria Assunta di Cairate, for example, displayed evidence of OA in their hands.[66] At San Lorenzo di Quingentole, males exhibited significantly more stress in their hands than females.[67] Most notably, evidence suggestive of RA was recorded at the site of Piazza Marconi in Cremona and possibly also at San Lorenzo di Desenzano, a rural cemetery with twenty-eight individuals dating from the seventh to eleventh centuries.[68] At the latter site, an arthropathy observed on the left ring finger of one individual could be due to RA or several other causes, including trauma.[69] The evidence from Cremona, on the other hand, is very convincing, in large part because it is seen repeatedly within the site, and the onset of RA is strongly linked to genetic and environmental factors.[70] These two sites present the only possible examples of erosive arthropathies (in addition to the cases of gout noted above) identified within the sites under consideration.

The general trend seen in the skeletal evidence suggests that OA and minor traumata of the ankles, feet, toes, and, to a slightly lesser extent, hands, were

62 Blockley, Caimi, Caporusso, Cattaneo, De Marchi, Miazzo, Porta, and Ravedoni, 'Campione d'Italia', 54–5.

63 Dal Poz, Ricci, Reale, Malvone, Salvadei, and Manzi, 'Paleobiologia della popolazione altomedievale di San Lorenzo di Quingentole', 151–95.

64 Ibid, 171–6.

65 Ibid.

66 Mattucci, Ravedoni, and Rettore, 'Analisi antropologica e paleopatologica', 523–4.

67 Dal Poz, Ricci, Reale, Malvone, Salvadei, and Manzi, 'Paleobiologia della popolazione altomedievale di San Lorenzo di Quingentole', 171–6.

68 Waldron, *Palaeopathology*, 46–53.

69 Canci, Chavarría Arnau, and Marinato, 'Il cimitero della chiesa altomedievale di San Lorenzo di Desenzano (BS)', 452–5.

70 Cattaneo and Mazzucchi, 'Popolazioni tardo antiche e dell'alto medioevo', 91–2.

widespread issues, affecting a sizable proportion of the population. In contrast, evidence of erosive arthropathies was extremely limited. Crucially, that evidence of various types of arthritic changes in the hands and especially the feet were observed and recorded with regularity—while signs of gout were not—indicates that evidence suggestive of gout has not been simply overlooked or underreported but that it is, in fact, lacking.

4.4 *Summary*

The skeletal evidence reveals that joint disease affected a significant percentage of the population. OA was the most prevalent condition reported, although possible cases of RA were also recorded at two sites. While the spinal column was almost always recorded as the most frequently affected area of the body, both large and small joints also exhibited signs of OA, testifying to the active lifestyles and physically demanding living conditions of many individuals. Before reassessing the relationship between gout and *podagra* with respect to this evidence, the treatments recorded for other arthropathies must be surveyed to provide the full picture of joint disease.

5 Textual Evidence for Joint Pain Beyond *Podagra*

In contrast to the big toe, pains associated with most other joints and joint areas, such as the back, shoulders, neck, elbows, and knees, have not been linked to a particular disease concept. Relatedly, and also unlike the case of *podagra*, a distinct, localised vocabulary has not emerged to address most other joint aches. That is, when pains related to the knees or shoulders, for example, are noted in recipes, they tend to be recorded in a simple, straightforward fashion, using phrases such as *ad geniculorum dolorem* ('for pain of the knees') and *ad scapularum dolorem* ('for pain of the shoulders').

The hips, however, present an important exception with some parallels to *podagra*. On the one hand, the use of the standard Latin term for hip, *coxa*, mirrors that of the aforementioned joints, appearing in expressions such as *ad coxarum dolorem* ('for pain of the hips'). On the other hand, two additional terms, *sciatica* and *nescia*, also refer to problems associated with the hips. Like *podagra*, these words a) have a Greek origin (in this case, both are Latinised descendents of ἰσχία (*ischia*), meaning 'hips' or 'hip joint'), and b) gave rise to a wider vocabulary of related words (e.g., *sciaticus*, describing someone suffering from *sciatica*).[71] Notably, in modern translations of classical and late antique medical texts, *sciatica* and *nescia* are often given as loosely defined hip conditions, with translators opting for broader interpretations of these terms rather than identifying them with a specific ailment.[72] A more open-ended interpretation recognises not only the complexity of past understandings of pain and disease, but also how they may differ from modern medical understandings—even when certain individual terms, such as 'sciatica', remain in use today. These more cautious translations highlight the need for a critical re-evaluation of *podagra*. The following analysis of the ways in which pain in joints beyond (or in addition to) the big toe appears in the recipe literature provides a framework for contextualising *podagra* and, ultimately, re-assessing the gout-*podagra* paradox.

Before reviewing the textual evidence, it is important to outline the terms and joints/joint areas under consideration. In this analysis, I consider major joints and joint areas that are linked to pain in recipes, including the neck, shoulders, lower back, hips, knees, and hands. I also consider recipes that refer to unlocalised joint aches and pains, tracing the appearance of terms such as *articulus*, 'joint', and *artriticus*, a condition defined by Isidore of Seville as 'an affliction of the joints'.[73] Rather than reading this term as 'arthritis' in a modern medical sense, I use Isidore's description of *artriticus* as 'an affliction of the joints', following the broader interpretations of *nescia* and *sciatica* noted above.

Likewise, this investigation takes an inclusive approach to the recipe literature.[74] While many treatments are explicitly focused on managing the aches

71 Isidore, *Etymologiae*, 4.7.29: *Sciasis vocata a parte corporis, quam vexat. Nam vertebrorum ossa, quorum summitas iliorum initio terminator, Graeci ἰσχία vocant*. See also: Isidore, *The Etymologies of Isidore of Seville*, trans. Barney, Lewis, Beach, and Berghof, 112.

72 Yvette Hunt, for example, translates *sciaticis* as 'sufferers of hip-disease', and notes that the condition is 'variously translated as hip-gout, hip-disease, and even sciatica despite its modern use relating to the sciatic nerve. It has been translated as "hip-disease" to allow the broadest possible understanding'; see *The* Medicina Plinii, trans. Hunt, 2.3 (and commentary at p. 176). Jutta Kollesch and Diethard Nickel translate *sciatica* as 'Hüftschmerzen', hip pain; for many examples, see Book 25 (on cures for lower back and hip pain) of Marcellus, *De medicamentis liber*, ed. Liechtenhan and Niedermann, trans. Kollesch and Nickel. Unusually, Hunt is similarly cautious with the term *podagra*; see *The* Medicina Plinii, trans. Hunt, 2.27 (and commentary at p. 215). Cf. Marcellus, *De medicamentis liber*, ed. Liechtenhan and Niedermann, trans. Kollesch and Nickel, Book 34, and Isidore, *The Etymologies of Isidore of Seville*, trans. Barney, Lewis, Beach, and Berghof, 4.7.31 (at p. 112).

73 Isidore, *Etymologiae*, 4.7.31: *Artriticus morbus ab articulorum passione vocabulum sumpsit*; translation from: Isidore, *The Etymologies of Isidore of Seville*, trans. Barney, Lewis, Beach, and Berghof, 112.

74 It is impossible to be entirely comprehensive in this analysis given the differences in how individuals feel, understand, and describe pain (and its causes). I have not, for example,

and pains of specific joints, the phrasing of some recipes can be more ambiguous. Consider, for example, recipes titled *Ad ceruicis dolorem*, 'For pain of the neck', and *Ad renum dolorem uel coxarum*, 'For pain of the kidneys or hips'.[75] The former is intended to treat neck pain and thus offers a remedy for a general joint area, the cervical spine. The latter, in contrast, claims to treat kidney and hip pain, a combination that raises the following question: should it be understood as a treatment for internal pains in the lower abdomen and pelvic region (including the kidneys, bladder, urinary tract, and so on) or a treatment for kidney pain as well as hip *joint* pain? In these types of cases, recipe titles (and any extra details contained within the recipes themselves) rarely provide a conclusive answer, and I include such recipes in the analysis if it appears possible that they were intended as treatments for joint pains alongside or in concert with other aims.

On this basis, I have identified 218 recipes that could be interpreted as targeting joint afflictions or pain other than or in addition to *podagra*. As in the preceding analyses, I have categorised these treatments by specificity, using the same parameters to divide them into non-specific, semi-specific, and highly specific groups (see Table 15). I have also investigated the distribution of target joint(s) and joint area(s) (see Table 16). The results of these analyses present both parallels to and divergences from the opening case study on *podagra*; I shall review how nonlocalised joint afflictions appear in the recipes before turning to individual joints and joint areas.

5.1 *General Afflictions of the Joints*

Within the sample, eighty-four recipes offer treatments intended for general 'joint afflictions' and joint pain. These recipes cover the full spectrum of specificity, and the non- and semi-specific treatments often target multiple joint issues, including *podagra*. In this discussion, I shall use 'general joint afflictions' as shorthand for recipes that mention either *artriticus* or problems affecting the *articuli*.[76] Of these eighty-four references to general joint afflictions,

---

included treatments for *omnem dolorem* ('all pain') in this study given that such a description is entirely open-ended, but it is, of course, possible that such recipes were intended to treat joint pains as part of their comprehensive coverage.

75 Examples of recipes entitled *Ad ceruicis dolorem* or *Ad dolorem ceruicis* can be found in codd. sang. 751, 759, and BAV pal. lat. 1088, while *Ad renum dolorem uel coxarum* is located in cod. sang. 44, p. 345. For an example of the former, see Appendix 2, entry 9.33; for the latter, see entry 5.19.

76 While the term *artriticus* appears more often, general problems with and pains of the *articuli* are sometimes mentioned, too; see, for example, cod. sang. 751, p. 404: *Ad uicia articulorum*. For the transcription, see Appendix 2, entry 9.11.

TABLE 15 Overview of the specificity of recipes for joint pain other than or in addition to *podagra*

Specificity	NSp	SSp	HSp	Total
# of Recipes	68	49	101	218
% of Total	31.2%	22.5%	46.3%	100%

thirty-six instances (42.9%) occur in non-specific panaceas, twenty-six (31.0%) represent semi-specific treatments targeting a range of similar conditions, and twenty-two (26.2%) are highly specific recipes focused exclusively on nonlocalised joint afflictions (see Table 17). These findings are fairly similar to the analysis of *podagra* recipes: in both cases, non-specific recipes make up the largest category, while the number of semi-specific and highly specific recipes represent between a quarter and third of the recipes.

By taking this analysis further and considering the specificity of treatments in relation to the different types of joint conditions named alongside general joint afflictions, a more nuanced picture emerges. In thirty-seven recipes, as shown in Table 16, *artriticus* and *articulus* are the only joint-related terms mentioned. To clarify, this is not to say that these are all highly specific recipes (according to the levels of specificity used in these analyses); rather, these are recipes in which the only joint-related condition listed concerns general joint afflictions, no matter the total number of conditions they claim to treat. The number of recipes in this category, therefore, is nearly twice that of specific recipes in this category (twenty-two, as seen in Table 17) because, although *artriticus* might be the only *joint* disease mentioned in some non-specific recipes, it is found alongside a host of other conditions, such as epilepsy, stomachache, and skin problems. On the other hand, over half of the recipes that include general joint afflictions as a target (forty-seven recipes, 56.0%) aim to treat additional, named joints and joint areas: *podagra* is included thirty-five times, while sixteen recipes list at least three different joints or joint areas. Of the thirty-five recipes that refer to both *artriticus* and *podagra*, nineteen (54.3%) are found in panaceas, whereas sixteen (45.7%) are semi-specific treatments, such as the *Potio contra artreticam siue nesciam uel podagram* of BAV pal. lat. 1088 or the *Unguentum acupo galastico* of cod. sang. 751, both noted above.[77]

77 BAV pal. lat. 1088, f. 65v: *Potio contra artreticam siue nesciam uel podagram*; cod. sang. 751, p. 319: *Unguentum acupo galastico ad omnem dolorem uel tumorem tam podagricis quam artetricis*. See Appendix 2, entries 16.25 and 9.2, respectively.

TABLE 16 Number and percentage of recipes for joint pain other than or in addition to *podagra* presented by target area[a]

a. General 'joint afflictions' (*artriticus, articulus*)				
	Total # of recipes with general 'joint afflications' as a target	# of recipes in which general 'joint afflictions' is the only joint pain mentioned	# of recipes in which general 'joint afflictions' & *podagra* are the only joint pain mentioned	# of recipes in which general 'joint afflications' are named with ≥ 2 other joint areas
#	84	37	35	16
% of 218	38.5%	17.0%	16.1%	7.3%
% of 83	100%	44.0%	41.7%	19.1%
b. Neck (*ceruix*)				
	Total # of recipes with the neck as a target	# of recipes in which the neck is the only joint area mentioned	# of recipes in which the neck & shoulders are the only joint areas mentioned	# of recipes in which the neck is named with ≥ 2 other joint areas
#	21	12	4	5
% of 218	9.6%	5.5%	1.8%	2.3%
% of 21	100%	57.1%	19.1%	23.8%

TABLE 16 Number and percentage of recipes for joint pain other than or in addition to *podagra* presented by target area (*cont.*)

c. Shoulders (*scapulae*)			
	Total # of recipes with the shoulders as a target	# of recipes in which the shoulders are the only joint area mentioned	# of recipes in which the neck & shoulders are the only joint areas mentioned
#	18	16	4
% of 218	8.3%	7.3%	1.8%
% of 18	100%	88.9%	22.2%

d. Lower back area (*lumbus*)			
	Total # of recipes with the lower back area as a target	# of recipes in which the lower back is the only joint area mentioned	# of recipes in which the back & hips are the only joint areas mentioned
#	15	6	10
% of 218	6.9%	2.8%	4.6%
% of 15	100%	37.5%	66.7%

TABLE 16 Number and percentage of recipes for joint pain other than or in addition to *podagra* presented by target area (*cont.*)

e. Hips (*coxae, nescia, sciatica*)					
	Total # of recipes with the hips as a target	# of recipes in which the hips are the only joint area mentioned	# of recipes in which *coxae* is used	# of recipes in which *nescia* is used	# of recipes in which *sciatica* is used
#	107	68	25	41	43
% of 218	49.1%	31.2%	11.5%	18.8%	19.7%
% of 107	100%	63.6%	23.4%	38.3%	40.2%
f. Knees (*genua, genicula*)					
	Total # of recipes with the knees as a target	# of recipes in which the knees are the only joint area mentioned	# of recipes in which the knees are named with ≥ 2 other joint areas		
#	18	9	5		
% of 218	8.3%	4.1%	2.3%		
% of 18	100%	50.0%	27.8%		

TABLE 16 Number and percentage of recipes for joint pain other than or in addition to *podagra* presented by target area (*cont.*)

g. Hands (*manus*)			
	Total # of recipes with the hands as a target	# of recipes in which the hands are the only joint area mentioned	# of recipes in which the hands are named with ≥ 2 other joint areas
#	5	1	4
% of 218	2.3%	0.5%	1.8%
% of 5	100%	20.0%	80.0%

h. Multiple targets (≥ 3 joints/joint areas)	
	Total # of recipes targeting ≥ 3 joints/joint areas
#	22
% of 218	10.1%
% of 22	100%

Note:

a The numbers of recipes in individual categories do not add up to their respective totals because a) the table presents a selection of the most important combinations of targeted joints/joint areas, and b) under 'e. hips', several individual recipes use two of the three terms, thereby elevating their totals.

TABLE 17 Recipes that target general joint afflictions by specificity

Specificity	NSp	SSp	HSp	Total
# of Recipes (% of Total)	36 (42.9%)	26 (31.0%)	22 (26.2%)	84 (100%)

Thirteen of the sixteen recipes that claim to treat at least three different joints and joint areas are non-specific, while just three are semi-specific. Thus, when general joint afflictions are listed alongside *podagra* or listed with multiple named joints and joint areas, the recipes tend to be non-specific panaceas, though semi-specific treatments that pair the pains of *podagrici* and *artritici* represent a significant minority within the sample.

When general joint afflictions are the only joint-related condition mentioned in a recipe, a different picture emerges: roughly three-fifths of the treatments are highly specific (twenty-two out of thirty-seven recipes, 59.5%). Examples include the *Unguentum ad artiticus* of BAV reg. lat. 1143 and *Gyma artreticis* of cod. sang. 759.[78] Five recipes (13.9%) are semi-specific, including two versions of a recipe entitled *Catarticum artreticis et ydropicis* intended to treat general joint pains and dropsy, while nine (25.0%) are non-specific, such as the *Oxira crocira* of BAV pal. lat. 1088, which claims to cure over fifteen different conditions, including general joint afflictions but also spleen, liver, and kidney problems, the bites of snakes and rabid dogs, and so on.[79] The ratio of these recipes' specificity contrasts with the *podagra* study, as illustrated in Table 14, where roughly half of the recipes are classified as non-specific and just thirty percent are highly specific.

Within the semi-specific treatments, the pairing of general joint afflictions with knee pain stands out as a recurring cluster. In three different treatments, these two joint issues—one general and one localised to a particular

78 BAV reg. lat. 1143, f. 169r: *Unguentum ad artiticus*; cod. sang. 759, p. 61: *Gyma artreticis*. See Appendix 2, entries 18.7 and 11.9, respectively.

79 Cod. sang. 44, p. 250: *Catarticum artriticis et idropicis*; cod. sang. 759, p. 58: *Catarticum artreticis ydropicis*; BAV pal. lat. 1088, f. 60r: *Oxira crocira facit epaticis, spleneticis, ad ypocondria, tensiones nefreticis, ad omnem neruorum tensiones, pleureticis, peripleumonicis, artriticis, sciaticis, et omnem neruorum contractiones, et luxas, et fracturas, et incisos neruos soluit, autem et omnes duritias, et ad serpentium morsus, et canis rabii morsum*. See Appendix 2, entries 5.10, 11.7, and 16.23, respectively.

joint—are grouped together. Consider, for example, the *Unguentum artitricis uel geniculorum dolorem* of cod. sang. 751, an ointment for those suffering from afflictions of the joints or knee pain, or the *Unguentum ad febrientes* of BAV pal. lat. 1088.[80] Although the latter recipe may not appear to offer a treatment for joint pain, the following phrase appears after its instructions for preparing the ointment: *similiter a genibus usque ad summum articulorum* ('similarly for knees and for all joints'), suggesting that the same preparation can also be used to alleviate afflictions of the knees and other joints.[81]

Recipes that target general joint afflictions thus present a complex picture: when this is the only type of joint issue recorded in a recipe, the treatment is often highly specific, presenting a recipe targeted at alleviating nonlocalised joint complaints. When paired with *podagra*, however, it is entirely non- or semi-specific, with many examples of cure-all panaceas. On the other hand, in the handful of cases where knee pain is the only other joint issue mentioned, the recipes tend to take a more targeted approach, claiming to offer both general and localised pain relief. Looking at this another way, out of the 218 recipes that may target joint diseases other than or in addition to *podagra*, sixty-eight are non-specific, and thirty-five of these (51.5%) involve general joint afflictions. Nonlocalised joint pains are thus mentioned in just over half of the non-specific remedies that treat joint disease other than or in addition to *podagra*. As seen in Table 15, I have classed forty-nine of the 218 recipes as semi-specific and 101 as highly specific. General joint afflictions are recorded in twenty-six and twenty-two recipes, respectively (53.1% and 21.8%), revealing that, broadly, as specificity increases, references to general joint afflictions decrease. There are still recipes that claim to target general joint issues exclusively, but, in the wider context, catch-all terms such as *artriticus* appear more frequently in non- and semi-specific treatments.

5.2 *Named Joints and Joint Areas: the Back, Neck, Shoulders, Hips, Knees, and Hands*

The back, neck, shoulders, hips, knees, and hands are mentioned as target areas in many recipes, whether individually or in combination with each other as well as the other joint-related terms discussed above. Having considered how nonlocalised joint afflictions appear in recipes, I shall now concentrate on the occurrence and distribution of aches and pains linked to these named

80 Cod. sang. 751, p. 320: *Unguentum artitricis uel geniculorum dolorem*; BAV pal. lat. 1088, f. 62r: *Unguentum ad febrientes*. See Appendix 2, entries 9.3 and 16.24.1.

81 BAV pal. lat. 1088, f. 62r: *Unguentum ad febrientes*. See Appendix 2, entry 16.24.1.

joints and joint areas. Out of the 313 recipes within the sample that appear to be intended to treat named joint aches and pains, 124 recipes remain when references to *podagra* and general joint afflictions are excluded (see Table 18). This selection presents a number of striking differences when compared to the previous analyses.

First, while nearly half of the recipes targeting *podagra* and over forty percent of those for general joint afflictions are classified as non-specific treatments, only twenty percent of these 124 recipes fall into the same category. The vast majority, approximately four-fifths, of these treatments are more specific in their focus.[82] Although these twenty-five non-specific recipes are much like the other non-specific treatments addressed above in that they claim to treat a vast range of ailments and are typically based on a large number of primarily exotic ingredients, they are unusual in one respect: in place of *podagra* and/or *artriticus* (terms seen so frequently in general antidotes and other panaceas), a specific joint area is named. The *Antidotus polichristus* of BAV reg. lat. 1143, for example, is recorded as a cure for hip pain as well as tooth pain, paralysis, vomiting blood, and so on.[83] As Table 18 illustrates, in all but one joint category, non-specific recipes comprise less than twenty percent of each group. The one exception, recipes that include the term *sciatica* (and related words), reverses this trend: nearly eighty percent of recipes that offer treatments for 'hip disease' using this word are non-specific. Indeed, if all recipes featuring *sciatica* and its related terms (twenty-three recipes) are removed from the sample, only seven of the remaining 101 recipes, or about five percent, are non-specific panaceas, highlighting the much more targeted nature of this recipe selection overall. That is, catch-all antidotes that list scores of individual diseases and ailments rarely list joint conditions other than *podagra*, *artriticus*, and *sciatica*. When other joints and joint areas are named in recipes, the treatments tend to be directed specifically at remedying the named joint(s) or joint area(s).

Semi- and highly specific recipes have been grouped together in Table 18 because many of the semi-specific treatments pair two neighbouring joints or joint areas, such as the neck and shoulders or the lower back and hips. Despite listing multiple areas, these recipes present very targeted treatments. Indeed, of the ten recipes that claim to offer relief for pain in the lower back and hips, for example, nine target this combination alone. The one exception is found in

82 As seen in Table 18, I have combined semi- and highly specific recipes in these cases because the semi-specific recipes generally present treatments that target two, nearby joint areas, such as the hips and lower back (as discussed below), and thus essentially offer highly specific treatments, even though two different joints or joint areas are named.

83 BAV reg. lat. 1143, ff. 161v–162v: *Antidotus polichristus*. See Appendix 2, entry 18.6.

TABLE 18 Number and percentage of recipes for joint pain with references to neither *podagra* nor general joint afflictions presented by specificity

a. Total number of recipes that mention joints without also referring to *podagra* and general joint afflictions (*artriticus, articulus*)			
Specificity	NSp	SSp/HSp	Total
# of Recipes	25	99	124
% of Total	20.2%	79.8%	100%
b. Neck (*ceruix*)			
Specificity	NSp	SSp/HSp	Total
# of Recipes	1	17	18
% of Total	5.6%	94.4%	100%
c. Shoulders (*scapulae*)			
Specificity	NSp	SSp/HSp	Total
# of Recipes	0	18	18
% of Total	0%	100%	100%
d. Lower back area (*lumbus*)			
Specificity	NSp	SSp/HSp	Total
# of Recipes	2	12	14
% of Total	14.3%	85.7%	100%
e. Hips (*coxae*)			
Specificity	NSp	SSp/HSp	Total
# of Recipes	2	18	20
% of Total	10.0%	90.0%	100%
f. Hips (*nescia*)			
Specificity	NSp	SSp/HSp	Total
# of Recipes	3	34	37
% of Total	8.1%	91.9%	100%
g. Hips (*sciatica*)			
Specificity	NSp	SSp/HSp	Total
# of Recipes	18	5	23
% of Total	78.3%	21.7%	100%
h. Knees (*genua, genicula*)			
Specificity	NSp	SSp/HSp	Total
# of Recipes	2	9	11
% of Total	18.2%	81.8%	100%
i. Hands (*manus*)			
Specificity	NSp	SSp/HSp	Total
# of Recipes	0	2	2
% of Total	0%	100%	100%

a small cluster of recipes in cod. sang. 751 under the heading *Ad laterum dolore*, 'For side pain'. The second treatment in this group extends to the hip and lower back: 'Likewise, burnt cabbage with grease, applied to the sides or the hips and lower back, heals wonderfully'.[84]

Moreover, when recipes are ordered according to the *a capite ad calcem* structure ('from head to heel'), there can be some ambiguity regarding the treatment targets. Consider, for instance, a group of recipes in BAV pal. lat. 1088 with the title, *Ad lumborum dolores*, 'For pain of the lower back'.[85] While the first recipe is limited to the lower back, the following treatment begins *Item ad lumborum uel coxarum dolores*, 'Likewise, for pains of the lower back or hips', while the third and final entry of the cluster is simply titled *Item*. In this case, I would suggest that the third recipe also targets both lower back and hip pain, though it is possible that it was intended just for lower back pain, the aim identified by this group's main title. A parallel case can be found in cod. sang. 44, while, in cod. sang. 751, a group of recipes located under the heading *Ad dolorem ceruicis*, 'For pain of the neck', are similarly expanded to include shoulder pain.[86] In line with the lower back examples, the second recipe starts *Item si escapulas doluerint*, 'Likewise, if the shoulders hurt', and the next two simply start with *Item*, 'Likewise'.[87]

While the pairing of individual joints and joint areas can thus be somewhat ambiguous, the majority of these recipes (sixty-nine of 101, 68.3%) represent highly specific treatments exclusively focused on a single joint/joint area. Of the eighteen recipes for shoulder pain, for instance, eight are semi-specific (including recipes that pair neck and shoulder pain) and ten are highly specific. Examples include three recipes under the heading *Ad scapularum dolorem*, 'For pain of the shoulders', in cod. sang. 44 and a recipe titled *Ad scabule dolorem* in BnF lat. 11218.[88] Intriguingly, the second recipe of the cluster in cod. sang. 44 has close parallels to the recipe in BnF lat. 11218, highlighting the shared sources of these different collections and the movement of medical

84 Cod. sang. 751, p. 461: *Item [Ad laterum dolore]. Caulae cumbustae cum exungia lateribus uel coxis et lumbis adpositus mire sanat.* See Appendix 2, entry 9.35.2.

85 BAV pal. lat. 1088, ff. 41r–41v: *Ad lumborum dolores*; *Item ad lumborum uel coxarum*; *Item.* See Appendix 2, entries 16.8.1–3.

86 Cod. sang. 44, p. 367: *Item ad lumborum uel coxarum dolorem*; cod. sang. 751, p. 457: *Ad dolorem ceruicis.* See Appendix 2, entries 5.31.2 and 9.33.1, respectively.

87 Cod. sang. 751, p. 457: *Item si escapulas doluerint*; *Item*; *Item.* See Appendix 2, entry 9.33.2–4.

88 Cod. sang. 44, pp. 361–2: *Ad scapularum dolorem*; BnF lat. 11218, f. 96v: *Ad scabule dolorem.* See Appendix 2, entries 5.27 and 3.6, respectively.

knowledge. Though not identical, both recommend applying a mixture of vervain and fresh beans cooked in wine with fat.

As noted above, recipes that claim to alleviate hip problems present a more complicated picture with respect to specificity. Treatments that include *sciatica* and related terms are exceptional among the subset of recipes that target named joints and joint areas: this particular terminology is seen much more often in wide-ranging antidotes and only rarely in highly specific remedies. On the other hand, as seen in Table 18, recipes that describe hip issues with words related to *coxa* and *nescia* are precisely the opposite: within the sample, no less than ninety percent of these recipes are semi- or highly specific. Notably, the recipes that include *coxa*-based words are fairly evenly split between semi- and highly specific treatments and include all instances of the lower back-hip pairing. In contrast, treatments for *nescia*, such as the *Potio ad nesciam* in BAV pal. lat. 1088, are almost entirely highly specific recipes that exclusively target this condition (thirty-two out of thirty-seven, 86.5%).[89] The different ways in which these three hip terms appear within the sample suggests some underlying distinctions in their use, including differences in how the terms were understood. The variation in vocabulary could also be linked to different sources, and tracing the transmission of each term may help to shed light on the movement of particular texts and traditions as well as the construction of new recipe collections in the early medieval west.

Overall, although each individual joint category examined in this section contains a lower number of recipes when compared to treatments for *podagra* or general joint afflictions, when viewed together, they indicate that treatments for named joints are often very targeted. While there are important exceptions, many of these recipes are intended exclusively for just one or two joints and/or joint areas in the same part of the body. These recipes and their contexts must now be reconsidered in the light of the skeletal evidence presented above.

6 Integrating the Evidence: a Return to the Gout-*Podagra* Paradox and the Question of Applicability

Having now reviewed the textual evidence for joint afflictions and pain in a variety of joints and examined the skeletal evidence for arthropathies in early medieval populations, it is possible to return to the gout-*podagra* paradox. Crucially, the following reappraisal is based on a comparative approach that

89 BAV pal. lat. 1088, f. 90r: *Potio ad nesciam*. See Appendix 2, entry 16.27.

employs looser, more flexible translations. This enables a broader approach to their interpretation, contrasting with the standard identification of *podagra* as 'gout'. After re-evaluating the relationship between gout and *podagra* with this new perspective on the appropriateness of this direct, one-for-one translation, I shall turn to the question of applicability, reflecting on all of the joints and joint areas addressed in this chapter.

6.1 *Gout Versus* Podagra*: Conflicting Evidence or a Modern Misnomer?*

This chapter's opening study presented a paradox: *podagra* is well-represented by textual sources, yet gout, according to current palaeopathological evidence, is nearly invisible in the osteological record. Does this disjuncture indicate that the medical recipes circulating in Carolingian manuscripts were, at least in this case, largely irrelevant to the populations who possessed them? As cautioned in Chapter 6, such a conclusion should not be automatically assumed since there are many reasons why probable cases of gout have not been observed in the osteological record. However, the fact that evidence for other types of joint diseases, including in the feet, is so frequently observed indicates that the lack of skeletal indicators suggestive of gout likely reflects that it was not a common condition—indeed, a low incidence of gout in the past, even at sites thought to have relatively high-risk populations, should not be surprising given that the disease only affects between one and four percent of people in the west today. Why, then, is *podagra* so frequently seen in pharmaceutical writings?

Instead of reading the disparity between the two bodies of evidence as a sign that recipes claiming to treat *podagra* were not widely applicable, I argue that, by considering the wider context, i.e., the evidence for arthropathies in other joints, a different conclusion should be drawn. Although *podagra* has traditionally been translated directly as gout, such a simple, one-for-one translation seems inappropriate on the basis of this chapter's findings—are the texts really describing a *single* condition? If the interpretation of *podagra* is broadened to include more generalised toe and foot joint pain, the skeletal evidence and written record begin to align. While it may be tempting to accept this broader understanding of *podagra* simply because it resolves the apparent mismatch in the data, a deeper analysis of the recipes that name *podagra* as well as other joints and joint areas alongside the osteological evidence supports this more flexible interpretation.

Unlike the assumed equivalence between the term *podagra* and the medical condition known today as gout, the descriptions of joint pain in most other areas of the body, such as the neck, shoulders, or knees, have not been linked to a single, distinctive disease entity, whether historically or in modern medicine. In other words, although *podagra* is consistently translated as gout, *lumborum dolores* is not read as a description of a particular pathology defined by modern medicine, such as spondyloarthritis affecting the lumbar vertebrae. Moreover, in cases where it might be tempting to link a Latin term to a modern medical condition, e.g., *sciatica* and sciatica, much scholarship today insists on more cautious, open-ended translations given the uncertainties of how these concepts were understood in the past.[90] The examples beyond big toe thus suggest that it would be useful to consider the potential breadth and flexibility of the term *podagra*. That is not to say that *podagra* could not have meant gout, a topic to which I shall return below, but that it may be misguided to assume that *all* references to *podagra* are equivalent to a modern medical definition of gout.

The prevalence of signs of other joint diseases in the lower extremities seen at many of the excavations under consideration strengthens this argument, suggesting that many *podagra* recipes may have been intended for a range of conditions and pains. More general joint pain due to the aging process and build-up of bio-mechanical stress represents one significant alternative given the extent to which OA is seen in the skeletal remains of individuals from this period. Furthermore, trauma, nerve pain, and other diseases can also cause pain in the joints of the feet and toes. The skeletal record thus suggests that a direct translation of *podagra* as gout may be too restrictive and that a variety of similar aches and pains could have been grouped under this term.

This more general understanding is further supported by the contexts in which the term *podagra* is found. Consider, for example, recipes where the term is listed alongside somewhat comparable conditions, such as the pain of *artriticus* or even joint dislocations and broken bones as recorded in the *Malagma aduersus dolores uel fracturas et podagra ad luxum* of cod. sang. 759.[91] Taking *podagra* to mean toe and foot joint pain, therefore, corresponds to many of the settings in which the term is found: treatments focused on pain management in the lower extremities more generally. At the same time, the relatively large number of highly specific recipes also fits a broader understanding of *podagra*. The prevalence of foot and toe pathologies in the archaeological record suggests that recipes targeting pain in these areas would always be in demand: the evidence reveals that essentially everyone who lived long enough would ultimately suffer from joint problems, much like populations today. Recipes claiming to treat a cluster of related symptoms concerning toe

---

90 For Hunt's comments on *sciatica*, see *The* Medicina Plinii, trans. Hunt, 176.

91 Cod. sang. 759, p. 63: *Malagma aduersus dolores uel fracturas et podagra ad luxum*. See Appendix 2, entry 11.11.

and foot pain, listed under the umbrella term *podagra*, would have been applicable to many individuals and could have been used in an attempt to help those suffering from OA, RA, gout, and other conditions.

Another angle strengthening this argument comes from recent research into other disease terms, such as Alessandra Foscati's work on *ignis sacer*.[92] This 'holy fire' has long been understood as the medieval Latin term for ergotism, 'Saint Anthony's fire', a fungal disease that results from the ingestion of rye, a common food product in medieval Europe, infected with *Claviceps purpurea*. As Foscati has convincingly argued, the unquestioning assumption that *ignis sacer* can be simply equated with ergotism misses 'the underlying complexity and semantic richness of the nosographic terms in question'.[93] Indeed, the 'polysemantic nature of the lexicon' that Foscati so clearly unpacks in the context of Saint Anthony's fire shares much in common with the gout-*podagra* paradox.[94] Most significantly, Foscati's framing of individual medical terms as 'semantic basins' in which multiple, changing, and often overlapping meanings accumulate has many resonances with the textual and osteological evidence presented in this chapter. I suggest that *podagra*, too, should be understood as a 'semantic basin' that has the potential to account for a wider range of aches and pains than those caused exclusively by gout.[95]

To be clear, this argument for breadth is not to say that references to *podagra* could not also represent true gout. As cited above, earlier sources, such as Hippocrates and Galen, did, in fact, provide accounts of a condition that fit extremely well with a modern medical description of the symptoms associated with gout, revealing that the disease was known as a distinct entity. Moreover, a handful of probable cases of gout have been identified in early medieval skeletal remains, indicating that recipes claiming to offer treatments for *podagra* in the more limited sense would still have been applicable, if only to a very small number of individuals. The presence and acknowledgement of true gout may help to explain the frequent inclusion of *podagra* in non-specific panaceas—it routinely appears as one of the standard, set pieces in cure-all antidotes. As seen in the examples above and discussed in Chapter 2, these cure-alls tend to name a large and varied set of conditions that they are intended to treat. Some

92 Alessandra Foscati, *Ignis sacer. Una storia culturale del 'fuoco sacro' dall'antichità al Settecento* (Florence: SISMEL Edizioni del Galluzzo, 2013); with an updated edition in English translation: Alessandra Foscati, *Saint Anthony's Fire from Antiquity to the Eighteenth Century*, trans. Francis Gordon (Amsterdam: Amsterdam University Press, 2020).

93 Foscati, *Saint Anthony's Fire*, 17.

94 Ibid, 18; for the shifting terminology over time, see Part I, 33–123.

95 Ibid, 20.

of these conditions are fairly generic, such as stomach pains and headaches, but many are extreme, ranging from snake bites to paralysis. *Podagra*, if interpreted broadly, could fit the former type of general condition, or, if taken to mean gout according to a modern definition of the disease, could fall into the latter category of rare, serious, and extreme conditions. That is, depending on how it is understood, the term could cover the entire spectrum of severity and/or urgency: on one hand, it could concern achy, arthritic joints (painful and problematic but ordinary), while on the other hand, it could refer to true gout, an excruciating, debilitating, and rare condition. In both cases, treatments would be highly desired.

Ultimately, while the prevalence of *podagra* in the texts contrasts with the general absence of gout in the skeletal remains, it does fit with the wider context: toe and foot joint pain would have been common issues. Moreover, contextualising recipes for *podagra* within their textual environment (i.e., observing the appearance of *podagra* in association with somewhat similar descriptions of foot, leg, and joint pain) supports a more general reading of the term and finds parallels with other recent research into the complex, 'polysemantic nature' of past disease lexicon.[96] Therefore, by reassessing the written record in the light of the osteological evidence, I argue that *podagra* should generally be interpreted as a collection of symptoms rather than a specific, modern diagnosis, potentially referring to gout but not limited to this disease exclusively. With this reframing of *podagra*, it is possible to return to the original question of applicability with respect to the chapter's entire textual and osteological sample.

6.2 *The Question of Applicability*

The variety of recipe styles, and especially their range in terms of specificity, demands an analysis of applicability at multiple levels. In particular, the divide between non-specific treatments and more targeted semi- or highly specific recipes must be considered separately. At first glance, non-specific panaceas may seem irrelevant, impractical, and inapplicable—and not simply based on their use of expensive, exotic ingredients (though this aspect was challenged in Chapter 3). These treatments' lack of a specific target raises the question, would anyone seek to use such recipes? The cure-all approach, however, seems not unlike certain modern 'home remedies', such as the heavy use of aspirin, acetaminophen, ibuprofen, or even antibiotics to treat a range of conditions that may or may not respond to the selected drug: a supposed panacea can

96 Ibid, 18.

offer an effective placebo.[97] The foreignness and expense of the ingredients involved in these complex recipes may have made them especially desirable, too: the higher the expense of the ingredients, the greater the perceived medical value. In fact, that antidotes such as the *Antidotum gira deacoloquintidis* of BAV pal. lat. 1088 incorporated exotic ingredients that were newly available in the west (in this case, camphor) suggests that these complex recipes were not simply for show but were actively integrating the latest pharmaceutical knowledge and substances (on which, see Chapter 3).[98] These features indicate that non-specific recipes may have been highly sought after, and especially in the elite contexts in which the surviving medical manuscripts are associated. The large number of panaceas in the literature must not, therefore, be automatically discounted as irrelevant to individuals in early medieval Europe.

The more specific recipes offer a different perspective on treatment. There is a high degree of overlap between the joints and joint areas named in texts and the areas of the body affected by OA, stress, and joint degeneration as observed in skeletal remains. The archaeological evidence revealed that the spine, from the neck to the lower back, often exhibited the most severe signs of arthritis, while the shoulders, hips, knees, elbows, feet, and hands were also affected. Indeed, at Seckenheim, a site with particularly good preservation, over 99% of the analysed individuals presented signs of spinal degeneration, and the frequency and severity with which individuals were affected by arthritic changes increased with age.[99] The skeletal evidence therefore suggests that the recipes intended to treat these specific joint areas, as well as treatments for 'general joint afflictions', would have been highly relevant to early medieval populations. Significantly, even burials at elite and/or monastic sites recorded evidence of arthritis and the accumulation of bio-mechanical stress, indicating that these conditions affected essentially everyone who lived long enough and not only those involved in tough agricultural labour or other physically demanding activities.

It is, however, interesting to note that foot- and toe-specific treatments are listed with much greater frequency than other joint-specific treatments. Consider, for example, that the sample includes 140 recipes that target *podagra*,

97 On the placebo effect in the context of early medieval English recipes, see Brackmann, '"It Will Help Him Wonderfully"'. On current trends in self-medication, see, for example, Rajasree K. Rajamma, Audhesh K. Paswan, and Lou E. Pelton, 'Flipping the script: Consumers' propensity for self-medication', *Journal of Marketing Theory and Practice* 29, no. 4 (2021): 448–62, https://doi.org/10.1080/10696679.2020.1870240.

98 BAV pal. lat. 1088, f. 90r: *Antidotum gira deacoloquintidis*. See Appendix 2, 16.26.

99 Navitainuck, Meyer, and Alt, 'Degenerative Alterations of the Spine', 179–83.

whereas pains of the neck are only named in twenty-one treatments. The lower back and shoulders, areas of the body that were often noted as showing signs of stress and degradation in the osteological evidence, appear at similarly low levels within the recipe sample. This may suggest that more general treatments for *artriticus* were intended for arthritic pains in most joints while pains in the lower extremities were conceived of as a separate entity, perhaps linked to the knowledge that these joints could experience different types of joint pain, such as that of true gout. Indeed, if the number of treatments targeting general joint afflictions are added to each of the other individual joint treatment categories, their recipe totals become much closer to the number of *podagra*-specific remedies. The hips are, again, an exception to the general pattern if all three terms are counted together; however, when each of the three hip terms is assessed individually, they present only slightly elevated numbers in comparison to other named joints and joint areas. The varied vocabulary used to describe hip ailments is certainly deserving of further study.

On the basis of these analyses, the overall picture is one of applicability. The skeletal remains of early medieval individuals reveal that joint pain would have been an issue for many people and suggest that the recipes examined in this chapter, whether intended to treat a specific sore, aching joint or more general joint pain, would have been highly relevant to communities in Carolingian Europe.

7 Conclusion

This chapter's reappraisal of recipes intended to alleviate the pains of *podagra* and analysis of treatments for other joints offers a more nuanced reading of the recipe literature reinforced by the osteological record. It underlines the importance of being cautious in interpreting early medieval medical terminology, especially when a certain word has been consistently and unquestioningly translated as a modern medical term. Moreover, the standard associations readers have with gout today, such as the stereotypes of who would have been affected by the disease in the past (namely, older, wealthy males—the royal, aristocratic, and ecclesiastical elite), have tended to reinforce the assumed equivalence between *podagra* and true gout when considering past populations. Yet, as the evidence discussed in this chapter illustrates, such a restricted interpretation of *podagra* may, in many cases, be inappropriate. Rather, it can be more helpful to understand *podagra* as a term that encompasses a wider collection of related symptoms relating to pain in the joints of the feet and toes. This wider interpretation does not exclude true gout but moves away from reading *podagra* exclusively as gout according to a modern medical definition of the disease. This chapter is not, therefore, arguing that true gout did not exist in the Carolingian world, but that *podagra* should not be solely equated with this definition.

In addition to highlighting the need for caution when analysing and interpreting the textual evidence, this chapter also confirms that reading recipes in combination with the osteological evidence offers valuable insights. If the recipe literature had been studied in isolation, the frequency to which *podagra* is referred could have been interpreted as a confirmation of the underlying assumptions about the prevalence of gout in potentially high-risk early medieval populations, reinforcing a circular argument. Similarly, given that other joints are recorded less frequently in recipes, a researcher working exclusively with textual evidence might have assumed that other arthropathies were less prevalent. Comparing the two sides of the story, the written record and the skeletal material, has thus helped to expose the complexity of the situation, casting fresh light on the health and lived experiences of individuals from the Carolingian period.

With this expanded understanding of the recipe literature and its applicability to joint diseases, the final case study of Part 2 now moves to the topics of trauma and surgery.

CHAPTER 9

Trauma and Surgery

Evidence of Undocumented Medical Practices?

1 Introduction: Interventions 'Without Iron'

> A plaster that breaks and opens wounds and scrofulous swellings without iron: Sal ammoniac, 1 pound; galena, 1 pound; oil, 1 pound; ashes of twigs, 1 pound; dove droppings, 3 ounces. Prepare [it] and use [it].[1]

The above recipe, a topical application made of various mineral, vegetable, and animal substances, claims to offer a non-surgical alternative to opening a wound or swelling: it presents a treatment that reputedly breaks them open *sine ferro*, 'without iron'. In a period before antibiotics and hygienic operating facilities, it is understandable that a substitute to surgical intervention would have been sought. Whether such a plaster would rupture a swelling or break open a wound is, of course, another matter and an investigation into the recipe's efficacy is beyond the scope of this book.

In pre-modern medicine, dietary and pharmaceutical treatments were generally preferred to surgical intervention. In most cases, surgery would have been the last resort, turned to when non-invasive treatments had failed or if surgery was the only possible course of action, as might have been the case with traumatic injuries that occurred in battle.[2] The general absence of early medieval surgical texts supports the idea that surgery was a rarity in this period, though exceptions, such as writings on the relatively minor surgical procedures of bloodletting, cautery, and scarification, are recorded. In contrast

1 Cod. sang. 44, p. 243: *Emplastrum qui sine ferro rumpit uulnera et scrofas et aperit. Salis ammoniaci lib I, mollibdine lib I, oleo lib I, cineris sarmentorum lib I, femus columbino ~ III, conficis et uteris*. See Appendix 2, entry 5.5.

2 Mitchell, *Medicine in the Crusades*, 184. The topic of wounds received in battle will be considered in more detail below; for more on wounds generally in the medieval period, see Larissa Tracy and Kelly DeVries, eds., *Wounds and Wound Repair in Medieval Culture* (Leiden: Brill, 2015). 'Periodic bloodletting', i.e., regular, and highly regulated, bloodletting, represents an important exception whereby a (minor) surgical procedure was actively sought; see Mary K. K. Yearl, 'Bloodletting as Recreation in the Monasteries of Medieval Europe', in *Between Text and Patient: The Medical Enterprise in Medieval and Early Modern Europe*, ed. Florence Eliza Glaze and Brian K. Nance (Florence: SISMEL Edizioni del Galluzzo, 2011), 217–43.

to the early medieval Latin evidence, treatises on more invasive surgeries did circulate in Antiquity, the medieval Islamicate world, and the later medieval west. Yet, just as the existence of dietary and pharmaceutical recipes is not, in itself, proof of their use in therapy, the inverse is true regarding surgery. That is, the lack of major surgical texts does not necessarily indicate that invasive surgery was not occurring in the early medieval west, but rather that, if such procedures were happening, knowledge of them was transmitted through non-textual means.[3] However, the recording of a non-invasive alternative to surgical intervention that emphasises this very feature suggests that surgery was to be avoided when possible. Do skeletal remains reveal signs of surgical practices unrecorded by the texts?

An investigation into whether evidence of surgical procedures can be observed in the osteological record is inherently linked to signs of weapon injuries, falls, and other trauma. Skeletal remains may provide indicators of the types of treatments that occurred during this period other than, or in addition to, surgery based on signs of healing (or lack thereof) recorded in the bones. It is necessary, therefore, to consider the evidence of more general traumata in both the written sources and osteological record. Accordingly, this chapter's recipe analysis explores the extent to which these texts attempted to heal and/or provide care for serious injuries, such as broken bones, rather than focusing on the examples of minor surgeries, including bloodletting and cautery, that occasionally appear alongside recipes or as part of treatments. The latter, given their superficial nature, are not recorded in the osteological record, whereas more significant injuries can be considered from both textual and skeletal perspectives.

In contrast to the conditions addressed in Chapters 7 and 8, trauma is usually the immediate result of a sudden event, such as a fall or blow. This direct cause and effect relationship has given rise to a fairly consistent understanding of the aetiology of traumatic injuries from Antiquity to the present day.[4] Despite this unusually high degree of consistency between the modern and medieval identification of the underlying mechanisms responsible for these types of pathologies, trauma remains a notoriously difficult concept to define. The *Oxford Concise Medical Dictionary*, providing a modern clinical perspective, defines trauma as 'a physical wound or injury, such as a fracture or blow',

---

3 Debby Banham and Christine Voth, 'The Diagnosis and Treatment of Wounds in the Old English Medical Collections: Anglo-Saxon Surgery?', in *Wounds and Wound Repair in Medieval Culture*, ed. Larissa Tracy and Kelly DeVries (Leiden: Brill, 2015), 153–74.

4 Margaret A. Judd and Rebecca Redfern, 'Trauma', in *A Companion to Paleopathology*, ed. Anne L. Grauer (Chichester: Wiley-Blackwell, 2012), 359–79, at p. 359.

taking a wide range of potential pathologies into account.[5] For palaeotrauma, however, there is neither a standardised definition of the concept nor an agreement on what exactly it covers. Margaret Judd and Rebecca Redfern's review of palaeopathology textbooks highlights 'that considerable variation exists in what conditions are regarded as having a traumatic origin or association, reflecting both changes within the discipline as a whole and the development of forensic anthropology'.[6] Among the main areas of debate are whether to differentiate between trauma and treatment; how to classify certain pathologies that may result from trauma but may also stem from other causes, such as osteomyelitis or repetitive microtraumata; and whether to include body modification, such as cranial deformation or foot binding, as trauma.[7] Given the complexities of defining palaeotrauma and the variations seen within existing classification systems, this study focuses on a subset of pathologies that are typically understood within the context of trauma, including fractures, dislocations, and signs of surgical intervention preserved in the skeletal record.[8]

Although evidence for invasive surgical procedures is lacking in the recipe literature, my analysis of this material indicates that non-invasive treatments for traumatic injuries are frequently recorded. The subsequent review of osteological evidence does, however, highlight a number of notable examples of major surgical procedures, such as trepanations. More generally, the high degree of healing observed in fairly standard traumata, such as broken bones, without signs of surgical intervention confirms the existence of non-invasive medical care. Re-evaluating the texts on the basis of the skeletal evidence, I argue that the non-invasive therapies presented in recipes would have been highly applicable to individuals in this period, and that they accord with the evidence preserved in the osteological record. At the same time, the limited evidence for more invasive surgeries seen in the skeletal remains provides a window onto medical knowledge that was transmitted through non-textual means during this period.

5 See 'trauma, n.' in Elizabeth A. Martin, ed., *Oxford Concise Medical Dictionary*, 9th ed. (Oxford: Oxford University Press, 2015), https://doi.org/10.1093/acref/9780199687817.001.0001.

6 Judd and Redfern, 'Trauma', 360.

7 Ibid, 359–62.

8 While the inclusion of surgery as a type of trauma has, as noted above, been debated, it is usually categorised as such.

2 Textual Evidence for Invasive Surgery and Trauma

2.1 *Surgery*

Given the ancient precedent of describing surgical procedures separately from pharmaceutical and dietary prescriptions, it might seem strange to look for evidence of surgery alongside recipes.[9] Yet, as explained in Chapter 2, the varied nature of early medieval medical compendia blurs such neat distinctions, and short, non-recipe excerpts and writings can be found in recipe collections. In a small recipe collection in cod. sang. 44, for example, entries such as *De uulneribus putridis* and *De cautere*, focus on superficial surgical procedures rather than recipes.[10] Moreover, as noted above, recipes occasionally mention fairly minor, superficial procedures, such as phlebotomy, cautery, and scarification, as a component of treatment—or even record treatments for the aftermath of these procedures. A poultice in cod. sang. 899 titled *Cataplasma ad tumorem brachii que ex fleubotomo contingit*, for example, is intended to combat swellings in the arm after bloodletting.[11] Old English recipe collections, too, record a handful of fairly superficial surgeries, such as the lancing and draining of an abscess and the removal of gangrenous flesh.[12] It therefore seems possible that *if* surgical techniques beyond the aforementioned minor procedures were recorded in the Carolingian world, they could have been located within this textual environment, either mentioned in recipes as part of a treatment or found as a discrete section of supplementary information within a larger collection. This, however, is not the case, and more complex surgical procedures are absent in the surviving texts.[13] These findings suggest that knowledge of more invasive surgeries, if in circulation, was transferred through non-textual means, such as apprenticeships and oral traditions. However, many treatments for open wounds and/or broken bones involved bandaging and suggest that the injury was protected and possibly immobilised, splinted, and/or manipulated; depending on the complexity of the injury, these processes could have involved some minor surgical procedures, though explicit details are absent.

---

9 Skinner, 'Visible Prowess', 92.

10 Cod. sang. 44, pp. 332–3: LXII. *De uulneribus putridis*; LXIII. *De cautere*.

11 Cod. sang. 899, p. 141: *Cataplasma ad tumorem brachii que ex fleubotomo contingit*. See Appendix 2, entry 14.4.

12 Banham and Voth, 'The Diagnosis and Treatment of Wounds', 154–6.

13 A small number of texts related to surgery, such as a list of surgical instruments, have survived. See Bliquez, 'Two Lists of Greek Surgical Instruments' and Fischer, '*Universorum ferramentorum nomina*'.

TABLE 19 Recipes that mention fractures and traumatic injuries

Specificity	Total	NSp	SSp	HSp
# of Recipes	184	26	17	141
% of Total	100%	14.1%	9.2%	76.6%

Exploring the broader category of trauma can offer more insights into the types of care recorded in the recipe literature for serious injuries.

2.2 *Trauma*

Despite the lack of references to invasive surgeries, serious traumatic injuries do appear with some frequency in the textual record. I have identified 193 recipes that claim to treat fractures, dislocations, cut tendons, and/or injuries caused by a specific type of trauma, such as a blow, puncture wound, fall, or named weapon. Recipes that only include general terms for wounds, ulcers, and sores, such as *uulnus and ulcus*, without further contextualisation are excluded from this chapter's analysis because they could not be linked to a traumatic injury. Likewise, recipes that use the non-specific *tumor*, which can range in meaning from swelling to tumour, without further clarification are not included. It should be noted, however, that three recipes for poultices in cod. sang. 899 combine this term with more details and suggest that they are treatments for swellings with bruising, and thus possibly linked to traumatic injuries. Two of these occur within a cluster of recipes under the heading *Cataplasma ad tumorem*; while the group of recipes cannot be taken as referring to bruising overall, these two recipes also include the words *liuor* (bruise) and *contusio* (contusion, bruise), pinpointing their target.[14] Finally, treatments for animal bites and stings as well as the trauma of childbirth are also excluded because signs of these injuries are often more difficult to see in the osteological evidence.

As seen in Table 19, the majority of these recipes (76.6%) are highly specific, while non- and semi-specific recipes only account for twenty-six (14.1%) and seventeen (9.2%) recipes, respectively. The non- and semi-specific categories follow the same criteria outlined in previous chapters, although I have

14 Cod. sang. 899, p. 141: *Item ad tumores, liuores, contusiones*; *Item ad liuorem tollendum*. See Appendix 2, entries 14.5.2–3.

classified any recipes that only concern traumatic injuries as highly specific, even in cases where multiple types of traumata are mentioned, such as fractures *and* dislocations. I shall briefly review the non- and semi-specific recipes before concentrating on those that target trauma exclusively.

The twenty-six non-specific recipes represent wide-ranging panaceas, eight of which correspond to just two antidotes that reoccur in multiple manuscripts. The *Oxira crocira* is found in codd. sang. 44, 761, BAV pal. lat. 1088, and reg. lat. 1143, and in each case the treatment claims to heal *luxum et fracturas*, 'dislocations and fractures' (the example in cod. sang. 761 also adds that it draws out thorns, *extrahit spinas*), alongside a host of other maladies.[15] Similarly, the *Apostolicon* plaster is seen in four manuscripts (codd. sang. 44, 751, 761, and BAV reg. lat. 1143) and consistently includes a phrase noting that it was intended to treat wounds caused by iron, glass, and other materials as well as embedded arrows.[16] The lengthy list of medical problems this plaster claims to treat then continues with the bites and stings of venomous animals before moving on to a range of other ailments. The non-specific recipes, as these two cases illustrate (and as has been noted in previous chapters), tend to treat a mixture of extreme and general medical issues; in this hybrid context, it is not surprising to see life-threatening wounds caused by traumatic injuries, such as arrows or sword blows, alongside serious and urgent (if also unusual) health problems, such as poisoning and snake bites.

Seventeen semi-specific recipes list traumatic injuries with or secondarily to other potentially related conditions. Several recipes, for instance, mention fractures while also noting wounds, pains, and/or infections. These other ailments could stem from a traumatic event and thus be directly connected with the fractures but, equally, they could represent unrelated conditions. As an example, cod. sang. 751 records a recipe that claims to heal putrid shins and all blows, *Qui facit ad tibias putridas et ad omnes plagas sanandas*.[17] While the putrid shins could reflect an open, infected sore that developed as a result of trauma, the limited description given in the recipe does not address whether

15 Cod. sang. 44, pp. 243–4: *Oxira crucira emplastrum*; cod. sang. 761, pp. 59–60: *Oxyra crocira*; BAV pal. lat. 1088, f. 60r: *Oxira crocira*; and BAV reg. lat. 1143, ff. 172r–172v: *Oxyra grocira*. See Appendix 2, entries 5.6, 12.2, 16.23, and 18.8, respectively.

16 Cod. sang. 44, pp. 238–9: *Emplastrum apostolicon*; cod. sang. 751, pp. 423–4: *Inplastrum apostolicon*; cod. sang. 761, pp. 65–6: *Emplastrum apostolicum*; and BAV reg. lat. 1143, ff. 133r–134r: *Apostolicon*. The shared phrase, with some variation between recipes, is: *ad … omnes plaga quae a ferro inciditur siue* [*sudibus*] *siue uitro siue canna, sagittas educendas infixas corpori*. See Appendix 2, entries 5.4, 9.24, 12.4, and 18.4, respectively.

17 Cod. sang. 751, pp. 367–8: *Qui facit ad tibias putridas et ad omnes plagas sanandas*. See Appendix 2, entry 9.5.

TABLE 20 Categories and subcategories of highly specific recipes that name traumatic injuries as the target of their treatment

Category	Subcategory	Number	% of HSp recipes (141)
Recipes that name a general type of traumatic injury	Fractures	26	18.4%
	Dislocations	15	10.6%
	Fractures & dislocations	1	0.7%
	Cut tendons	6	4.3%
	Total	48	34.0%
Recipes that name a source/cause of traumatic injury	Blows	61	43.3%
	Punctures	22	15.6%
	Blows & punctures	1	0.7%
	Falls	2	1.4%
	Total	86	60.1%
Recipes that name both types and sources of trauma		7	5.0%

the conditions might be linked. Sores on the shins could also fit with haematogenous osteomyelitis, for example, and have no relation to a traumatic injury. Three of these recipes, such as the *Malagma aduersus dolores fracturas et podagra ad luxum* of cod. sang. 759, include *podagra* alongside fractures and dislocations and, as elaborated in Chapter 8, may be linked to more general joint and/or pain treatments of the lower extremities.[18] Given these ambiguities, the following analysis concentrates on the 141 highly specific recipes.

As shown in Table 20, the highly specific recipes can be divided into two main categories: forty-eight recipes (34.0%) name a general type of traumatic injury, such as fractures and dislocations, as the target of their treatment, while eighty-six (61.0%) note the source or cause of a traumatic injury, such as a blow or puncture. There are also seven recipes (5.0%) that mention both injury type(s) *and* cause(s) of trauma. I have further divided the two primary categories into more specific subunits, as seen in Tables 20–22, based on the recipes' titles and any additional information contained within them.

18 Cod. sang. 759, p. 63: *Malagma aduersus dolores uel fracturas et podagra ad luxum*. See Appendix 2, entry 11.11.

TABLE 21 Breakdown of highly specific recipes that name a general type of traumatic injury

Category	Total	Fracture	Dislocation	Fracture & dislocation	Cut tendons
# of recipes	48	26	15	1	6
% of total (48)	100%	61.4%	15.9%	2.3%	13.6%

Of the forty-eight highly specific recipes that are intended to treat general injuries, twenty-six (54.2%) focus exclusively on fractures (see Table 21). Twenty of these recipes provide treatments for broken bones generally, bearing titles such as *Ad fracturas ossorum*, *Ad osa fracta in corpore*, and *Ad osso fracto* across a variety of manuscripts, including codd. sang. 751, 759, BnF lat. 11218, and BAV pal. lat. 1088. Two of the entries in cod. sang. 751 reveal the extent of variation seen among the trauma treatments recorded in the texts: on the one hand, the recipe entitled *Ad osso fracto*, 'for a broken bone', recommends that the patient drink sulphur with wine and water for nine days, whereas the preparation *Ad ossa si fuerint fracta in testa* provides instructions for treating broken bones of the skull that involve the application of a powder directly on the injured area and, if the skin is broken, washing and bandaging.[19] In cod. sang. 759, the two recipes listed under the heading *Ad fracturas ossorum*, 'for fractures of bones', likewise present multiple approaches: the first suggests both a topical application as well as a drink, while the second offers only a topical treatment.[20]

Six recipes intended for fractures, like the treatment for fractures of the skull seen in cod. sang. 751, name specific areas of the body. One treatment in BnF lat. 11218 titled *Ad costas fractas*, 'For broken ribs', recommends a preparation made of glass, pitch, and vinegar.[21] The other five recipes are all intended exclusively for cranial fractures, two of which, *De simplices uulneribus ad capitis*

19 Cod. sang. 751, p. 378: *Ad osso fracto. Solfor bibat per die VIIII terciam partem dinarium pinsantem ieiunus cum uino et aqua*; p. 432: *Ad ossa si fuerint fracta in testa. De pipinella puluis facis super teola exsiccas et super puluere ponis, si reticolus fuerit ruptus lana de papiro super reticulo ponis, et inde aceto et mel lauabis*. See Appendix 2, entries 9.6 and 9.25, respectively.

20 Cod. sang. 759, p. 52: *Ad fracturas ossorum*. See Appendix 2, entry 11.6.

21 BnF lat. 11218, f. 97r: *Ad costas fractas. Uitro, pice, acito resoluis in patena, bene adiuuat*. See Appendix 2, entry 3.7.

fracturam of BAV pal. lat. 1088 and *Ad capitis fractura* of cod. sang. 751, appear to be derived from a treatment found in *De herba vettonica liber*, though the recipe of cod. sang. 751 is somewhat abbreviated.[22] Notably, the longer recipe in BAV pal. lat. 1088 (as well as the original in *De herba vettonica liber*) includes a comment on removing bone fragments: *ossa fractura extrahit*. While it may be tempting to read this as evidence for some degree of surgical intervention, perhaps even linked to trepanation (a technique which, as discussed below, has been observed in early medieval skeletal remains), it would be inappropriate to jump to such a conclusion based on the recipe's limited description. The other recipes addressing cranial fractures, also found in cod. sang. 751, do not belong to the *De herba vettonica liber* tradition and make no reference to bone fragment removal: the remedy *Ad capitis fractura* offers fairly detailed instructions for the preparation of an ointment that contains exotic, aromatic ingredients, such as mastic and colophony resin, whereas a treatment titled *Ossa in capite si fracta fuerint*, 'Bones in the head, if they were broken', recommends a simple topical application made from agrimony and old grease.[23]

As shown in Table 21, fifteen recipes target dislocations, such as the recipes titled *Ad luxum*, 'For a dislocation', in cod. sang. 751 or *Ad luxatura*, also meaning 'For a dislocation', in cod. sang. 44.[24] The ankle, *talus*, is specifically mentioned in several treatments, such as a recipe under the heading *Ad talorem dolorem quis luxauerit ut dolor pausit* in cod. sang. 759, suggestive of a sprained ankle.[25] Moreover, one recipe in cod. sang. 1396 and six in BAV pal. lat. 1088 pair dislocation with bruising; this coupling is very fitting since discolouration and swelling often complement injuries such as sprains and dislocations. The six treatments in BAV pal. lat. 1088 are found under the heading *Ad contussionem*

22 BAV pal. lat. 1088, f. 44v: *De simplices uulneribus ad capitis fracturam. Uittonica contussa et super uulnus inposita mira celeritate gluttinat eo quide sanabis si tertio quoque die recentiorem frequentius inposueris donec sanescat etiam et ossa fractura extrahit*; cod. sang. 751, p. 408: *Ad capitis fractura. Uerba uittonica contusa in capitę in plaga inpositam rase celeritate gluttinatur*. For full transcriptions, see Appendix 2, entries 16.9 and 9.14, respectively. Cf. Pseudo-Antonius Musa, *De herba vettonica liber*, ed. Howald and Sigerist, no. 1: *Ad capitis fracturam. Herba uettonica contusa et super capitis ictum inposita uulnus mira celeritate glutinatum sanabit; eo quidem efficacius, si tertio quoque die refectam, id est recentiorem, frequentius inposueris, donec sanat. Eius potestas tantam habere fertur utilitatem, ut ossa quoque fracta ui sua extrahat*.

23 Cod. sang. 751, pp. 405–6: *Ad capitis fractura*; p. 437: *Ossa in capite si fracta fuerint*. See Appendix 2, entries 9.13 and 9.28.

24 Cod. sang. 751, p. 405: *Ad luxum*; p. 440: *Ad luxum*; cod. sang. 44, p. 348: *Ad luxatura*. See Appendix 2, entries 9.12, 9.29, and 5.20, respectively.

25 Cod. sang. 759, p. 72: *Ad talorem dolorem quis luxauerit ut dolor pausit*. See Appendix 2, entry 11.15.

uel luxatura de praesenti, 'For bruising or dislocation of the present', while the one in cod. sang. 1396 is titled *Ad luxum uel contussim*; all provide instructions for topical applications.[26] Just over half of the recipes that are intended to treat dislocations provide more information about the injury, such as the presence of bruising or that the ankle is the area concerned. This contrasts with the fracture treatments, where the majority of recipes (twenty out of twenty-six) do not supply additional details about the nature of the break or its location. Furthermore, although the treatments for fractures and dislocations are usually separate, one recipe, the *Unguentum ad fractura uel luxatura*, mentions both types of injuries. Located in cod. sang. 759, this ointment uses the fat of a wether, wax, old olive oil, laurel oil, and flax seeds to create a topical application.[27]

Finally, 'cut tendons' are the focus of six recipes, four of which are found together in BAV pal. lat. 1088 under the heading *Ad neruos incisos*.[28] All four of these present simple topical applications: the first two recommend a preparation made with earthworms, the third sage, and the fourth a mixture of snails (with their shells) and frankincense. Intriguingly, although this general type of injury appears much less frequently in the recipe sample under analysis than either fractures or dislocations, cut tendons receive comparatively more coverage in classical and late antique sources. The *Medicina Plinii*, for example, devotes a fairly substantial chapter to *Recentibus vulneribus et nervis incisis* ('For recent wounds and cut tendons') that features over twice as many prescriptions as its later chapter on broken bones, *Ossibus fractis*.[29] Indeed, the first and last of the four recipes for cut tendons in BAV pal. lat. 1088 share much in common with two of the opening treatments found in the *Medicina Plinii*.[30]

Unlike the previous examples of recipes that name a general type of traumatic injury, eighty-six recipes name a source or cause of trauma that resulted in the injury. As seen in Tables 20 and 22, I have grouped these treatments into four subcategories: a) recipes for wounds sustained by blows or strikes,

---

26 BAV pal. lat. 1088, f. 45v: *Ad contussione uel luxatura de praesenti*; cod. sang. 1396, p. 20: *Ad luxum uel contussim*. See Appendix 2, entries 16.12 and 15.2, respectively.

27 Cod. sang. 759, p. 75: *Unguentum ad fractura uel luxatura*. See Appendix 2, entry 11.17.

28 BAV pal. lat. 1088, f. 45r: *Ad neruos incisos*. See Appendix 2, entry 16.11.

29 *Plinii Secundi Iunioris qui feruntur De medicina libri tres*, ed. Önnerfors, 3.3 and 3.25. For the English translation, see *The* Medicina Plinii, trans. Hunt, 72–5, 94–5.

30 *Plinii Secundi Iunioris qui feruntur De medicina libri tres*, ed. Önnerfors, 3.3.1–2: *Vermes terreni triti conglutinant, adeo ut etiam neruos incisos solident die septimo ... cochleae cum suis testis tusae cum myrrha et ture pari pondere etiam praecisos neruos sanant.*

TABLE 22 Breakdown of highly specific recipes that name a source/cause of traumatic injury

Category	Total	Blows	Punctures	Blows & punctures	Falls
# of recipes	86	61	22	1	2
% of total (86)	100%	70.9%	25.6%	1.2%	2.3%

b) puncture wounds, c) wounds caused by both blows and punctures, and d) injuries that occurred due to a fall. The majority of these recipes concern injuries related to general physical violence, including those caused by unspecified blows and strikes (*plaga*, *percussus*, etc.) as well as those caused by weapons, such as swords or arrows. Very few of the named traumata are related to non-violent incidents, such as falls or puncture wounds caused by something other than a weapon. It must be remembered, however, that a weapon injury does not necessarily indicate intentional violence but could have been the result of a hunting accident or even 'horseplay'. The *Annals of St. Bertin* record, for example, that in the year 864 Charles the Child, the grandson of Louis the Pious, 'was struck in the head with a sword by a youth named Albuin. The blow penetrated almost as far as the brain, reaching from his left temple to his right cheekbone and jaw', though 'he only meant to enjoy some horseplay with other young men of his own age'.[31]

Sixty-one recipes mention blows and strikes of various kinds, totalling over two-thirds (70.9%) of the treatments that name a source of trauma. Most of these recipes provide only general descriptions of the cause of the injury they intend to heal, using terms such as *plaga* or *percussus*, as noted above. Cod. sang. 751, for example, contains ten general treatments for blows in which forms of the word *plaga* are given and three with *percussus* and related terms, BAV pal. lat. 1088 includes thirteen and eight, respectively, and so on.[32] Several of the recipes in cod. sang. 751, such as the three entitled *Potio ad plaga*, provide

31 *Annales Bertiniani*, ed. Waitz, entry for 864 (at p. 67): *Karolus iuvenis … noctu rediens de venatione in silva Cotia, iocari cum aliis iuvenibus et coaevis suis putans, operante diabolo ab Albuio iuvene in capite spatha percutitur pene usque ad cerebrum*; translation from *The Annals of St Bertin*, trans. Nelson, 111–12.

32 Cod. sang. 751, recipes with *plaga*: pp. 39 (two cases), 392, 399, 405, 407, 410, 435, 451 (two cases); recipes with *percussus*: pp. 404, 439, 471; BAV pal. lat. 1088, recipes with *plaga*: ff. 39r, 44r–45r (one cluster of five recipes, one cluster of six recipes), 50v.

instructions for producing a potion that would be drunk. As might be expected for these kinds of injuries, others suggest topical applications, such as an entry contained within *De mandragora*, a small cluster of recipes that use mandrake as the primary ingredient. The instructions state: 'grind up mandrake root and boil [it] with oil and apply [it] on the wound; it heals wonderfully'.[33] While none of the recipes in cod. sang. 751 is identical, a number of ingredients, such as agrimony, betony, and milfoil, are named repeatedly. In contrast to these preparations that tend to use fairly common and potentially local plant products, a powder for healing wounds in BAV pal. lat. 1088 incorporates a range of non-local aromatics, including myrrh, frankincense, and mastic.[34] Although this recipe provides little guidance on how to administer the powder, others supply more detail about the context of the injury and the treatment process. A cluster of five treatments in BAV pal. lat. 1088, for example, describe the wounds as being caused by iron (*a ferro*).[35] Recipes for powders found in cod. sang. 759 and BnF lat. 11219 refer to injuries that may involve shattered bones (*si ossa habet minuata*).[36]

Puncture wounds alone are mentioned on twenty-two occasions, as seen in Table 22. While most of the recipes offer general treatments for puncture wounds (*punctas*), one recipe in BAV pal. lat. 1088 is intended to treat wounds caused by poisoned arrows, *Ad eos qui cum toxicata sagittasi sunt*, and a recipe in cod. sang. 751 offers a cure for a foot (or any other body part) pierced by a thorn, *Si spina in pede uel in alico membro fuerit*.[37] Clusters of five and three recipes to treat puncture wounds of the side can be found in BAV pal. lat. 1088 and cod. sang. 44, respectively, while another recipe for side punctures, *Ad puncta que in lateribus superuenit*, is located in BnF lat. 11218.[38] The three recipes of cod. sang. 44 parallel the first three recipes of those listed in BAV pal. lat. 1088, and the recipe in BnF lat. 11218 also appears to be loosely

33 Cod. sang. 751, p. 392: *De mandragora … Ipsa radice teris et dequoquis cum oleo et super plaga pone mirum sanat*. See Appendix 2, entry 9.7.1.

34 BAV pal. lat. 1088, f. 50v: *Puluera ad plagam assucandam et stringendam et celerius sanandam et carnem mortuam manducat*. See Appendix 2, entry 16.18.

35 BAV pal. lat. 1088, f. 44v: *Ad alia uulnera uel plagas ubicumque a ferro aut quolibet*. See Appendix 2, entry 16.10.

36 Cod. sang. 759, p. 61: *Puluis qui facit ad implire placas etiam et si ossa minuta habuerit excutit*; BnF lat. 11219, f. 225ra: *Puluis ad implere plagas et si ossa habet minuata discutit*. See Appendix 2, entries 11.10 and 4.3, respectively.

37 BAV pal. lat. 1088, ff. 46v–47r: *Ad eos qui cum toxicata sagittasi sunt*; cod. sang. 751, p. 396: *Si spina in pede uel in alico membro fuerit*. See Appendix 2, entries 16.13 and 9.9, respectively.

38 Cod. sang. 44, pp. 364–5: *Ad punctas qui in latere superueniunt*; BAV pal. lat. 1088, ff. 39v–40r: *Ad punctas que lateribus superueniunt*; BnF lat. 11218, f. 97r: *Ad puncta que in lateribus superuenit*. See Appendix 2, entries 5.29, 16.6, and 3.8, respectively.

related to the first recipes in these clusters as all three treatments name southernwood (*abrotano*) as their primary ingredient.[39] Like some of the examples seen above, the overlapping information presented in different manuscripts illustrates not only the shared sources of pharmaceutical information that circulated in early medieval Europe, but also their individuality. That is, although two of the recipe collections in which these particular examples are found belong to the *Teraupetica-Tereoperica* family of texts, they contain many differences that point to a complex process of transmission and adaptation over time.[40] A recipe in cod. sang. 759, *Remedium ad punctas*, likewise highlights how recorded medical knowledge was shifting during this period; in this case, beer is listed as an ingredient, suggesting that the recipe may have been influenced by local knowledge and/or adapted to suit readily available products (on which, see Chapter 4).[41]

The single example of a highly specific recipe that refers to both blows and punctures, *Medicamen mirabile ad placas ad sagita percusso*, is found in cod. sang. 759.[42] Unlike most other subcategories, the majority of recipes that mention multiple forms of named trauma are non-specific recipes. The only other grouping in which non-specific recipes predominate is the 'fractures and dislocations' subcategory, suggesting that antidotes and other panaceas, in their tendency to list particularly extreme medical problems, feature multiple weapon-based injuries—if such injuries are listed at all—rather than an arrow wound *or* a sword blow individually. Recipes that mention falls are only recorded twice (see Table 22); along with treatments for thorns, these recipes are unusual in naming traumatic injuries that do not necessarily stem from a violent act (whether intentional or accidental). These two recipes are found under the title *Si homo de arbore uel de equo ceciderit*, 'If a person has fallen

39 The first recipes of the clusters and the single recipe in BnF lat. 11218 are as follows: BAV pal. lat. 1088, f. 39v: *Ad punctas que lateribus superueniunt. Aprotano trito in aqua colatum medium calicem tepidum bibat, admiscis modicum sal*; cod. sang. 44, p. 364: *Ad punctas qui in latere superueniunt. Abrotano trito in aqua colato medio calice tepidum bibat, admiscis modicum sal*; BnF lat. 11218, f. 97r: *Ad puncta que in lateribus superuenit, hoc est defecciones se in febre acute superuenit. Abrotanum in aqua tritum et euaporacione ne adhibeatur propere omnia et agriamen uetandum est*. For full transcriptions, see Appendix 2, entries 16.6.1, 5.29.1, and 3.8, respectively.

40 Ferraces Rodríguez, 'Un recetario médico altomedieval'; Ferraces Rodríguez, 'Reutilización de fuentes en recetarios medicos de la antigüedad tardía'.

41 Cod. sang. 759, p. 68: *Remedium ad punctas lias de ceruisa recentis colas n<...> das et alio tando buter simul miscis et bibe dabis statim sanabitur*. See Appendix 2, entry 11.14 for the full transcription.

42 Cod. sang. 759, p. 67: *Medicamen mirabile ad placas ad sagita percusso*. See Appendix 2, entry 11.13.

from a tree or a horse', in cod. sang. 751.[43] The first provides instructions for a topical application and linen wrap, while the second produces a potion to drink.

The final category, recipes that mention both general injuries as well as a named source of trauma, includes seven highly specific treatments. Although two recipes from cod. sang. 751 have titles that would suggest a single target, *Ad luxum*, 'For a dislocation', and *Potio ad plaga*, 'A potion for blows', additional information appears within the recipe itself. In the first, *Ad luxum* is written in red capitals and then followed by *ad luxum uel quolibet casum si percussum fuerit ut liuorem faciat*, a phrase that reveals that the recipe is intended to treat not only dislocations but also cases in which a strike has caused bruising.[44] While this is similar to the dislocation recipes that mentioned bruising noted above, it differs in specifying that a blow, *percussum*, was involved. In contrast, a recipe from cod. sang. 878, Walahfrid Strabo's *vademecum*, titled *Ad fracturam uel uulnera ferri*, 'For a fracture or wounds of iron', more clearly indicates the multipurpose nature of the treatment in its title and recommends a mixture of 'barley flour, boar fat, and stinging nettle' with no further instructions regarding the preparation or administration fo the treatment.[45] Unusually, each of the ingredients in this recipe has been glossed in Old High German.[46] These additions, however, date to the eleventh century and therefore cannot be taken as evidence for how this recipe was read in the Carolingian period.

3 Osteological Evidence for Trauma and Surgery

3.1 *Identifying and Understanding Trauma in the Osteological Record*

When assessing evidence for palaeotrauma, the nature of the wound and extent of bone remodelling can provide important information about the trauma that caused the injury, whether medical intervention occurred, and whether the patient survived the incident. Fractures are the primary source of evidence for trauma in the skeletal record, though dislocations, especially of the shoulder, may also be observable in some cases. The type of break and its location on the body provide a framework for understanding the injury

43 Cod. sang. 751, p. 395: *Si homo de arbore uel de equo ceciderit*. See Appendix 2, entry 9.8.

44 Cod. sang. 751, p. 400: *Ad luxum*. See Appendix 2, entry 9.10.

45 Cod. sang. 878, p. 333: *Ad fracturam uel uulnera ferri. Farina ordeacia, adeps aprinus uel uerrinus, urtica minor*. See Appendix 2, entry 13.1.

46 For the glosses, see von Steinmeyer and Sievers, *Die althochdeutschen Glossen*, vol. 4, 455.

and may suggest whether the traumatic event was accidental or intentional.[47] A fall, for example, could result in a crush fracture (a fracture of a vertebra due to compression) or a Colles fracture (a fracture of the distal radius due to landing on an outstretched hand). A blow to the head often causes a depressed fracture (a fracture of the skull where the bone is forced inwards), whereas a strike to a long bone may result in a linear cutmark (due to a sharp, slicing weapon, such as a sword) or a transverse fracture (a fracture at right angles to the bone's long axis).[48]

Although the latter example, a transverse fracture, can be caused by many different types of traumata and should not be automatically interpreted as the result of interpersonal violence, the location of the injury can be instructive. Fractures that occur on the shaft of the radius and/or ulna, for example, are often referred to as 'parry fractures' since it is plausible 'that the individual was using his or her arm to ward off a blow aimed at the head'.[49] Yet, despite the information provided by the injury's location and form, it must be remembered that the interpretation of the traumatic incident always remains a case of speculation.[50] While a 'parry fracture' is *suggestive* of an individual parrying a blow to the head, it is possible that this was not the case. Furthermore, as noted above with the example of 'horseplay' from the *Annals of St. Bertin*, it is important to keep in mind that some weapon-based injuries in the past may have been accidental.[51]

Regardless of the question of intent, it may still be possible to deduce the means by which certain fractures occurred: cranial injuries located in the left frontoparietal region, for instance, suggest a 'face-to-face encounter' where 'the weapon inflicting these wounds [was] held in the right hand'.[52] When considering trauma due to weapons, the appearance of the fracture may also

47 Tosi, Badino, and Pezzoni, 'Medical Conditions Observed in Osteoarchaeological Remains', 29–34.

48 Waldron, *Palaeopathology*, 139–41.

49 Ibid, 151.

50 For a discussion of the need for caution when interpreting signs of violence in the past (and examples of overzealous readings of the skeletal evidence), see M. R. Geldof, '"And to describe the shapes of the dead": Making Sense of the Archaeology of Armed Violence', in *Wounds and Wound Repair in Medieval Culture*, ed. Larissa Tracy and Kelly DeVries (Leiden: Brill, 2015), 57–80.

51 *Annales Bertiniani*, ed. Waitz, entry for 864 (at p. 67); translation from *The Annals of St Bertin*, trans. Nelson, 111–12.

52 Jochen Weber and Alfred Czarnetzki, 'Brief Communication: Neurotraumatological Aspects of Head Injuries Resulting from Sharp and Blunt Force in the Early Medieval Period of Southwestern Germany', *American Journal of Biological Anthropology* 114, no. 4 (2001): 352–6, https://doi.org/10.1002/ajpa.1047, at p. 354.

offer insights into the type of weapon used. Swords or knives tend to leave a distinct cutmark whereas a projectile, such as an arrow or spear, results in a small piercing or indentation.[53] Sticks, stones, maces, and other large items will typically result in a blunt force trauma, such as a depressed fracture.[54]

The presence or absence (and, if present, extent) of remodelled bone at the site of injury can shed light on the timing of the traumatic event and healing process. If there is no sign of remodelling, then the injury occurred at or very near to the individual's death.[55] In some cases, it can be difficult to distinguish between peri- and post-mortem trauma, though the fragmentation of bones due to soil weight or any damage incurred during the excavation process are often recognisable based on the appearance of the fracture edge.[56] If the individual survived the initial trauma, bone repair begins almost immediately (evidence of remodelling can be seen within roughly two days of the incident) and may continue for several years.[57] The gradation of remodelling seen at the site of injury can therefore provide a timeframe for understanding the healing process: did the individual make a full recovery or die within a few days or weeks after sustaining the trauma? If there are only early signs of bone repair, it suggests that the individual survived the initial traumatic incident but died relatively soon after, perhaps due to complications associated with the injury.[58]

When an individual survives a traumatic incident, it may also be possible to see evidence of treatment. The successful healing of a broken bone requires immobilisation and, depending on the location and type of fracture, returning the bone to its normal anatomical position.[59] A number of complications may result if this does not occur, if it is done poorly, or if the individual begins to use the injured bone before it is fully healed, such as non-union, shortening, and/or angulation.[60] Broken bones, and especially open fractures where the skin has also been broken, are susceptible to infection, and the development of osteomyelitis may be visible in the skeletal remains.[61] The complete remodelling

53 Tosi, Badino, and Pezzoni, 'Medical Conditions Observed in Osteoarchaeological Remains', 30; Weber and Czarnetzki, 'Neurotraumatological Aspects of Head Injuries', 352.

54 Tosi, Badino, and Pezzoni, 'Medical Conditions Observed in Osteoarchaeological Remains', 30; Weber and Czarnetzki, 'Neurotraumatological Aspects of Head Injuries', 352.

55 Tosi, Badino, and Pezzoni, 'Medical Conditions Observed in Osteoarchaeological Remains', 30.

56 Waldron, *Palaeopathology*, 138; Tosi, Badino, and Pezzoni, 'Medical Conditions Observed in Osteoarchaeological Remains', 30.

57 Waldron, *Palaeopathology*, 148.

58 Ibid.

59 Ibid, 142.

60 Ibid, 143.

61 Ibid, 143–4.

of bone at the site of injury would indicate that the individual survived for at least several years after the trauma occurred and suggests that some type of medical care was involved in their recovery. Poorly healed fractures, such as those exhibiting a pseudoarthrosis ('a fibrous joint formed between the broken ends of the bones' resulting from non-union), do not necessarily indicate that medical care was absent since this bone formation may have resulted from the use of the injured bone before healing was complete.[62]

Finally, the limits of osteological evidence must be remembered. Skeletal remains will only record evidence of traumatic injuries that have affected the skeleton, meaning that many forms of trauma will not be preserved in the archaeological record: while a sword blow might produce an obvious cutmark in a bone, a dagger might only pierce the soft tissue and leave no trace of the injury. The resulting underrepresentation of traumatic injuries in the skeletal record is therefore essential to keep in mind in the following review of skeletal evidence and will be revisited in the discussion that follows. Similarly, the lack of evidence for soft tissue trauma is also important to note in relation to the limited textual evidence for surgical intervention. Although, as mentioned above, surgery is rarely seen in the early medieval written record, a number of superficial procedures, most frequently bloodletting, do appear in medical texts as well as other documentary evidence. The *Plan of St Gall*, for example, includes a room in the medical area specifically designated as the monastery's site for phlebotomy.[63] Information regarding certain times to avoid bloodletting, such as lists of Egyptian Days (days thought to be unlucky, especially with respect to phlebotomy), also appears in and alongside calendrical texts.[64] While the practice is occasionally mentioned in medical recipes as a component of a treatment, there are also writings that focus specifically on bloodletting, including epistles and other treatises that provide guidance on the best (or worst) days and times to phlebotomise, describe the different veins involved, and so on.[65] Within the manuscript sample involved in this book, examples of calendars that include information on bloodletting can be seen in codd. sang. 751 and 878, while BnF lat. 11218, BAV reg. lat. 1143, codd. sang. 44,

62 Ibid, 144.

63 Cod. sang. 1092. The label reads: *fleotomatis hic gustandum uel potionariis*; see Horn and Born, *The Plan of St. Gall*, 184–8.

64 On the relationship between calendars and medicine, see Wallis, 'Medicine in Medieval Calendar Manuscripts'; on Egyptian Days, see Don C. Skemer, '*Armis Gunfe*: Remembering Egyptian Days', *Traditio* 65 (2010): 75–106.

65 For a list of texts on bloodletting, see Beccaria, *I codici*; see also Sabbah, Corsetti, and Fischer, *BTML*, nos. 185–8, 234–41; Fischer, *BTML 1*, no. A-100.

217, and 751 all contain versions of an *Epistula de phlebotomia*.[66] These types of superficial surgical procedures, however, are not investigated in the present study since they only affect soft tissues and thus leave no skeletal indicators.

3.2 *Evidence for Trauma in Early Medieval Skeletal Remains*

Although fractures, wounds, and other injuries appear less frequently in the skeletal record than the oral pathologies and joint diseases addressed in previous chapters, there is still extensive evidence of trauma. Based on the criteria for assessing fractures outlined above, such as the type and location of the wound or degree of bone remodelling, it is also possible to consider the types of traumatic incidents that caused these injuries and whether the individuals survived. In some cases, these variables can shed light on the wider context in which the trauma occurred. At the northern Italian site of San Martino di Ovaro, a cemetery containing thirty-one individuals, skeletons exhibited evidence of a variety of types of injuries, including fractures suggestive of both accidental traumata and intentional violence. Radial fractures typical of a fall can be seen on two individuals, for example, whereas signs of a significant attack were observed on another skeleton.[67] The skull of this individual showed evidence of two major peri-mortem blows with a heavy cutting weapon (probably a sword), one across the jawbone and one from above.[68] Roughly a fifth of this population also exhibited signs of osteomyelitis. While the development of an infection of the bone could stem from an open wound, it is also possible that these cases resulted from an existing infection that spread haematogenously.[69] At the Corso Roma cemetery in Acqui Terme, a site in use from the seventh to ninth centuries that contained thirty-three individuals, fractures were observed in three skeletons: one male and one female had ulnar fractures, while another individual had broken their fifth metatarsal.[70] Periostitis, inflammation of the periosteum, was also recorded in the humerus

66 Cod. sang. 751, p. 428: untitled lunar calendar; cod. sang. 878, pp. 366–7: *Conservatio fleotomiae et dies caniculares*. BnF lat. 11218, ff. 34v–37r: *Epistola fleobotomie*; BAV reg. lat. 1143, ff. 94v–96v: *Epistola fleopotomiae*; cod. sang. 44, pp. 191–4: *Epistula de phlebotomia*; cod. sang. 217, pp. 252a–252b, 255a–255b; cod. sang. 751, pp. 359–61: *Epistula de fleotomia Gallieni*, pp. 455–6: *Epistula de phlebotomia*, and pp. 456–8: *Epistula de phlebotomia*.

67 Amoretti, 'Analisi paleobiologiche dei resti scheletrici', 513–15.

68 Ibid.

69 Aufderheide and Rodríguez-Martín, *The Cambridge Encyclopedia of Human Paleopathology*, 172.

70 Mallegni, Bedini, Vitiello, Paglialunga, and Bartoli, 'Su alcuni gruppi umani', 233–61.

of one individual and can, like osteomyelitis, result from either an existing infection or an injury that became infected.[71]

A mixture of traumatic injuries was also reported at the cemetery excavated at La Perosa in Rivoli. This cemetery includes thirty-seven individuals and dates from the sixth to eighth centuries.[72] A radial fracture was seen on one male, while another male exhibited cranial injuries.[73] Although the fracture of the radius is not described in detail, the authors note that the fractured cranium showed no signs of remodelling and that this blow was almost certainly the direct cause of the individual's death.[74] Traumatic injuries were observed on a number of the individuals uncovered during restoration work at the Carolingian church of Sant'Agostino in Caravate.[75] For example, a 'small quadrangular perforation' was observed on the skull of one individual, a female aged approximately forty to fifty years old at death, and interpreted as the result of a blow from 'a pointed weapon with a pyramidal trunk head', such as an arrow.[76] Bone remodelling was present at the site of the injury, indicating that this individual survived the incident.[77] A second individual, a male of roughly the same age, exhibited a fractured fibula, depressed cranial fracture, and deviated septum. While the direct cause of the fibular fracture is unclear, the depressed fracture was the result of blunt force trauma. According to the authors, the deviated septum 'is probably the result of a traumatic event', though a congenital origin is also possible.[78] In the case of both fractures, complete bone

71 Mallegni, Bedini, Vitiello, Paglialunga, and Bartoli, 'Su alcuni gruppi umani', 233–61; Aufderheide and Rodríguez-Martín, *The Cambridge Encyclopedia of Human Paleopathology*, 179.

72 Mallegni, Bedini, Vitiello, Paglialunga, and Bartoli, 'Su alcuni gruppi umani', 233–61.

73 Ibid.

74 Ibid.

75 Marta Licata, Mario Ronga, Paolo Cherubino, and Giuseppe Armocida, 'Different Types of Traumatic Lesions on Mediaeval Skeletons from Archaeological Sites in Varese (North Italy): Diagnosis on *ante mortal* Fractures Using Macroscopic, Radiological and CT Analysis', *Injury* 45, no. 2 (2014): 457–9, https://doi.org/10.1016/j.injury.2013.10.013; Marta Licata, Melania Borgo, Giuseppe Armocida, Luca Nicosia, and Elena Ferioli, 'New Paleoradiological Investigations of Ancient Human Remains from North West Lombardy Archaeological Excavations', *Skeletal Radiology* 45 (2016): 323–31, https://doi.org/10.1007/s00256-015-2266-6.

76 Licata, Ronga, Cherubino, and Armocida, 'Different Types of Traumatic Lesions', quotation from p. 458; further discussion in Licata, Borgo, Armocida, Nicosia, and Ferioli, 'New Paleoradiological Investigations', 327.

77 Licata, Ronga, Cherubino, and Armocida, 'Different Types of Traumatic Lesions', 458.

78 Ibid, 458–9.

remodelling was evident, revealing that the individual made a full recovery (at least in terms of the skeletal processes involved in healing).[79]

At the rural monastic site of Santa Maria Assunta di Cairate, which includes three distinct burial areas, relatively little trauma was recorded in the more privileged burial groups found within the church (Groups A and B), though it must be noted that the majority of these individuals were female and thus perhaps less likely to participate in the types of activities that tend to result in traumatic injuries, such as hunting or fighting.[80] One exception, however, stands out: a particularly tall female found in Group B (which, as noted in Chapter 7, has been interpreted as an elite family unit) suffered a compound fracture of her left tibia.[81] Evidence of extensive bone remodelling is visible, suggesting that this individual lived for at least several years after the traumatic incident occurred. In contrast, many more injuries are observed in Group C, a collection of sixty-eight individuals thought to represent the general population who lived in the surrounding area during this period. Fractures of the clavicle, ribs, ulna, and tibia were recorded.[82] While the presence of remodelled bone in these cases indicates that the injured individuals survived the traumatic incidents that caused these injuries, evidence of periostitis, especially in the bones of the lower limbs (the femur, tibia, and fibula), was also frequently noted.[83] Although it often remains unclear if this inflammation was due to an infected wound or the spread of an existing infection, in some of these cases, such as the female with the compound tibial fracture, the periosteal reaction can be convincingly linked to a traumatic injury.

Similarly, at the Saint Servatius complex in Maastricht, one instance of osteomyelitis observed on a skeleton dated to the site's final phase of use 'was most likely secondary to a fracture of the femur'.[84] Among the individuals dated to this period, nearly twenty percent exhibit evidence of fractures, all of which show signs of healing.[85] This is not the case, however, for trauma caused by sharp-bladed or pointed objects. In a study of a larger sample of

79 Licata, Ronga, Cherubino, and Armocida, 'Different Types of Traumatic Lesions', 458–9; Licata, Borgo, Armocida, Nicosia, and Ferioli, New Paleoradiological Investigations', 327.

80 Monica Motto, 'Sepolture nel monastero di Cairate: tipologia e organizzazione delle aree cimiteriali, uno sguardo di sintesi', in *Un monastero nei secoli. Santa Maria Assunta di Cairate: scavi e ricerche*, ed. Valeria Mariotti (Mantua: SAP, 2014), 501–17; Mattucci, Ravedoni, and Rettore, 'Analisi antropologica e paleopatologica', 519–32.

81 Ibid, 523.

82 Ibid, 521–4.

83 Ibid, 523.

84 Panhuysen, 'Demography and Health in Early Medieval Maastricht', 197.

85 Ibid, 181.

early medieval skeletons from Maastricht, 228 individuals dated from the fifth to tenth centuries were analysed, and seven individuals displayed evidence of violent wounds due to sharp-edged weapons.[86] One individual showed signs of multiple blows (to the skull, torso, and hand), five had cranial fractures, and one exhibited a blow to the tibia.[87] In three cases, no evidence of bone remodelling was present, indicating that these were peri-mortem injuries and probably the cause of death.[88]

Both the urban cemetery excavated at Piazza Marconi in Cremona (in use from the seventh to tenth centuries) and the rural necropolis excavated at Bolgare (in use during the seventh and eighth centuries) contain large skeletal assemblages exhibiting evidence of traumatic injuries. Some of these skeletal markers, such as radial fractures, suggest episodes of interpersonal violence or injuries derived from occupational activities, not unlike many of the other sites reviewed above.[89] Yet, in contrast with other excavations, trauma was most frequently noted in the lower limbs of individuals buried in these cemeteries; this prevalence, however, appears to be linked to the use of a broad definition of trauma at these sites.[90] For example, fractures are recorded primarily on leg bones at Cremona, a result heightened by the inclusion of osteochondritis dissecans, a type of fracture 'caused by direct trauma or repetitive microtrauma', while small fractures in the phalanges due to repeated microtraumata were often reported at Bolgare.[91] Overall, this evidence for lower limb and foot injuries inclusive of microtraumata, relates more to long-term processes of wear and tear (see Chapter 8) than to a sudden traumatic incident.

A somewhat similar combination of fractures and signs of stress was observed among adult males at San Cassiano.[92] The eight tombs found inside the church contained seven adult males and one child; although these burials, dated to the late sixth or seventh centuries, predate the Carolingian period,

86 Raphaël G. A. M. Panhuysen, 'Het scherp van de snede: Sporen van geweld in vroegmiddeleeuws Maastricht', *Archeologie in Limburg* 92 (2002): 2–7; Robert C. Woosnam-Savage and Kelly DeVries, 'Battle Trauma in Medieval Warfare: Wounds, Weapons and Armor', on *Wounds and Wound Repair in Medieval Culture*, ed. Larissa Tracy and Kelly DeVries (Leiden: Brill, 2015), 27–56, at p. 35.

87 Panhuysen, 'Het scherp van de snede', 2–7; Woosnam-Savage and DeVries, 'Battle Trauma in Medieval Warfare', 35.

88 Ibid.

89 Cattaneo and Mazzucchi, 'Popolazioni tardo antiche e dell'alto medioevo', 87–98.

90 Ibid.

91 Cattaneo and Mazzucchi, 'Popolazioni tardo antiche e dell'alto medioevo', 87–98; Waldron, *Palaeopathology*, 153–4.

92 Chavarría and Marinato, 'Frammentazione e complessità', 61–8.

it is useful to consider these skeletons from a comparative perspective. The signs of trauma at San Cassiano, both micro and macro, have been connected with horseback-riding and the use of weapons. The legs, for example, revealed evidence of repeated stress linked to habitual horseback-riding, while the location and types of fractures observed within this small burial group are suggestive of injuries sustained from falling off a horse.[93] These findings suggest that the males buried at San Cassiano were a fairly elite group and contrast with the pattern of leg fractures and stress indicators seen at Cremona and Bolgare, pathologies linked to labour that repeatedly over-loaded the back and legs, such as hard agricultural work and heavy lifting.[94]

Moving to southwest Germany, Jochen Weber and Alfred Czarnetzki conducted a study of head injuries based on the skeletal remains found in four early medieval cemeteries (Kirchheim am Ries, Neresheim, Nusplingen, and Schretzheim) that were in use from the sixth to the eighth centuries.[95] Thirty-three of the 304 skulls analysed (11%) exhibited cranial fractures, twenty-nine of which were judged to be male and four female.[96] Twenty-one skulls had linear fractures caused by a strike from a sharp-edged weapon, such as a sword, whereas depressed fractures due to blunt force were observed on nine skulls; three skulls show evidence of both types of fractures.[97] Of the twenty-one skulls with evidence of sword blows, six recorded multiple fractures, and in all six of these cases, no sign of bone remodelling was present, suggesting that these individuals probably died as a result of their injuries.[98] Two of the skulls exhibiting sharp fractures also showed no signs of healing, but some degree of bone remodelling was observed on the remaining twenty-five skulls.[99] In other words, over three-quarters of the individuals with cranial fractures survived the initial traumatic incident. Furthermore, three skulls exhibited signs of trepanation, 'the deliberate removal of pieces of bone from the skull', evidenced by scratching or cutmarks around a circular opening, and, incredibly, all of these wounds showed signs of healing.[100] While the evidence of healed

93 Ibid.

94 Chavarría and Marinato, 'Frammentazione e complessità', 61–8; Cattaneo and Mazzucchi, 'Popolazioni tardo antiche e dell'alto medioevo', 87–98.

95 Weber and Czarnetzki, 'Neurotraumatological Aspects of Head Injuries', 352–6.

96 Ibid, 353.

97 Ibid.

98 Ibid.

99 Ibid.

100 Waldron, *Palaeopathology*, 161; Weber and Czarnetzki, 'Neurotraumatological Aspects of Head Injuries', 353.

fractures at many sites speaks to some level of medical care, these three cases of trepanation present definite evidence of surgical intervention.

Comparative evidence from earlier sites in continental Europe as well as contemporary sites in the British Isles provide additional examples of surgery. Charlotte Roberts and Jacqueline McKinley, for example, highlighted nineteen cases of trepanation in Insular contexts from the fifth to ninth centuries, while more recent studies have identified further examples.[101] An excavation from Hemmaberg, Austria, has produced one of the most remarkable cases of early medieval surgery and medical intervention. Twenty-nine individuals dated to the sixth century were found in a small cemetery associated with the early medieval church of St Hemma and Dorothea; though pre-dating the Carolingian period, stratigraphic evidence combined with grave goods and burial customs 'place [these individuals] firmly within the Frankish cultural sphere'.[102] One of the skeletons, a male aged 35 to 50 years old at death, was missing the left foot and distal joints of the left tibia and fibula. While it might be assumed that this was due to poor preservation, the skeleton was otherwise well-preserved and the point where the tibia and fibula ended was marked by extensive bone remodelling.[103] Furthermore, 'a sub-circular iron band with a diameter of 6.8–7.3 cm' was found in place of the lower leg and foot, highly suggestive of a prosthetic attachment.[104] Ultimately, the osteological analysis of the tibia and fibula indicated that the foot and distal portion of the tibia and fibula had been amputated and that, despite suffering from osteomyelitis, this individual eventually recovered. Full remodelling of the bones indicates that the wound completely healed and the individual survived for at least some years after the surgery.[105] Although there is not enough evidence to deduce the cause of the amputation, the existence of this case of surgical intervention followed by long-term medical care—as illustrated by the individual's survival of

101 Charlotte A. Roberts and Jacqueline McKinley, 'A Review of Trepanations in British Antiquity Focusing on Funerary Context to Explain Their Occurrence', in *Trepanation: History, Discovery, Theory*, ed. Robert Arnott, Stanley Finger, and C. U. M. Smith (Lisse: Swets & Zeitlinger Publishers, 2003), 55–78; S. A. Mays, 'A Possible Case of Surgical Treatment of Cranial Blunt Force Injury from Medieval England', *International Journal of Osteoarchaeology* 16, no. 2 (2006): 95–103, https://doi.org/10.1002/oa.806.

102 M. Binder, J. Eitler, J. Deutschmann, S. Ladstätter, F. Glaser, and D. Fiedler, 'Prosthetics in Antiquity—An Early Medieval Wearer of a Foot Prosthesis (6th Century AD) from Hemmaberg/Austria', *International Journal of Paleopathology* 12 (2016): 29–40, https://doi.org/10.1016/j.ijpp.2015.11.003, at pp. 30–1.

103 Binder, Eitler, Deutschmann, Ladstätter, Glaser, and Fiedler, 'Prosthetics in Antiquity', 31–2.

104 Ibid, 32.

105 Ibid, 33–9.

the initial surgery and the resulting infection as well as his use of a prosthetic lower leg after recovery—is noteworthy, not least because this cemetery has been linked to an early Frankish context.

Overall, the above examples indicate that standard traumatic injuries, such as broken bones, were not infrequent; while some may have been caused by interpersonal violence, others could have been due to accidents, such as a fall. There are, however, a number of spectacular cases that bear witness to surgical inventions, such as multiple trepanations and the Hemmaberg amputation. Most significantly, the evidence of healing in many examples reflects effective (and often long-term) medical care.

4 Reading Recipes in the Light of Osteological Evidence for Trauma and Surgery

The skeletal evidence presented above preserves signs of trauma from a variety of sources, including violent incidents involving weapons, injuries caused by falls or occupational hazards, and, rarely, examples of surgical intervention. Bone remodelling indicates that large numbers of early medieval individuals survived not only an initial traumatic incident but also made full recoveries (at least in terms of the skeletal healing process). Evidence of healed fractures is highly suggestive of medical care, even if this care remains otherwise invisible in the skeletal record. Although many of the examples of surgery listed above, such as the trepanations from early medieval England, are from sites beyond the Frankish Empire or, as in the case of the amputation, pre-date the Carolingian period, there are occasional signs of surgery in potentially Carolingian contexts, including the handful of trepanations in southwest Germany which may date to the eighth century.

While the textual evidence lists treatments for a similar range of traumatic injuries, there are no clear signs of trepanation, amputation, or other surgical procedures beyond superficial surgeries, such as bloodletting and cautery, in the recipes under analysis. The reference to the removal of bone fragments comes closest to providing a possible hint of more complex and potentially invasive surgical practices (and is especially intriguing given that it occurred in the context of cranial fractures), yet it offers no direct comments on surgery. Reassessing the recipe literature in view of the skeletal evidence thus indicates that the surviving written sources do not provide a complete picture of contemporary medical approaches since surgical procedures, as documented by the skeletal remains, were clearly performed—if only rarely.

This finding, however, should not diminish the significant parallels observed between the osteological record and the recipes with respect to fractures, dislocations, and various wounds inflicted by weapons. Indeed, these parallels take on increasing significance given that signs of healing were observed in skeletal remains with some frequency. Overall, the evidence for traumatic injuries, whether general (such as fractures) or more specific (such as wounds caused by particular weapons), corresponds with the types of injuries named in recipes, thereby indicating that much of the recorded knowledge would have been applicable to early medieval populations. The osteological evidence, moreover, suggests that surgical intervention may not have been needed in many cases: immobilisation of the injured bone, reduction of inflammation, and pain management would have often been the necessary course of action. These more basic, non-invasive treatments fit with the information offered by recipes. Although I cannot begin to address the possible efficacy of these treatments with regard to inflammation reduction or pain management, the large number of healed fractures in the skeletal record is striking. The inclusion of instructions for bandaging in some recipes suggests that these treatments could have been used in conjunction with knowledge passed on through alternative means, such as oral traditions, regarding bone setting or splinting techniques. Like the preceding chapters, the skeletal evidence provides a crucial counterbalance to the written record, offering a means to reassess the recipe literature and dig deeper into the recipes' potential applicability to individuals in early medieval Europe.

With these two bodies of evidence in mind, several areas of analysis can be pressed further in relation to the question of applicability.

4.1 *Type of Injury: Conflicting Evidence?*

Puncture wounds appear with some frequency in the recipe sample, with arrows (*sagittae*), thorns (*spinae*), and other non-specified punctures (*punctae*) mentioned on over twenty occasions. The skeletal remains, however, provide relatively little evidence of such injuries: the vast majority of weapon injuries appear to be linked to either sharp-edged weapons or blunt force trauma. The female skull with a probable arrow wound as well as a male excavated at Saint Servatius with evidence of a similar injury represent some of the few exceptions.[106] Does this disjuncture suggest that the textual record, at least with respect to this type of injury, had little relevance to early medieval populations? While this could be the case, like the example of gout in the preceding

106 Panhuysen, 'Demography and Health in Early Medieval Maastricht', 183–4.

chapter, the absence of evidence should not be read as evidence of absence. Instead, it is highly probable that the archaeological record provides a very skewed picture of puncture wounds because these types of injuries are much less likely to leave a trace of their impact on skeletal remains. Consider, for example, a stab wound in the viscera: major traumatic injuries need not affect the skeleton. Therefore, despite the few cases of puncture wounds observed in the archaeological record, the medical texts' focus on puncture wounds should not be dismissed as irrelevant.

Injuries that could be classified as 'non-violent', such as falls, seem to present the opposite situation with respect to the two bodies of evidence. Among the recipes that named specific causes of traumatic injuries, over ninety-five percent listed a violent action or weapon as responsible for the wound in question.[107] The two recipes for falling off a horse or out of a tree and two treatments for punctures from thorns represent the only exceptions. Surely falls and injuries from occupational hazards occurred more frequently than this record suggests; indeed, some of the reports consulted in this study argued that the osteological evidence exhibited not only markers of horseback-riding but also injuries related to falls. While this could represent a disconnect between the textual and skeletal evidence, again, I argue that a deeper analysis of the texts reveals a different story. Unlike an arrow wound or a sword blow, which may need fairly specialised treatments, a fall could result in a broken bone, a dislocation, a sprain, major bruising, and so on. Many of the recipes for general injuries, such as fractures, dislocations, and bruising, could apply to these types of general accidents. Given the varied nature of the resulting injuries, it would be more appropriate to treat the specific issue with which the patient presents rather than 'a fall'. With this in mind, the lack of recipes explicitly intended for falls and other accidents makes more sense and supports the applicability of the general injury treatments to individuals in the Carolingian world.

4.2 *The Question of Surgery*

As noted in the textual analysis, several parts of the body, including the head, were mentioned repeatedly. The recipes' emphasis on this area fits with the archaeological evidence: cranial fractures were among the most frequently observed traumatic injuries in the skeletal record. While the trepanations observed in the osteological record reveal that some surgical methods were used to treat head conditions (though it is often unclear if the underlying

107 Although it must be remembered that some of these injuries may have been accidental, the method of inflicting damage (blows, strikes, cuts, etc.) can be described as violent.

cause(s) of a trepanation were related to trauma), the majority of healed head injuries seen in the osteological record appear to have healed as a result of non-invasive medical treatment. This finding further strengthens the argument that the recipe literature was highly applicable to individuals in early medieval Europe since not only do the types of trauma recorded on the skeletons and in the texts consistently overlap, but the methods of treatment also appear to have a high degree of correspondence. That is, the skeletal evidence suggests that, although surgical procedures were practised, non-invasive treatments were preferred—a finding that is not unexpected in an age without modern antibiotics and anaesthetics.

Yet, some invasive, complex surgeries did occur, if only rarely. Given the relative pausity of surgical information in the texts, especially with respect to complex, invasive surgeries, such as amputation and trepanation, where did the individuals who performed these surgeries acquire their knowledge? Debby Banham and Christine Voth have argued that oral traditions and practical training may have played a significant role in the transmission of surgical knowledge in the Insular world, and it appears that continental Europe experienced a similar phenomenon.[108] This is not to say that *much* surgery was occurring during this period, but to acknowledge that texts were certainly not the exclusive source of medical knowledge at this time. Here, it is important to remember that the Hemmaberg amputation as well as several trepanations occurred within a Frankish context. Though largely pre-dating the Carolingian period, these cases of surgical intervention offer a glimpse into earlier Frankish medical practices, suggesting that knowledge of surgery, perhaps drawing on Frankish traditions or medical practices picked up through contact with the Roman military, was passed on outside of the written record. The potential links between military medicine and surgical practice in relation to the particularly violent traumata of warfare will be considered in the following section.

4.3 *Evidence for Trauma Beyond Medical Texts*

Finally, a comment must be made on the wider context and the evidence for trauma as documented by textual sources beyond the medical manuscripts, such as capitularies, law codes, annals, histories, and poetry. Records of warfare and violence represent perhaps the most obvious source of information regarding traumatic injuries recorded by non-medical texts. Einhard's *Life of Charlemagne*, for example, emphasised the brutality of the Saxon Wars,

108 Banham and Voth, 'The Diagnosis and Treatment of Wounds', 153–74.

noting that Charlemagne would repeatedly 'avenge [the Saxon's] treachery and demand a fitting punishment until everyone who was accustomed to resist was crushed and brought back under his control'.[109] In addition to territorial expansion and defence, internal conflicts, such as the civil wars of the early 840s fought between Charlemagne's grandsons, were another source of largescale violence. The Battle of Fontenoy (841) was famously memorialised by Angelbert, a follower of Lothar who survived the battle. While his verses do not provide details about the specific injuries sustained in battle, the general description of the death toll and suffering of survivors paints a vivid picture of the carnage: 'There has been no worse massacre on the field of battle. / Christian law is violated; blood flows in waves; / and in hell the maw of Cerberus opens with glee'.[110] Although such emotionally charged lines may have an element of dramatisation, it certainly suggests that much blood was shed. The epic *Waltharius*, despite presenting an even more theatrical perspective, depicts scenes of hand-to-hand combat. When battling a series of Franks, the hero Walter killed Eleuthir by splitting his 'brain in two and, cutting through the neck itself, opened up his chest'.[111] Soon he 'turned his anger toward [Tanastus] and tore his shoulder from its joint and sliced through his side with iron, spilling his guts'.[112] While the historical accuracy of the *Waltharius* cannot be taken at face value, its portrayal of the characters' attitudes towards violence and illustration of the type of trauma that might have been expected in combat provide a useful cultural framework in which to understand warfare and injury in the Carolingian period.[113]

---

109 Einhard, *Vita Karoli Magni*, ed. O. Holder-Egger, MGH SS *Rer. Germ.* 25 (Hanover: Hahn, 1911), Chapter 7 (at p. 10): *Nam numquam eos huiuscemodi aliquid perpetrantes inpune ferre passus est, quin aut ipse per se ducto aut per comites suos misso exercitu perfidiam ulcisceretur et dignam ab eis poenam exigeret, usque dum, omnibus qui resistere solebant profligatis et in suam potestatem redactis.* Translation from Einhard, *Life of Charlemagne*, in *Two Lives of Charlemagne*, trans. David Ganz (London: Penguin Books, 2008), Chapter 7 (at p. 23).

110 Angelbert, *Versus de bella quae fuit acta Fontaneto*, ed. Ernst Dümmler, MGH *Poet.* 2 (Berlin: Weidmann, 1884), 138: *Caedes nulla peior fuit campo nec in Marcio; / fracta est lex christianorum; sanguinis proluvio, / unde manus; inferorum, gaudet gula Cerberi.* Translation from Angelbert, *The Battle of Fontenoy*, in *Poetry of the Carolingian Renaissance*, trans. Peter Godman (London: Duckworth, 1985), 263.

111 Ekkehard I of St. Gall, *Waltharius*, ed. and trans. Abram Ring (Leuven: Peeters, 2016), 124–5: *Huic galeam findens cerebrum diffudit et ipsam / Cervicem resecans pectus patefecit, at aegrum.*

112 Ekkehard, *Waltharius*, ed. and trans. Ring, 128–9: *Hinc indignatus iram convertit in ipsum / Waltharius humerumque eius de cardine vellit / Perque latus ducto suffudit viscera ferro.*

113 Jan M. Ziolkowski, 'Fighting Words: Wordplay and Swordplay in the *Waltharius*', in *Germanic Texts and Latin Models: Medieval Reconstructions*, ed. Karin E. Olsen, Antonina

Studies of Carolingian arms and armour based on documentary, iconographic, and archaeological evidence offer another perspective on the nature of the wounds sustained in battle. Simon Coupland's analysis of military equipment, for example, has confirmed the importance of mounted warfare and the use of lances, swords, and bows in battle, fitting with the signs of horseback-riding seen in the osteological record and suggesting that treatments for injuries due to falls would have been readily applicable.[114] Coupland also highlights that Carolingian swords were highly sought-after by the Franks' neighbours and that, despite the court's attempts to prevent them from falling into the wrong hands, 'archaeological evidence suggests that export embargoes were unsuccessful'.[115] Significantly for this discussion, the use of similar weapons across a range of contexts (internecine wars, borderland conflicts, Viking raids, etc.) would have resulted in comparable injuries. Despite this varied body of evidence on Carolingian warfare derived from literary, documentary, iconographic, or archaeological sources, evidence for medical practice and practitioners in such military environments remains very limited. The extent of this lacuna is striking when compared to the surviving evidence for military medicine in classical and late antique Rome as well as later medieval Europe.[116] On the basis of this comparative evidence and taking into consideration the severity and urgency of the medical care needed on the battlefield, it seems likely that surgical procedures would have also been practised in context of combat in the Carolingian world.

The frequency with which Carolingian rulers attempted to regulate violence beyond the battlefield, however, reveals that traumatic injuries due to interpersonal violence could occur outside of warfare. In the *Capitulary of Herstal* of 779, for example, counts and bishops acting as judges were prohibited 'from maiming men through hatred or ill-intent', while the *Admonitio generalis* of 789 banned revenge killings.[117] Notably, Charlemagne's capitularies specifically

---

Harbus, and Tette Hofstra (Leuven: Peeters, 2001), 29–51; Jan M. Ziolkowski, 'Blood, Sweat and Tears in the *Waltharius*', in *Insignis Sophiae Arcator: Medieval Latin Studies in Honour of Michael Herren on his 65th Birthday*, ed. Gernot R. Wieland, Carin Ruff, and Ross G. Arthur (Turnhout: Brepols, 2006), 149–64.

114 Simon Coupland, 'Carolingian Arms and Armor in the Ninth Century', *Viator* 21 (1990): 29–50.

115 Coupland, 'Carolingian Arms and Armour in the Ninth Century', 44.

116 On Roman military medicine, see, for example, Ido Israelowich, 'Medical Care in the Roman Army during the High Empire', in *Popular Medicine in Graeco-Roman Antiquity: Explorations*, ed. William V. Harris (Leiden: Brill, 2016), 215–30. For medicine in the Crusades, see Mitchell, *Medicine in the Crusades*.

117 Warren C. Brown, *Violence in Medieval Europe* (Harlow: Pearson Education Limited, 2011), 71–8; *Capitulare Haristallense*, ed. Alfred Boretius, MGH *Capit.* 1, no. 20 (Hanover: Hahn,

targeted eliminating violence in ecclesiastical communities on a number of occasions: pronouncements in 802 and 811 forbad the clergy from bearing arms and maintaining armed followers.[118] Perhaps the potential for violent encounters helps to explain Walahfrid's inclusion of a treatment for 'fractures and wounds from iron' in his *vademecum*, cod. sang. 878.[119] On the other hand, early medieval law codes shed light on the use of legitimised violence, such as corporal punishment. Take, for example, *Rothair's Edict* from the Lombard Kingdom in the middle of the seventh century.[120] While the majority of the 388 laws offer financial penalties, some present physical punishments, such as the amputation of a hand:

> 242. Concerning the illegal minting of coins: He who mints gold or strikes money without the king's command shall have his hand cut off.
> 243. On forged charters: He who forges a charter or other kind of document shall have his hand cut off.[121]

An understanding of the wider Carolingian context in which violence occurred helps to situate the evidence of trauma preserved in the archaeological record as well as approaches to traumatic injuries seen in the recipe literature. The archaeological sites reviewed above do not appear to represent battlegrounds given that, although trauma was evident, it was not recorded in the majority of individuals, as might be the case with a mass grave of war dead. Similarly, there is no evidence to suggest that the collections of recipes under consideration were written with either warfare or judicial punishments in mind. Instead,

---

1883), c. 1; *Admonitio generalis*, ed. Alfred Boretius, *MGH Capit.* 1, no. 22 (Hanover: Hahn, 1883), c. 8.

118 Brown, *Violence in Medieval Europe*, 75; *Capitula a sacerdotibus proposita*, ed. Alfred Boretius, *MGH Capit.* 1, no. 36 (Hanover: Hahn, 1883), c. 18; *Capitulare missorum item speciale*, ed. Alfred Boretius, *MGH Capit.* 1, no. 35 (Hanover: Hahn, 1883), c. 37; *Capitula de causis cum episcopis et abbatibus tractandis*, ed. Alfred Boretius, *MGH Capit.* 1, no. 72 (Hanover: Hahn, 1883), c. 4.

119 Cod. sang. 878, p. 333: *Ad fracturam uel uulnera ferri*; see Appendix 2, entry 13.1.

120 *Edictus Rothari*, in *Leges Langobardorum*, ed. Friedrich Bluhme, *MGH LL* 4 (Hanover: Hahn, 1868), 1–90; *Rothair's Edict*, in *The Lombard Laws*, trans. Katherine Fischer Drew (Philadelphia: University of Pennsylvania Press, 1973), 39–130; on early medieval law codes more generally, see Katherine Fischer Drew, *Law and Society in Early Medieval Europe: Studies in Legal History* (London: Variorum, 1988).

121 *Edictus Rothari*, ed. Bluhme, 242 (at p. 60): *Si quis sine iussionem regis aurum figuraverit aut moneta confinxerit, manus ei incidatur*; 243 (at p. 60): *De cartola falsa. Si quis cartolam falsam scripserit aut quodlibet membranum, manus ei incidatur*. Translation from *Rothair's Edict*, trans. Fischer Drew, 100.

given the parallels seen in the osteological and textual evidence, I suggest that these collections would have been applicable to the day-to-day healthscapes of many individuals in early medieval Europe—not so relevant to those on military campaigns, but highly relevant to those in, for example, a monastic community or an aristocratic household. The non-medical written sources, and especially Charlemagne's capitularies, indicate that violence occurred not simply in military settings but also in these domestic environments, if at a lower level. This finding fits with the degree and frequency of injuries seen in the skeletal remains. It must also be remembered that some individuals may have survived the injuries they sustained in warfare and these wounds may account for some of the cases of trauma observed in the archaeological record.

Overall, the types of recipes recorded in the medical texts appear to have been highly applicable to many individuals in the Carolingian world, offering basic treatments for standard injuries. Indeed, the recipe literature seems particularly suited to those individuals who would have had access to the texts, such as the members of ecclesiastical communities and elite households. Warfare, however, represents violence on a different scale given the severity, urgency, and sheer number of injuries that would have occurred in battle.[122] When entire limbs could be removed in a single blow, a topical plaster could only do so much.[123] I suggest, therefore, that medical practitioners involved in military campaigns relied on an additional body of knowledge unrecorded by the written sources, and one that quite possibly included surgery. This information must have been primarily transmitted through non-textual knowledge exchange, such as oral traditions and practical experience.

5 Conclusion

Traumatic injuries, despite their seemingly straightforward cause-and-effect relationship, remain a challenging subject to investigate in past populations. This chapter has revealed that there is a fairly high degree of overlap between the textual evidence and skeletal record, especially with respect to fractures and wounds sustained from various types of blows. This suggests that much

122 Banham and Voth, 'The Diagnosis and Treatment of Wounds', 169.

123 As illustrated by Walter's attack on Gunther: Walter 'pried Gunther's shield away on the right, made a mighty and amazing blow, and tore off his leg up to the knee, all of it below the thigh' (*Impetit et scuto dextra de parte revulso / Ictum praevalidum ac mirandum fecit eique / Crus cum poplite adusque femur decerpserat omne*); Ekkehard, *Waltharius*, trans. Ring, 152–3.

of the knowledge recorded in the texts was applicable to early medieval populations, at least in certain contexts. Warfare, however, would have resulted in traumata on an entirely different level, and the treatments recorded in the recipes analysed in this study would not have suited such an environment.

Despite the general parallels between the two bodies of evidence, there are particular areas that might, at first glance, seem to present conflicting results. Yet, an in-depth analysis of the evidence has revealed that these more challenging topics are not necessarily incompatible with the bigger picture: with respect to puncture wounds or non-violent traumatic injuries, by contextualising the evidence, the seemingly contradictory results were reconciled. Surgery and warfare, however, are special cases, offering an important reminder that, although there is much evidence to support the use of the recipes recorded in Carolingian manuscripts in the practice of medicine, alternative sources of medical knowledge, such as oral traditions, remained vitally important during this period.

Conclusion

CHAPTER 10

Putting Knowledge Into Practice

1 Introduction: Revisiting the Case of Terenti(an)us

In view of the evidence presented in the preceding chapters, I shall return to the case of Terenti(an)us with which this book opened and reconsider these two recipes, the *Antidotum podagricum* of cod. sang. 751 and the *Potio ad podagra* of cod. sang. 759.[1] These recipes served as a useful entry point into the question of whether medical knowledge recorded in eighth- and ninth-century manuscripts was used *in* the practice of medicine given their inclusion of Terenti(an)us' seemingly personal comments regarding his experience of using this treatment. The recipes' codicological contexts radically alters the picture: the different scripts seen in codd. sang. 751 and 759, combined with the distinct textual environments in which the recipes are found, indicates that the two treatments were based on an earlier source. Terenti(an)us' claims cannot be read, therefore, as direct evidence linking medical knowledge and practice in the Carolingian period. Most importantly, this example illustrates how the written record can be over-interpreted when individual texts are analysed in isolation, highlighting the need for new approaches to the study of the relationship between medical knowledge and practice. Having explored this relationship through the prisms of practicality and applicability and considered both textual and osteological evidence, what can now be said about the potential use of these two recipes?

While it remains impossible to be certain if either one of these treatments was consulted in the context of therapy, the evidence examined throughout the preceding chapters suggests that, broadly, the recipe literature recorded in the early medieval Latin west was intended to be used in medical practice. In reassessing the particularities of the Terenti(an)us case, the findings from several of this book's case studies are especially relevant. First, consider the practicality of these treatments with respect to the *materia medica* they name. The detailed instructions of both recipes list a mixture of ingredients that could have been growing locally, such as centaury (*centauria*) and birthwort (*aristolocia rotunda*), as well as exotic products, including myrrh (*mirra*) and cardamom

1 Cod. sang. 751, pp. 489–90: *Antidotum podagricum*; cod. sang. 759, p. 60: *Potio ad podagra*. See Chapter 1 for a more detailed review of the recipes and Appendix 2, entries 9.38 and 11.8, respectively.

(*cardamomo*, only listed in cod. sang. 759).[2] Although the recipes include neither the newly recorded non-local substances discussed in Chapter 3 nor any of the notably local alcohols highlighted in Chapter 4, similar combinations of local and imported ingredients have been seen repeatedly. While the inclusion of exotic ingredients has historically raised red flags regarding recipes' practicality, the evidence presented in Chapter 3 demonstrates that these types of non-local substances were periodically available in the Frankish Empire—if only in limited quantities and restricted to the elite. Other aspects of these recipes' instructions, however, appear to be less practical: Terenti(an)us reports that he used the potion for 365 days and suggests that longer may be necessary. The daily consumption of such a potion over the course of an entire year does not seem viable. In sum, although the use of the ingredients named in these recipes does not make them inherently impractical, the treatments' recommended long-term use would certainly pose challenges and suggests that the recipes would have been exceedingly difficult to use in practice.

The recipes' applicability, however, is more promising. As shown in Chapter 8, few cases of gout have been recorded in skeletal remains dated to the Carolingian period. Yet, the relatively high frequencies of more general foot and ankle arthropathies suggest that treatments claiming to help *podagra* should often be interpreted more broadly. If the Terenti(an)us recipes are therefore taken to address foot and toe joint pain, including OA, RA, gout, and other diseases or injuries affecting the toes and feet, the treatments appear to be highly applicable.

This re-evaluation of the opening recipes reflects the mixed picture of the recipes overall: while the case studies pursued in the preceding chapters have highlighted examples of practical and applicable treatments, there remain counterexamples, i.e., recipes that would have been difficult, if not impossible, to put into practice and/or that would not have been applicable to individuals in early medieval Europe. Collectively, however, the findings presented in this book point to a general picture of practicality and applicability, suggesting that pharmaceutical information was often recorded with the intention of being used in the context of therapy—though such a use may have been combined with others. The analysis of a large sample of recipes, in conjunction with the integration of osteological evidence, has made these conclusions possible.

2 Note: while *cardamomum* is often interpreted as 'cardamom', it is sometimes taken to mean 'cress' (which could have been a potentially local product); see, for example, Monica Green's comments in *The* Trotula*: A Medieval Compendium of Women's Medicine*, ed. and trans. Monica H. Green (Philadelphia: University of Pennsylvania Press, 2001), 275.

I shall briefly review the results of Parts 1 and 2 to flesh out and expand on these findings and their implications.

2 Bringing Together the Case Studies

As seen in this book's opening chapters, although there is only limited evidence documenting the existence of medical practitioners in early medieval Europe, there is even less evidence regarding the specifics of their practices, and especially the degree to which—if at all—these practices relied on the pharmaceutical knowledge recorded in the manuscripts of the period.[3] The present study has therefore investigated the relationship between medical knowledge and practice in the Carolingian world from a new angle, taking a dual approach that brings together both textual and osteological evidence. Chapter 1 established the conceptual framework that underpins this book. A review of early work in the field showed that, traditionally, many scholars have worked on individual texts (or families of texts) in isolation and prioritised writings tied to classical and late antique traditions. Although the field is changing, the longstanding lack of scholarship on recipes located outside of the established texts demands more analyses of this material. Simultaneously, the potential pitfalls of studying such texts in isolation, highlighted by the opening example of Terenti(an)us, contributed to the selection of a large sample of understudied recipes from twenty-four manuscripts. Although a revisionist wave of scholarship overturned many negative stereotypes concerning early medieval medicine, it has also led to the generation (and repetition) of new assumptions regarding the use of medical texts. My reassessment of the question of practicality has aimed to move beyond the circular arguments seen in some of this work. Finally, by focusing on the potential applicability of pharmaceutical writings to individuals in early medieval Europe, this book also draws on evidence from the osteological record, building on and contributing to scholarship that has called for an investigation into past population health alongside traditional studies of the history of medicine.

Chapter 2 opened Part 1 with an introduction to and contextualisation of the recipe literature under analysis. This chapter laid the groundwork for the following three chapters that explored the question of practicality. Chapters 3 and 4 analysed a selection of the *materia medica* listed in recipes, asking if

3 Flint, 'The Early Medieval 'Medicus'', 127–45; Skinner, *Health and Medicine in Early Medieval Southern Italy*; Pilsworth, *Healthcare in Early Medieval Northern Italy*; Pilsworth, 'Could you just sign this for me John?', 363–88; Park, 'Medicine and Society', 67–9; Leja, *Embodying the Soul*.

these substances could have been obtained in the Frankish world during the eighth and ninth centuries. Chapter 3 initiated the case studies by analysing the introduction of a cluster of ingredients from the east, tracing their inclusion in recipes individually, and considering evidence for the movement of these substances (in addition to the arrival of pharmaceutical information pertaining to them). I argued that recipes involving these non-local ingredients were practical, even if the ways in which they were practical differ from typical perceptions of practicality (as exemplified by the local *materia medica* examined in the following chapter). The evidence indicates that the substances in question would have been available, but only sporadically, in small quantities, and at great expense. I suggest, therefore, that recipes listing these types of ingredients store 'latent knowledge', offering information that could be used when the necessary substances were available. This may help to explain why there are so many different recipes that claim to treat the same symptom(s) or condition(s): each recipe provides a treatment option and could have been used depending on what ingredients were on hand. Based on these findings, I also argued that the inclusion of newly introduced eastern *materia medica* revealed that scribes were adapting the recipe literature and incorporating 'cutting-edge' information. These modifications—that is, the integration of the latest pharmaceutical information—strengthen the idea that this body of knowledge was intended to be used in the practice of medicine.

Turning to the opposite end of the 'localness' spectrum, Chapter 4 concentrated on the appearance of beer and mead (*medus*) in eighth- and ninth-century recipes. When considered alongside evidence for the production of these beverages in the Frankish Empire, it suggests that the scribes responsible for these recipe collections incorporated ingredients suited to local conditions. I argued that the inclusion of these alcohols represents a practical addition to the recipe literature and indicates that scribes were actively engaging with this body of knowledge, updating it to rely on more accessible ingredients. These features likewise support the idea that many recipes were recorded with the intention of being used in therapy.

Chapter 5 then moved from an examination of ingredients to an analysis of other features within recipes. I investigated the appearance of a vernacular unit and the inclusion of instructions for substituting ingredients if a desired substance was unavailable. The use of the Latinised vernacular unit *staupus* and the addition of information on substituting *materia medica* represent two highly practical features. The former points to user-friendly adaptations made to suit a changing linguistic landscape. While the latter is similarly practical, it should not be overemphasised since, in many cases, it may reflect information derived from earlier sources rather than the experiences of Carolingian medical practitioners.

Collectively, the three chapters connected different yet complementary perspectives on the practicality of the recipe literature. Based on this combination of evidence, I argued that many recipes were practical in terms of both their design and potential useability: on the one hand, they contain modifications that would have aided an individual consulting the texts and, on the other hand, they often present several treatment options that would have enabled a reader to select a recipe based on their available ingredients and other variables.

Building on the assessment of practicality, Part 2 turned to the question of applicability. Chapter 6 provided the foundation for the case studies of Chapters 7–9, outlining the challenges of bringing together textual and osteological evidence and reviewing the sites involved in the following chapters. Chapter 7's focus on dental disease exhibited many examples of overlap between the two bodies of evidence: the signs of poor dental health seen in the skeletal remains, such as cavities, tooth loss, and the accumulation of dental calculus, corresponded to many of the descriptions of dental problems recorded in the recipes. These treatments thus appear to have been highly applicable to individuals in early medieval Europe. Moreover, while the potential utility of a number of treatment subcategories, such as cosmetic dentifrices, may have seemed questionable at first, a more detailed examination suggested that such recipes would have been particularly relevant to the individuals who likely had access to these texts, namely, elite members of aristocratic households and ecclesiastical communities.

Chapter 8 concentrated on joint diseases, beginning with a study on gout. Although I identified many examples of recipes claiming to treat *podagra*, few cases of gout have been observed in early medieval skeletal remains. In contrast to the relative absence of gout, evidence for general arthropathies, such as OA, was frequently noted. After reviewing recipes for more general joint disease in the light of the osteological record, I reassessed the gout-*podagra* paradox and argued that the apparent lack of correspondence between the evidence for gout and *podagra* reflects an inappropriately rigid translation of the medieval Latin terminology rather than a simple mismatch in the evidence. Understanding the medieval usage of *podagra* as more generalised foot pain instead of the modern medical definition of gout not only aligns more closely with the osteological evidence, but also demonstrates the dangers of applying modern medical definitions to medieval medical terms. Overall, based on the frequency with which arthritis and signs of stress were observed in the skeletal remains, recipes intended to treat joint pain—from the cervical spine to the big toe—would have been applicable to essentially everyone who lived long enough to develop these pathologies.

Lastly, Chapter 9 investigated surgical intervention and trauma. Given the relative lack of treatises on surgery in the early medieval west, this chapter assessed how the non-invasive treatments recorded in the recipes compared to the evidence seen in the osteological record and explored whether there is evidence to suggest that surgical practices unrecorded by written sources were being practised during this period. While signs of surgery, such as trepanation, were observed in skeletal remains, these types of invasive practices were reported very rarely. Meanwhile, given the evidence for healed fractures and other injuries that do not bear signs of surgical intervention, the recipe literature's non-invasive treatments for traumatic injuries seem to fit with the osteological record. An examination of texts beyond the medical corpus, however, revealed that the skeletal evidence considered in this study did not appear to record the extremely severe injuries of warfare. Although the recipes under analysis would not have suited the context of military medicine, it does appear that they would have been highly applicable in other settings, such as an elite household or monastery.

While it must be remembered that each of these case studies represents a single type of condition, all three chapters provided evidence that broadly supports the applicability of the recipe literature to individuals in early medieval Europe. Bringing Parts 1 and 2 together, it appears that a large proportion of these treatments were both practical and applicable, though, as the case of Terenti(an)us illustrates, this assessment is far from universal. The individual factors relating to a recipe's practicality and applicability remain highly complex and often context specific. Thus, in arguing that the recipe literature was largely practical and applicable, I do not mean that recipes were *always* and/or *uniformly* practical and applicable, but rather that they were potentially practical and applicable given the right circumstances. These recipes offer treatments that, though they might not have been consistently useful or usable, *could* have been used when an individual presented with Disease X or Injury Y and when Ingredient A, B, and C were available. Consider, for example, the injuries discussed in Chapter 9: the osteological evidence suggests that fractures were not an exceedingly common problem but that they did occur. It would therefore make sense to have information regarding potential treatments ready to be deployed when such an injury happened, even if the need for these treatments was relatively rare. Likewise, the frequency with which multiple treatment options were recorded suggests that a recipe could be selected on the basis of the available ingredients. Cynehard's complaints about his lack of non-local *materia medica* clearly illustrates that certain ingredients were difficult to source during this period. Yet, since many of these types of ingredients appear to have been occasionally available, if only in limited quantities and at a high price, a recipe incorporating such ingredients stored knowledge that had the potential to be used in practice. Ultimately, even if many recipes were not (or only rarely) consulted in therapy, it is their *potential* for use in this context that is a key conclusion of this book's analyses.

The question of the recipes' intended use(s) is inherently linked to this finding. As discussed in Chapter 1, medical texts could have been used in a variety of different, if often overlapping, ways.[4] That many recipes were potentially practical and applicable in early medieval Europe does not necessarily mean that they were recorded with the intention of being used in medical practice, but simply that they *could* have been used in this context. The addition of user-friendly features in many recipes' instructions, the increasing appearance of locally producible ingredients, as well as, paradoxically, the inclusion of previously unrecorded products from the far east all suggest, however, that recipes, on the whole, were recorded with the intention of being used in therapy. These particular elements reveal not only that recipes were adapted in ways that would have facilitated their use in treatment but also that scribes incorporated the latest pharmaceutical knowledge.

Even if the recipes' potential useability in medical practice was often the primary motivation that lay behind their collection and documentation, it is important to emphasise that this was by no means the only motivation. BnF lat. 13955, a manuscript not considered in the present study, contains an assortment of texts related to the liberal and mechanical arts as well as recipes and was, therefore, perhaps intended primarily for educational purposes. That being said, it could have served both pedagogical and therapeutic functions; indeed, many of the recipes examined in this study could have had multiple purposes and/or their uses could have changed over time.

A consideration of the ways in which the recipes were used necessitates a comment on the environments in which these uses occurred. As argued in Chapter 9, the recipe literature analysed in this study is unlikely to have been suitable for the extreme conditions of warfare. It appears, however, that the monastic setting in which many of these manuscripts were produced would have had a better fit. Yet, the osteological evidence indicates that many recipes would have been applicable to individuals living in a wide range of communities, so the potential for medical practice must be considered in additional contexts. Given that there is evidence documenting the existence of medical

4 Horden, 'Prefatory Note', 1–6.

texts in both monastic and lay libraries, royal and aristocratic households also represent likely locations for the practice of medicine related to the information contained in these medical texts.[5] But what can be said about the potential use of these writings outside of the most privileged strata of society? Based on the skeletal record, it appears that the recipe literature would have been widely applicable in non-elite contexts, as well. Despite the relevance of the treatments to individuals from all levels of society, however, I suggest that the use of these texts in relation to medical practice would have been largely limited to elite communities since the consultation of medical writings is predicated on literacy. There is, however, evidence of monks practising medicine beyond the cloister walls and the possibility that local communities surrounding elite sites or pilgrims passing through ecclesiastical institutions could have benefitted from medical care at these locations.[6] Furthermore, the addition of medical recipes to a number of 'priests' handbooks', a phenomenon noted by Carine van Rhijn in a selection of manuscripts not considered in the present study, likewise suggests that medical knowledge was moving beyond the cloister and circulating in local communities.[7] The application of the texts in non-elite contexts should not, therefore, be ruled out, though, given the need for literacy, the individuals using such material are likely to have come from an elite establishment.

The cost of treatments must also be considered when addressing the contexts of medical practice—could people with more limited resources have afforded the ingredients listed in recipes or would their high prices suggest a very restricted clientele? Although some recipes rely on expensive, imported *materia medica*, others combine a mixture of local and non-local substances. A significant proportion, moreover, tend to use only a handful of products—if not a single ingredient—that could have been obtained locally, whether grown (such as the many plants also listed in texts on gardens and gardening), foraged (including berries, mushrooms, and ferns), or produced (such as beer, *medus*, and cheese). This range in ingredients suggests that the use of certain recipes is likely to have been restricted to individuals within those communities which had sufficient wealth to import *exotica* and/or the necessary connections to be involved in the gift-giving economy that operated within royal, aristocratic, and ecclesiastical networks. The 'shopping list' from Corbie, however, shows

5 On the evidence for the circulation of medical manuscripts, see Glaze, 'The Perforated Wall', 69–79; on lay medical book ownership, see Glaze, 'The Perforated Wall', 13–14, n. 6.

6 Horden, 'What's Wrong with Early Medieval Medicine?', 12–13; Park, 'Medicine and Society', 68–9.

7 van Rhijn, *Leading the Way to Heaven*, 195–202.

that some non-local imports, at least by the second half of the ninth century, might have been within the reach of a wider proportion of the population. On the other hand, many recipes may have been more generally accessible due to their reliance on 'kitchen table medicine', i.e., ingredients that could have been growing or produced locally and would have been more easily obtainable across all levels of society.[8] In fact, with respect to recipes that rely on local products, and especially newly recorded local products, the texts may offer a glimpse into the medical practices beyond the literate elite by documenting previously unrecorded pharmaceutical knowledge. Taking these factors into account, I maintain that the texts were used primarily in elite contexts, such as the royal court, aristocratic households, and monastic communities given a) the literacy needed to engage with this material, b) the resources required to source certain ingredients, and c) the intellectual environments and networks necessary to produce or obtain the manuscripts in which this information was recorded. The knowledge they transmit, however, was likely circulating more widely.

3 Moving Forward: Final Remarks and Future Directions

Ultimately, this book has offered an innovative approach to investigating the relationship between early medieval medical knowledge and practice, providing insights into this topic with implications for understanding how and by whom these texts may have been used. This research underlines the valuable contribution that 'miscellaneous' recipes may make to the study of early medieval medicine as well as the benefits of reading this material in conjunction with evidence from skeletal remains. Further work in both of these areas—and, of course, their integration—is much needed. While this book has analysed a substantial number of relatively understudied recipes, thousands more have yet to be explored. Based on the case studies analysed in this book, additional research into such recipes is likely to uncover further influences on the medical knowledge recorded in eighth- and ninth-century manuscripts. This work is therefore intrinsically linked to both the local and global Middle Ages, and the history of health and medicine is ideally suited to participate in discourses surrounding global, regional, and local knowledge networks and their points of intersection.

8 My thanks to Carine van Rhijn for the phrase 'kitchen table medicine'.

Part 1 has also drawn attention to a variety of other medical texts, and especially those that are often found within recipe collections, such as treatises on weights and measures and substitution lists, that remain chronically understudied. A better understanding of these types of writings would help to contextualise the recipe literature more generally. Similarly, medical glossaries and *hermeneumata* are deserving of more research, presenting additional entry points into the question of practicality. Are any of the newly recorded exotic substances explained in glossaries or *hermeneumata*, for example? Were these complementary texts being updated alongside the recipes, keeping up with the expansion of pharmaceutical knowledge?

Looking beyond the texts, excavations of additional sites, the increasing number of publications that address skeletal remains, and the development of new techniques provide many exciting directions for future work incorporating osteological evidence. In particular, as noted by Piers Mitchell, alongside the study of larger samples due to growing numbers of excavated and published burial sites, 'we can also improve the way we study [skeletal remains]. Progressive use of bioarchaeological techniques in partnership with other scientific specialisms allows much greater information to be gleaned from modern excavations'.[9] Recent advances in proteomics and genomics, for example, are revolutionising the study of health in the past and offering new points of intersection with historical research. Consider the emerging field of biocodicology, the study of biological information contained within manuscripts. This new research area has revealed the importance of studying a manuscript's biological record as a means to gain insights into both the physical object itself (its materials, production, and conservation) as well as its users and the environments in which it was used. The development of non-invasive biomolecular sampling techniques is making such research increasingly feasible by reducing costs and complementing conservation work.[10] Protein analyses can reveal substances on the surface of parchment leaves while an examination of ancient DNA (aDNA) can uncover pathogens.[11] This has immense potential for helping to elucidate the specific contexts in which manuscripts were handled

9 Mitchell, *Medicine in the Crusades*, 243.

10 Sarah Fiddyment, Matthew D. Teasdale, Jirí Vnouček, Élodie Lévêque, Annelise Binois, and Matthew J. Collins, 'So you want to do biocodicology? A field guide to the biological analysis of parchment', *Heritage Science* 7 (2019), https://doi.org/10.1186/s40494-019-0278-6; Matthew D. Teasdale, Sarah Fiddyment, Jirí Vnouček, Valeria Mattiangeli, Camilla Speller, Annelise Binois, Martin Carver, et al., 'The York Gospels: A 1000-year biological palimpsest', *Royal Society Open Science* 4, no. 10 (2017), https://doi.org/10.1098/rsos.170988.

11 See, for example, M. D. Teasdale, N. L. van Doorn, S. Fiddyment, C. C. Webb, T. O'Connor, M. Hofreiter, M. J. Collins, and D. G. Bradley, 'Paging through history: parchment as a

and, crucially, could provide more definitive answers to some of the questions underpinning this book. Indeed, a recent study of an early modern birthing girdle has identified proteins found in cervico-vaginal fluid, thereby confirming the use of this girdle as part of the birthing process.[12] With respect to the early medieval manuscripts analysed in this book, is there evidence, for example, of any of the ingredients listed *in* the recipes *on* the pages in which they are recorded? While this question must be saved for a future study, it reveals one of the many new doors that are opening in this field and the ever-increasing potential for interdisciplinary research: the study of Carolingian medical knowledge and practice has a bright future.

---

reservoir of ancient DNA for next generation sequencing', *Philosophical Transactions of the Royal Society B* 370 (2015), https://doi.org/10.1098/rstb.2013.0379.

12 Fiddyment, Goodison, Brenner, Signorello, Price, and Collins, 'Girding the loins?'.

Appendices

APPENDIX 1

The Manuscript Sample

This appendix provides a general overview of each of the twenty-four manuscripts that contributed recipes to the analysis, including information on their dating, origins, and contents.

Manuscripts from the Bibliothèque Nationale de France

Paris, BnF lat. 2849A

BnF lat. 2849A is a composite manuscript made up of two distinct codicological units later bound together; medical material is only found in the first section.[1] Bernhard Bischoff has suggested that this part of the manuscript, ff. 1r–23v, can be dated to the third quarter of the ninth century, but he was not certain where to place the manuscript's origins, noting that it was most likely produced in France or Italy.[2] Medical texts, including a cluster of unattributed recipes and a monthly regimen, occur on ff. 16v–23v; the small recipe collection (ff. 18v–23v) yielded fifty-four recipes.

Paris, BnF lat. 2858

BnF lat. 2858, a manuscript dated to the third quarter of the ninth century, contains the only surviving copy of the letters of Lupus of Ferrières.[3] Bischoff considered this manuscript to be a product of Lupus' circle and located its origins to either Fleury or Auxerre.[4] While Lupus' letters make up the majority of the manuscript (ff. 1r–63v), two recipes appear in the final section of the volume (on f. 67v and f. 68r, respectively) alongside an excerpt from Boethius and various other letters.[5] Given the unexpected context of this medical material, the manuscript appears to have been unknown to Augusto Beccaria, though Ernest Wickersheimer included it in his catalogue.[6]

1 Bischoff, *Katalog der festländischen Handschriften*, vol. 3, no. 4253; Beccaria, *I codici*, no. 19; Wickersheimer, *Les manuscrits*, no. 49.
2 Bischoff, *Katalog der festländischen Handschriften*, vol. 3, no. 4253.
3 Bischoff, *Katalog der festländischen Handschriften*, vol. 3, no. 4255; Bernhard Bischoff, 'Caritas-Leider', in *Mittelalterliche Studien. Ausgewählte Aufsätze zur Schriftkunde und Literaturgeschichte*, ed. Bernhard Bischoff (Stuttgart: Hiersemann, 1967), vol. 2, 56–76, at p. 66.
4 Bischoff, *Manuscripts and Libraries in the Age of Charlemagne*, trans. Gorman, 123.
5 Wickersheimer, *Les manuscrits*, no. 50.
6 Ibid.

Paris, BnF lat. 5543

According to Bischoff, BnF lat. 5543 was produced in a writing centre in France; its appearance in Fleury by the tenth century may suggest that it was written at this site.[7] Although the manuscript's place of origin is somewhat uncertain, Bischoff pinpointed its production to the year 847.[8] The manuscript contains a diverse mixture of texts that primarily focus on computistical, calendrical, and astronomical themes, including computus tables and calendars, an illustrated catalogue of stars, and a selection of writings by Bede and Isidore of Seville.[9] While some medical material can be found within this textual environment (for example, Egyptian Days (*dies aegyptiaci*), or particular days of the year that were thought to be unlucky and often noted as days to avoid bloodletting, are included in some of the calendars), the manuscript opens with a small section of recipes on ff. 1r–3r. It appears, however, that some pages have been lost, since it begins in the middle of a prescription. Although Beccaria did not include BnF lat. 5543 in his catalogue, like the preceding manuscript, it was known to Wickersheimer.[10] In total, the surviving folia yielded sixty-five recipes.

Paris, BnF lat. 6882A

BnF lat. 6882A is a composite manuscript made up of medical texts written in the ninth, twelfth, and thirteenth centuries.[11] The ninth-century material, dated more specifically to the first half of the ninth century by Bischoff, is situated at the beginning of the manuscript (ff. 1–26). Bischoff suggested that it may have been composed in southwest France.[12] Within this section of the manuscript, excerpts from the Pseudo-Galenic *De succedaneis liber* and Isidore's *Etymologiae* can be found alongside information on weights and measures, instructions for phlebotomy, *hermeneumata*, and, according to Beccaria, miscellaneous recipes and extracts ('miscellanea di estratti e di ricette').[13] A contents list on ff. 1v–8v suggests that the manuscript once included a large, early medieval pharmaceutical compilation, but the collection itself has not survived. A number of individual recipes, however, were added to the margins of the

7 Bischoff, *Katalog der festländischen Handschriften*, vol. 3, no. 4367; Marco Mostert, *The Library of Fleury. A Provisional List of Manuscripts* (Hilversum: Verloren, 1989), no. 1058f.

8 Wickersheimer, *Les manuscrits*, no. 56; Bischoff, *Katalog der festländischen Handschriften*, vol. 3, no. 4367.

9 On links between calendars, computus, and medicine, see Wallis, 'Medicine in Medieval Calendar Manuscripts'.

10 Wickersheimer, *Les manuscrits*, no. 56.

11 Beccaria, *I codici*, no. 26; Wickersheimer, *Les manuscrits*, no. 63.

12 Bischoff, *Katalog der festländischen Handschriften*, vol. 3, no. 4419; Wickersheimer, *Les manuscrits*, no. 63.

13 Beccaria, *I codici*, no. 26.

contents list and are also found in small groups on ff. 11r–11v, 18r–18v, 19r–19v, and 21r–24r. My transcription of these folia resulted in a total of sixty-one recipes.

Paris, BnF lat. 7021

According to Bischoff, BnF lat. 7021 can be dated to the first or possibly second quarter of the ninth century and may have been written at a centre in the vicinity of Paris.[14] Hippocrates' *Aphorisms* represents the primary text of this manuscript, covering ff. 1r–118r out of 119 folia.[15] I transcribed the only other text found within the codex, a single antidote located on ff. 118v–119r.[16]

Paris, BnF lat. 9332

BnF lat. 9332, an early ninth-century manuscript from western France (most probably Fleury), contains excerpts from three well-known classical and late antique medical texts: Oribasius' *Synopsis* (ff. 1va–138va), Alexander of Tralles' *Therapeutica* (ff. 138vb–242vb), and Dioscorides's *De materia medica* (ff. 243ra–321va).[17] The earliest surviving copy of the *Epistula vulturis*, a short treatise on the medico-magical uses of vulture body parts, was inserted into the text of *De materia medica* on f. 251va–251vb.[18] In addition to these writings, unattributed recipes are located on ff. 69rb, 233vb, and 321va. My transcriptions of the material added to these pages produced nine recipes.

Paris, BnF lat. 11218

Bischoff noted a number of early Caroline hands in BnF lat. 11218, dating the 126-folia manuscript to the late eighth or early ninth centuries and suggesting Burgundy as a possible location for its composition.[19] Its contents are entirely medical, and include a diverse range of texts, such as excerpts from the Hippocratic and Galenic corpora, several texts by Vindicianus (fl. fourth century), a selection of Isidore's *Etymologiae*, instructions on phlebotomy, a variety of prognostic and calendrical works, as well as many groups of recipes that have not been associated with an individual classical or late antique source.[20] Regarding the latter, these are listed by Beccaria as miscellaneous

---

14 Bischoff, *Katalog der festländischen Handschriften*, vol. 3, no. 4420; Wickersheimer, *Les manuscrits*, no. 64.

15 Beccaria, *I codici*, no. 27.

16 Cf. Wickersheimer's transcription of this recipe in *Les manuscrits*, no. 64.

17 Bischoff, *Katalog der festländischen Handschriften*, vol. 3, no. 4569; Bischoff, *Manuscripts and Libraries in the Age of Charlemagne*, trans. Gorman, 31, 144; Beccaria, *I codici*, no. 31; Wickersheimer, *Les manuscrits*, no. 71. Note: this manuscript is also linked to Bern, Burgerbibliothek, A 91.7, a manuscript not under analysis in the present study.

18 Loren C. MacKinney, 'An Unpublished Treatise on Medicine and Magic from the Age of Charlemagne', *Speculum* 18, no. 4 (1943): 494–6, https://doi.org/10.2307/2853665, at p. 494.

19 Bischoff, *Katalog der festländischen Handschriften*, vol. 3, no. 4669.

20 Beccaria, *I codici*, no. 34; Wickersheimer, *Les manuscrits*, no. 76.

recipes and extracts (again, 'miscellanea di estratti e di ricette') or as series of recipes lacking any order ('una serie di ricette senza ordine').[21] In total, the sections of the manuscript I transcribed, ff. Av, 10v–12r, 15v, 24r–26r, 32v, 43r–52r, 56r–100r, 101r, 102r, 107v–110v, and 113r–126r, produced 803 individual recipes.

Paris, BnF lat. 11219

BnF lat. 11219 is thought to have been produced at Saint-Denis.[22] Like BnF lat. 11218, its texts are entirely focused on medicine and cover a wide range of medical writings. These include a number of epistolary texts and excerpts from classical and late antique authors, a series of treatises on phlebotomy, several *hermeneumata*, a dietetic calendar, writings on prognostication, as well as collections of recipes.[23] While a primary hand, dated to the middle of the ninth century, is responsible for the majority of these texts, a series of other hands can be found throughout the manuscript. Many of these, such as those responsible for glosses in Old High German, have been dated to the tenth century and later; Bischoff dates these vernacular additions, for example, to the twelfth century.[24]

Near the end of the manuscript, ff. 221va–229vb contain unattributed recipes and present a complex mixture of these different hands. Past scholarship has tended to interpret this material as a series of later additions.[25] A close palaeographical study and re-examination of the order in which the hands appear, however, suggests that, at least in this section of the manuscript, the various hands date to the very end of the present study's date range.[26] It is particularly noteworthy that many of these individual hands appear to be closely related, possibly representing teachers and students. As such, the manuscript bears witness to the addition of material over time and to the continued engagement with the manuscript itself over several generations of scribes. While its latest hands in the sections of recipes relevant to this study may extend into

21 Beccaria, *I codici*, no. 34.

22 Bischoff, *Katalog der festländischen Handschriften*, vol. 3, no. 4670; Jean Vezin, 'Le point d'interrogation, un élément de datation et de localisation des manuscrits. L'exemple de Saint-Denis au IXe siècle', *Scriptorium* 34, no. 2 (1980): 181–96, at pp. 191–2; Jean Vezin, 'Les manuscrits copiés à Saint-Denis en France pendant l'époque carolingienne', *Paris et Île-de-France. Mémoires* 32 (1981): 273–87, at p. 283.

23 Beccaria, *I codici*, no. 35; Wickersheimer, *Les manuscrits*, no. 77. See also Sabbah, Corsetti, and Fischer, *BTML*; Fischer, *BTML 1*; and Fischer, *BTML 2*, entries on 'Dynamidia (Hippocratis)' and 'Pseudo-Galenus: *Prognostica* (*Inc.* Frons rubet)'.

24 Bischoff, *Katalog der festländischen Handschriften*, vol. 3, no. 4670.

25 Beccaria, *I codici*, no. 35.

26 My thanks to Rosamond McKitterick and Anna Dorofeeva for their assessments of these folia. While McKitterick posits that the folia in question contain hands primarily from the mid-to late ninth century, Dorofeeva suggests a slightly later dating, moving into the tenth century but emphasises the relatedness of the hands.

the tenth century, their close relationship to the earlier material and the overall ambiguity of the manuscript's date range make it appropriate to include these recipes in the following analyses. My transcriptions produced 121 recipes.

Manuscripts from the Stiftsbibliothek St. Gallen[27]

Cod. sang. 44

Cod. sang. 44 is a composite manuscript made up of two distinct halves. A bible given to St Gall in *c.* 780 covers pp. 1–184 while a compilation of over twenty individual medical texts can be found on pp. 186–368.[28] The medical half of the manuscript, a distinct 'medical manuscript' prior to its union with the bible, has been dated to the second half of the ninth century, and Bischoff has suggested that it was written in northern Italy.[29] Its texts include a wide range of medical topics and genres of writing, such as excerpts from the Hippocratic and Galenic corpora, letters of Vindicianus, the *Herbariencorpus*, and prognostic and calendrical texts.[30] Three major early medieval recipe collections can also be found within the manuscript, covering pp. 228–60, 337–54, and 354–68, each of which were transcribed and published in the early twentieth century: Henry Sigerist included the first in *Studien und Texte zur frühmittelalterlichen Rezeptliteratur* and Julius Jörimann addressed the second two in *Frühmittelalterliche Rezeptarien*.[31]

While some research into their content has been pursued (John Riddle's study of non-local *materia medica*, for example, uses Sigerist's transcriptions), rarely have the three recipe collections been discussed together or with other texts within the medical half of the manuscript.[32] Some of these individual components, however, have been recognised as related to material in other codices; the third of the large early medieval recipe collections (pp. 354–68), for example, has been noted as sharing much in common with a recipe collection in BAV pal. lat. 1088 (also part of this study's sample), and Arsenio Ferraces Rodríguez has linked both to the *Teraupetica-Tereoperica* tradition

27 Manuscripts held in St Gall are paginated not foliated.
28 Beccaria, *I codici*, no. 129; Bischoff, *Katalog der festländischen Handschriften*, vol. 3, nos. 5529a-30.
29 Bischoff, *Katalog der festländischen Handschriften*, vol. 3, nos. 5529a-30; Bischoff, 'Italienische Handschriften', 177–8.
30 Beccaria, *I codici*, no. 129. Meg Leja considered this manuscript in relation to her analysis of the *Lorscher Arzneibuch*, see Leja, 'The Sacred Art', 17–18.
31 *Studien und Texte*, ed. Sigerist, 78–99; *Frühmittelalterliche Rezeptarien*, ed. Jörimann, 37–61.
32 Riddle, 'The Introduction and Use of Eastern Drugs'.

that ultimately descends from Theodorus Priscianus' (fl. fourth century) *Euporista*.[33] These two collections, though clearly related, appear to be several steps removed from each other and earlier texts (and, crucially, contain numerous entirely distinct recipes), and thereby merit inclusion in this study.

Overall, I take a more comprehensive approach to the manuscript's 'miscellaneous' and unattributed recipes, considering not only the early medieval recipe collections (for which I have produced new, revised transcriptions), but also including individual marginal remedies noted by Beccaria (pp. 195, 197, and 215), as well as small groups of recipes either unmentioned by Beccaria or labelled 'miscellaneous' (pp. 186, 276–80, 282–6, 304, and 330–6), in my analyses. In total, the manuscript contributed 917 recipes to the study, and a selection of these recipes can be seen in Figures 3 and 7.

Cod. sang. 217

Cod. sang. 217 is thought to have been written in northern Italy and has been dated to the early ninth century by Bischoff.[34] This is a particularly complex manuscript, containing at least two distinct works that were later bound together. This subsequent binding has resulted in the reordering of quires as well as the loss of certain sections, some of which are also still held in St Gall and will be addressed below in the discussion of cod. sang. 1396.[35]

While the Stiftsbibliothek's earliest surviving copy of Gregory's *Regula pastoralis* comprises much of the manuscript (pp. 1–249), a varied collection of medical texts makes up the final quarter of the codex (pp. 252–341). Small groups of recipes are interspersed between the *St. Galler Botanicus* and *St. Galler Bestiarius*, neither of which follow their intended order. Monica Niederer has published an edition and translation of the *Botanicus*, a text that stems from the classical and late antique herbal tradition.[36] Within this re-bound environment, I transcribed the recipes found on pp. 253–74 and 332–8, putting the pages in the following order: 255, 256, 253, 254, 259, 260, 257, 258, 261–74, 335–8, and 332–4. Although Peter Köpp has also published a transcription of these pages, a revised transcription was needed. Furthermore, in my transcriptions of recipes from cod. sang. 217, just as in cod. sang. 44, I have included not only material

33 Ferraces Rodríguez, 'Un recetario médico altomedieval'; Ferraces Rodríguez, 'Reutilización de fuentes en recetarios medicos de la antigüedad tardía'.

34 Bischoff, *Katalog der festländischen Handschriften*, vol. 3, nos. 5662a-63; E. A. Lowe, *Codices Latini antiquiores: A Palaeographical Guide to Latin Manuscripts Prior to the Ninth Century*, 11 vols. (Oxford: Clarendon Press, 1934–66), vol. 8, no. 926; Beccaria, *I codici*, no. 131. Both Clare Pilsworth and Meg Leja have considered this manuscript in their analyses of medical manuscripts, see Pilsworth, *Healthcare in Early Medieval Northern Italy*, 78–81 and Leja, 'The Sacred Art', 16–17.

35 *Vademecum eines frühmittelalterlichen Arztes*, ed. and trans. Köpp, 15.

36 *Der St. Galler* Botanicus, ed. and trans. Niederer.

from recipe collections, but also individual recipes or small clusters found between the primary textual units.[37] In total, the manuscript contributed 316 recipes to the study.

Cod. sang. 397

Although it contains the hands of approximately forty different scribes, cod. sang. 397 has been identified as the *vademecum* of Grimald, Abbot of St Gall (841–72). As such, it can be dated to the middle of the ninth century, specifically from the 830s to the 860s, and tied to locations where Grimald was active, such as Aachen and St Gall.[38] Grimald's connections to the court (as Louis the German's arch-chaplain, chancellor, and a *missus Dominicus*) resulted in his movement around the Frankish Empire, so it is likely that the manuscript was added to over time and at a number of different locations.[39]

The codex consists of a vast and varied assemblage of different texts, such as information about the St Gall area, poems, liturgical writings, and material relating to many different branches of the natural world, including medicine. Given the relatively minor role played by medical writings within the *vademecum* as a whole, it is not surprising that Beccaria appears to have been unaware of this manuscript and thus did not describe it in his catalogue. The short texts concerning medicine and healthcare, which range from a list of Egyptian Days to a word list defining places of care (such as *xenodochium* and *nosochomium*), occur throughout the manuscript.[40] Within this mixture of medical material, I identified and transcribed two recipes on p. 22.

Cod. sang. 550

Dated to the second and third quarters of the ninth century (with some later additions, too), Bischoff has suggested that cod. sang. 550 was likely produced in a Swiss writing centre.[41] The manuscript contains hagiographical texts, the *formulae* of Reichenau and Murbach, a penitential of Pseudo-Cummean, and ends with a series of grammatical

37 *Vademecum eines frühmittelalterlichen Arztes*, ed. and trans. Köpp.

38 Bischoff, *Katalog der festländischen Handschriften*, vol. 3, no. 5741. The manuscript is also linked with a series of folia in BAV reg. lat. 421 (ff. 21–25), a manuscript not under analysis in the present study.

39 Bernhard Bischoff, 'Bücher am Hofe Ludwigs des Deutschen und die Privatbibliothek des Kanzlers Grimalt', in *Mittelalterliche Studien. Ausgewählte Aufsätze zur Schriftkunde und Literaturgeschichte*, edited by Bernhard Bischoff (Stuttgart: Hiersemann, 1981), vol. 3, 187–212, at pp. 199–201.

40 For the Egyptian Days, see cod. sang. 397, p. 26; on Egyptian Days more generally, see, for example, Skemer, '*Armis Gunfe*'. For the list of places of care, see p. 38; the terms include: *xenodochium, ptochotrophium, nosochomium, orphanotrophium, gerontochomium*, and *brephotrophium*.

41 Bischoff, *Katalog der festländischen Handschriften*, vol. 3, no. 5761; Bischoff, 'Bücher am Hofe Ludwigs des Deutschen', 194–5.

exercises. A small medical section appears on pp. 54–5, representing a single folio separating the *Inventio Michaelis archangeli* (pp. 39–53) and the following *formulae* (pp. 56–161). My transcription of these pages produced three recipes. Like the preceding example, Beccaria does not include this manuscript in his catalogue.

Cod. sang. 751

A massive codex primarily focused on medical writings, cod. sang. 751 consists of several dozen different texts within its 500 pages.[42] This manuscript, first noted in Chapter 1 in relation to the case of Terenti(an)us, appears to have been produced in a northern Italian writing centre, though it probably arrived in St Gall soon after its compilation.[43] Dated to the first half of the ninth century, the compendium contains medical glossaries, the *Liber Esculapii*, prognostic and calendrical texts, a version of the *Physica Plinii*, passages from the *Herbariencorpus*, Galenic and Hippocratic texts, selections from Vindicianus' writings, instructions for bloodletting, and works on diet.[44]

Beccaria described many of the short sections of text between these better known medical writings and excerpts simply as 'various recipes', 'other recipes and extracts', or 'miscellaneous recipes and extracts' (e.g., pp. 37–9, 172–5, 304–8, 318–24, 362–9, 377–414, 414–24, and 430). Furthermore, a significant number of folia in the final one hundred pages of the manuscript (namely, pp. 431–45, 448–52, 455–63, 467–75, 478–91, and 494) are unmentioned in the catalogue.[45] However, two numbered contents lists indicate the planned nature of the assortment of texts included within the manuscript. The first contents list, found on pp. 341–7, corresponds to the material on pp. 355–414 (which includes the 'miscellaneous' sections on pp. 362–9 and 377–414), while the second, found on pp. 424–28, outlines much of the rest of the manuscript. Both of these discrete compilations contain hundreds of individual recipes, though they also contain additional texts largely orientated around pharmacy (e.g., on weights and measures). In total, the manuscript contributed 1187 recipes to the study, and a selection of these treatments can be seen in the book's cover image as well as in Figure 2.

42 Beccaria, *I codici*, no. 133.

43 Bischoff, *Katalog der festländischen Handschriften*, vol. 3, no. 5844.

44 Beccaria, *I codici*, no. 133. See also Sabbah, Corsetti, and Fischer, *BTML*; Fischer, *BTML 1*; and Fischer, *BTML 2* (entry on 'Dynamidia (Hippocratis)') regarding material on pp. 339–40, 365, 416–17.

45 Beccaria, *I codici*, no. 133: 'ricette varie', 'altre ricette ed altri estratti', or 'miscellanea di ricette e di estratti'.

Cod. sang. 752

Cod. sang. 752 is thought to have been composed at St Gall itself.[46] Paralleling codd. sang. 44 and 217, the codex represents a composite manuscript made up of two distinct units. In this case, both textual units focus on medicine and have been dated to *c.* 900.[47] The first section of the manuscript, pp. 1–80, contains the *Medicina Plinii*.[48] In the several pages between the end of this text and the start of Gargilius Martialis' (fl. third century) *Medicinae ex oleribus et pomis* (which is often found together with the *Medicina Plinii*), a diverse group of medical writings appears. These include a dietetic calendar, a group of recipes for darkening the hair, and the *Spera Apulei Platonici*, a medico-mathematical prognostic device used to predict the outcome of an illness.[49] The second half of the manuscript, pp. 161–326, contains an excerpt from Isidore of Seville's *Etymologiae* and one of the few surviving copies of the *Oxea et chronia passiones Yppocratis, Gallieni et Urani*. I transcribed material on pp. 5, 81–82, and 158–9, totalling fifteen recipes. Two of these recipes can be seen in Figure 5.

Cod. sang. 759

The opening Terenti(an)us example also features cod. sang. 759. Bischoff suggests that this early ninth-century manuscript was composed in Brittany; the text is written in an Insular script that shows continental influences.[50] The 94-page codex contains a variety of medical texts, such as extracts of Oribasius and Galen, dietetic calendars, and information on weights and measures.[51]

The second half of the manuscript, pp. 53–94, contains a large recipe collection, although a number of pages of the collection have been lost. While its contents list records 446 entries, only entries 1–137 and 271–353 survive, or roughly half of the collection (220 out of a possible 446 entries). I transcribed the surviving portions of this collection as well as two smaller groups of recipes on pp. 1–8 and 45–6. In total, the manuscript contributed 451 recipes, a selection of which can be seen in Figures 1 and 6.

---

46 Beccaria, *I codici*, no. 134; Bischoff, *Katalog der festländischen Handschriften*, vol. 3, no. 5845.

47 Beccaria, *I codici*, no. 134; Bischoff, *Katalog der festländischen Handschriften*, vol. 3, no. 5845.

48 For a recent English translation, see *The* Medicina Plinii, trans. Hunt.

49 Roy Michael Liuzza, 'The Sphere of Life and Death: Time, Medicine, and the Visual Imagination', in *Latin Learning and English Lore: Studies in Anglo-Saxon Literature for Michael Lapidge*, ed. Katherine O'Brien O'Keeffe and Andy Orchard (Toronto: University of Toronto Press, 2005), vol. 2, 28–52, at p. 29. For a transcription of the *Spera* (both text and image), see Sigerist, '"The Sphere of Life and Death" in Early Medieval Manuscripts', 294–6.

50 Bischoff, *Katalog der festländischen Handschriften*, vol. 3, no. 5846; Bischoff, *Manuscripts and Libraries in the Age of Charlemagne*, trans. Gorman, 30.

51 Beccaria, *I codici*, no. 135.

Cod. sang. 761

Cod. sang. 761, another manuscript written in an Insular script, appears to have been composed in the early ninth century.[52] Bischoff located the manuscript's origins to Fulda, a writing centre known to have had scribes writing in a 'continental Insular' script until the middle of the ninth century.[53] The codex contains extensive selections of Oribasius' *Synopsis* and *Euporista* as well as excerpts from the Hippocratic and Galenic corpora.[54] In addition to these established textual traditions, the manuscript contains a relatively small collection of recipes on pp. 51–66 that are unattributed to a single classical or late antique source. From this collection, I transcribed forty-six recipes.

Cod. sang. 878

Cod. sang. 878, a manuscript thought to have been Walahfrid Strabo's *vademecum*, contains a wide variety of writings, ranging from works on computus to Priscian's (fl. c. 500) *Institutiones grammaticae*.[55] Texts relating to health and medicine are interspersed throughout the codex. In particular, Hippocrates' *Epistula ad Antiochum regem*, Anthimus' *De observatione ciborum*, a treatise on phlebotomy, and several pages of 'miscellaneous recipes and extracts' ('miscellanea di ricette e di estratti') are found in clusters over pp. 327–93.[56] I transcribed the so-called miscellaneous sections (pp. 331–4, 372–7, and 392–3), resulting in seventeen recipes.

Although the manuscript has been linked to Walahfrid, a number of different hands can be seen within its pages. The Old High German glosses on p. 333, for example, certainly cannot be attributed to Walahfrid since they appear to date to the eleventh

52 Bischoff, *Katalog der festländischen Handschriften*, vol. 3, no. 5847.

53 Bischoff, *Katalog der festländischen Handschriften*, vol. 3, no. 5847; Bischoff, *Manuscripts and Libraries in the Age of Charlemagne*, trans. Gorman, 118, 149; Herrad Spilling, 'Angelsächsische Schrift in Fulda', in *Von der Klosterbibliothek zur Landesbibliothek. Beiträge zum zweihundertjährigen Bestehen der Hessischen Landesbibliothek Fulda*, ed. Artur Brall (Stuttgart: Hiersemann, 1978), 47–98.

54 Beccaria, *I codici*, no. 136.

55 Cod. sang. 878; Bischoff, *Katalog der festländischen Handschriften*, vol. 3, no. 5862. For more on cod. sang. 878 and its connection to Walahfrid Strabo, see Bischoff, 'Eine Sammelhandschrift Walahfrid Strabos', 34–51; Bischoff, *Manuscripts and Libraries in the Age of Charlemagne*, 101; Richard Corradini, 'Pieces of a Puzzle: Time and History in Walahfrid's *Vademecum*', *Early Medieval Europe* 22, no. 4 (2014): 476–91, https://doi.org/10.1111/emed.12083; and Richard Corradini, 'Wissenschaft und Zeitdiagnose. Zur Transformation antiken Wissens in Walahfrid Strabos Vademecum', in *Neue Wege der Frühmittelalterforschung: Bilanz und Perspektiven*, ed. Walter Pohl, Maximilian Diesenberger, and Bernhard Zeller (Vienna: Österreichischen Akademie der Wissenschaften, 2018), 287–308.

56 Beccaria, *I codici*, no. 139.

century.[57] Regarding the three medical sections I transcribed, Bischoff has suggested that Walahfrid was responsible for the ninth-century material on pp. 331–4 and 372–7, though the text on pp. 392–3, a collection of antidotes, belongs to a different, roughly contemporary hand (named scribe 'P' by Bischoff).[58]

Cod. sang. 899

According to Bischoff, cod. sang. 899 was produced at St Gall at the very end of the ninth century.[59] Largely a poetry anthology, it includes works such as Ausonius' (fl. fourth century) *Mosella* and Walahfrid Strabo's *Versus Strabi de beati Blaithmaic vita et fine* as well as poems by Paul the Deacon (d. before 800), Peter of Pisa (d. before 800), and Theodulf of Orléans (d. 821).[60] The codex also contains writings on the liberal arts, a notable number of Greek and latinised Greek words, and several medical sections.[61] Given this mixture of genres, largely non-medical in their areas of focus, the manuscript appears to have been unknown to Beccaria. My transcriptions of the medical writings on pp. 83–4, 131, and 137–42 produced a total of forty-two recipes, a selection of which can be seen in Figure 4.

It is significant to note a link between this manuscript and two others in the present study, codd. sang. 397 and 752, all of which can be directly associated with St Gall. These three codices share a distinct unit of medical information: two recipes that contain an unusual (and hence highly recognisable) cluster of ingredients named in the vernacular and explained in Latin (the version of these recipes in cod. sang. 752 can be seen in Figure 5).[62] In cod. sang. 899, the second recipe ends with the phrase *de libro*

57 von Steinmeyer and Sievers, *Die althochdeutschen Glossen*, vol. 4, 455.

58 More specifically, Bischoff considers the writing on pp. 331–4 to represent 'W III', the penultimate phase of Walahfrid's script, whereas he has labelled the text on pp. 372–7 as 'W IV', thereby dating this section of the manuscript to the final years of Walahfrid's life. Bischoff, 'Eine Sammelhandschrift Walahfrid Strabos', 34–51; my thanks also to Richard Corradini for discussing these sections of the manuscript.

59 Bischoff, *Katalog der festländischen Handschriften*, vol. 3, no. 5865. Like cod. sang. 397, the manuscript is also connected to a series of folia in BAV reg. lat. 421 (ff. 20, 27–8, and possibly 33), a manuscript not under analysis in the present study.

60 Bernhard Bischoff, 'Übersicht über die nichtdiplomatischen Geheimschriften des Mittelalters', in *Mittelalterliche Studien. Ausgewählte Aufsätze zur Schriftkunde und Literaturgeschichte*, ed. Bernhard Bischoff (Stuttgart: Hiersemann, 1981), vol. 3, 120–48, at p. 138; Bischoff, 'Bücher am Hofe Ludwigs des Deutschen', 201, 210.

61 Significant sections of Greek words can be found on pp. 57, 83–4, and 107, for example. Bernhard Bischoff, 'Das griechische Element in der abendländischen Bildung des Mittelalters', in *Mittelalterliche Studien. Ausgewählte Aufsätze zur Schriftkunde und Literaturgeschichte*, ed. Bernhard Bischoff (Stuttgart: Hiersemann, 1967), vol. 2, 246–74, at pp. 256, 268.

62 The recipes are located in cod. sang. 397, p. 22; cod. sang. 752, p. 158; and cod. sang. 899, p. 131; see Chapter 5.

grim tuli; a mark of abbreviation above the 'm' in *grim* suggests that this should be expanded to 'Grimald', thereby indicating that this material was copied from cod. sang. 397, Grimald's *vademecum*.

Cod. sang. 1396

Cod. sang. 1396, unlike the manuscripts reviewed above, represents a collection of fragments that the Stiftsbibliothek St. Gallen keeps together as a single unit.[63] Within this diverse assemblage, there is a section of fragmentary medical writings, several of which date to the Carolingian period. A number of these folia have been linked with cod. sang. 217. As noted above, during a later binding of cod. sang. 217, several sections of text were lost from the original manuscript, some of which remain in St Gall and now form part of cod. sang. 1396; the pages in question are labelled pp. 9–16 and 19–22 in cod. sang. 1396.[64] These folia belong to the same group of recipes I transcribed from cod. sang. 217, meaning they, too, originated in a northern Italian centre in the early ninth century. My transcription of these fragments produced an additional 118 recipes.

Manuscripts from the Biblioteca Apostolica Vaticana

BAV pal. lat. 187

Although BAV pal. lat. 187 begins with a psalter (ff. 1v–6v, incomplete), the majority of the manuscript is medical in focus: f. 7r contains two unattributed recipes and ff. 8r–66v represents the oldest surviving (though incomplete) copy of *The Alphabet of Galen*.[65] Surprisingly, the manuscript is not featured in Beccaria's catalogue. The places of origin and dates of the manuscript's three constituent parts are still debated. While E. A. Lowe dated all three units to the eighth century and suggested that it was produced in northern Italy on the basis of the cursive seen on f. 7r, Bischoff revised the dating to the late eighth and early ninth centuries and identified eastern France as a possible area of origin.[66] Nicholas Everett has proposed an earlier dating of all parts of

63 Bischoff, *Katalog der festländischen Handschriften*, vol. 3, nos. 5886–93 (note that the medical sections under consideration here are covered by no. 5889); Beccaria, *I codici*, no. 140.

64 On the original order of the pages in cod. sang. 217, see *Vademecum eines frühmittelalterlichen Arztes*, ed. and trans. Köpp, 15.

65 Lowe, *CLA*, vol. 1, nos. 80–1; Bischoff, *Katalog der festländischen Handschriften*, vol. 3, no. 6474; The Alphabet of Galen*: Pharmacy from Antiquity to the Middle Ages*, ed. and trans. Nicholas Everett (Toronto: University of Toronto Press, 2012), 121–3.

66 Lowe, *CLA*, vol. 1, nos. 80–1; Bischoff, *Katalog der festländischen Handschriften*, vol. 3, no. 6474; Bischoff, *Die Abtei Lorsch im Spiegel ihrer Handschriften*, 60, 118–19.

the manuscript, pointing to parallels with sixth- and seventh-century medical writings in terms of both content and palaeography, and supports its production at an northern Italian centre.[67] While I am inclined to follow Bischoff's dating, and have therefore included the two recipes from f. 7r in the present study, like Everett and Lowe, I suggest that a northern Italian origin (and then subsequent move north) seems most plausible.

BAV *pal. lat. 1088*

BAV pal. lat. 1088, a medical manuscript written in the area of Lyon in the middle or third quarter of the ninth century, consists entirely of medical texts.[68] Excerpts of Galen, Quintus Serenus (fl. second century), and Vindicianus, several groups of recipes unattributed to a particular source, as well as two larger early medieval recipe collections are contained within its 121 folia.[69] Glosses in Old High German can be seen in some of the recipes.[70] As noted above, the recipe collection on ff. 31r–50r, which includes a contents list on 31r–33rc, has many parallels to the third recipe collection of cod. sang. 44 (pp. 354–68). While their similarities highlight the movement of knowledge and dissemination of shared of sources during this period, the ways in which the individual compilations differ simultaneously speak to the fluidity of such collections: scribes could add, remove, and adapt material as their conditions allowed.

In addition to transcribing the collection on ff. 31r–50r, I also transcribed the smaller recipe collection on ff. 50r–66r since, according to Beccaria, it represents another example of a 'miscellanea di ricette e di estratti'.[71] An edition of this recipe collection has recently been published by Arsenio Ferraces Rodríguez, but this was not available when I transcribed and analysed the text.[72] Taking into account these two recipe collections as well as a number of individual recipes inserted on ff. 94r–95r and 107v, the manuscript contributed 835 recipes to the analysis.

BAV *reg. lat. 598*

BAV reg. lat. 598 represents a collection of fragments written at different times and covering a variety of topics.[73] Two sections of the manuscript concern medicine and have been dated to the Carolingian period: ff. 26r–33r and 124r–125r. While the first section contains a selection of excerpts from known texts, such as Quintus Serenus' *Liber medicinalis* and Hippocrates' *Epistula ad Antiochum regem*, the second medical

67 The Alphabet of Galen, ed. and trans. Everett, 121–3.

68 Bischoff, *Katalog der festländischen Handschriften*, vol. 3, no. 6574; Beccaria, *I codici*, no. 103.

69 Beccaria, *I codici*, no. 103.

70 von Steinmeyer and Sievers, *Die althochdeutschen Glossen*, vol. 4, 363–5 and 367–8.

71 Beccaria, *I codici*, no. 103.

72 Ferraces Rodríguez, 'Un recetario médico altomedieval', 41–80.

73 Beccaria, *I codici*, no. 104.

section (ff. 124r–125r), consists of a brief collection of unattributed recipes written in *c.* 900. This cluster produced twelve individual recipes. Intriguingly, these folia appear to be particularly understudied; although Bischoff addressed the other codicological units of the manuscript in his *Katalog der festländischen Handschriften*, he did not comment on this passage.[74]

BAV *reg. lat. 1143*

BAV reg. lat. 1143 is an early ninth-century manuscript made up of three codicological sections: a) ff. 1–85 and 201–202, b) ff. 86–189, and c) ff. 190–200.[75] At least four quires are missing (V–VI and XIII–XIV), and the manuscript has been damaged by humidity. Bischoff has suggested that the codex was composed in the area around Mainz.[76] The surviving texts are entirely related to health and medicine and include a selection of Theodorus Priscianus' *Euporista*, the end of book III of Alexander of Tralles' *Therapeutica*, Vindicianus' *Epistula ad Pentadium*, Hippocrates' *Epistula ad Antiochum regem*, as well as a large number of recipes and extracts labelled 'miscellaneous' by Beccaria (e.g., ff. 80v–86r, 105v–109v, 118r–125r, 129v–134v, 141r–187v, 188r–189r, 190r–193r, and 196r–200r).[77] In total, the manuscript contributed 312 recipes to the study.

BAV *vat. lat. 5951*

Dated to the first quarter of the ninth century, Bischoff has suggested that BAV vat. lat. 5951 was produced in Italy or possibly southern Burgundy.[78] Certain elements in the script and particular notes might reflect a connection to Nonantola.[79] The manuscript mostly consists of Celsus' (fl. second century) *De Medicina*, although Book I of Muscio's *Gynaecia* (*c.* 500) was inserted on ff. 65r–65v in the twelfth century. In addition to these two texts, recipes have been added as marginal notes on ff. 1r, 1v, 2r, 66v, and 68v. These additions have been written by several different hands, some of which appear to date to the ninth century, while others, including the cough recipe on f. 68v added by a certain 'Iohannes Calabri' (quite possibly John Philagathos, the tenth-century antipope John XVI), were added in the tenth century and later.[80] Unfortunately, some of the manuscript's margins have sustained damage, such that, of the ninth-century additions, only a single recipe could be transcribed.

---

74 Bischoff, *Katalog der festländischen Handschriften*, vol. 3, nos. 6718–22.

75 Bischoff, *Katalog der festländischen Handschriften*, vol. 3, nos. 6766–7.

76 Ibid.

77 Beccaria, *I codici*, no. 106.

78 Bischoff, *Katalog der festländischen Handschriften*, vol. 3, no. 6927.

79 Bischoff, *Manuscripts and Libraries in the Age of Charlemagne*, trans. Gorman, 151; Beccaria, *I codici*, no. 102.

80 My thanks to Silvia Maria Marchiori for sharing unpublished work on the early medieval Latin tradition of Celsus' *De medicina* and John Philagathos.

APPENDIX 2

Recipe Transcriptions

The following appendix includes full transcriptions of the individual recipes which are named in the text. As noted in Chapter 2, some manuscripts contain many more recipes than others and thus contributed more material to the study (e.g., codd. sang. 44, 751, BAV pal. lat. 1088, and BnF lat. 11218). Individual recipes from five manuscripts (BnF lat. 2858, 6882A, 7021, and 9332 as well as BAV pal. lat. 187) were not used as specific examples in the above chapters and are therefore absent from this appendix, though the recipes were part of the general analyses. The recipe numbering is structured as follows:

- The first number corresponds to a particular manuscript, starting with the first manuscript involved from the Bibliothèque nationale de France (i.e., 1 is BnF lat. 2849A) and ending with the final manuscript from the Biblioteca Apostolica Vaticana (i.e., 19 is BAV vat. lat. 5951). The order is outlined below.
- The second number corresponds to the order in which the recipe appears in the manuscript. For example, entry 3.5 addresses the antidote titled *Antidotum qui dicitur acharistus* found on ff. 57v–58r of BnF lat. 11218 and entry 3.6 addresses the next recipe in this manuscript that is also discussed in the present study, which, in this case, is the recipe titled *Ad oris uicia* found on ff. 89r–89v.
- Some entries have a third number; this is to signify the different, individual recipes that are sometimes found under a single title. The recipes of entry 2.2 provide one such example: entry 2.2 corresponds to a recipe group titled *Contra artetricos*; this heading covers two recipes on f. 2v of BnF lat. 5534. These two recipes are labelled 2.2.1 and 2.2.2.

For transcription conventions, see the 'Note on Transcription and Translation'; for metrological conventions, see the 'Note on Weights, Measures, and Their Symbols'.
Manuscript order:

Bibliothèque nationale de France

1. Lat. 2849A
2. Lat. 5543
3. Lat. 11218
4. Lat. 11219

Stiftsbibliothek St. Gallen

5. Cod. sang. 44

6. Cod. sang. 217
7. Cod. sang. 397
8. Cod. sang. 550
9. Cod. sang. 751
10. Cod. sang. 752
11. Cod. sang. 759
12. Cod. sang. 761
13. Cod. sang. 878
14. Cod. sang. 899
15. Cod. sang. 1396

Biblioteca Apostolica Vaticana
16. Pal. lat. 1088
17. Reg. lat. 598
18. Reg. lat. 1143
19. Vat. lat. 5951

Bibliothèque Nationale de France

1 *Lat. 2849A*

1.1 *De dentes dolores*, f. 19r

De dentes dolores . Ius de edre frequenter in nare inponat de illa parte ubi indolit et de illa radice que dicitur spana inter duas dentes qui dolent ibidem mittat cum cira cludat ipso pertuso quod illa radices exinde non exeat et haec per dies tres facere debes.

2 *Lat. 5543*

2.1 *Cura ad omnes apostomas*, ff. 1v–2r

2.1.1 Cura ad omnes apostomas . mel (.) ii . butiro (.) i . uino uetere . (.) i . marrubio *fasc* i . felterre . similiter . betonica . similiter . hec omnia mitte in olla rude . et coquis lente igne . ut ueniat ad (.) ii . cum refrigerauerit . tepidum linteo extorques addes piper puluerem ∻ i . exinde ieiunus accipiat coclearia v . aut vii . post cenam iii.

2.1.2 Item <........> (.) iii . coliandro ∻ i . piper grana . c . marrubio *fascl* i . ruta . si<militer> in olla rude coque ut adsunt . perueniat . et cum oleo bibat.

2.1.3 Item . cinere de uite alba . exinde lixiuia calices viiii . de uino uetere commisces . bibat cum oleo.

2.1.4 Item ex rafano . galoxinas . iii . in uino uetere mitte et cum oleo bibat.

2.1.5 Item aloxinum cum melle et absintio . sufficienter bene compositum ex uino uetere . coque . usque ad ii . partes.

2.1.6 Item marrubio . ius calices iii . apio . iii . betonica . similiter . mel . similiter . uinum uetus calices \staupos/ viiii . coque . lento igne in olla rude . usque ad staupos xii.

2.1.7 Item uite betonica . et gamandrea . et apio . ius *cal* vi . per triduo bibat cum oleo.

2.1.8 Item adipe porcino *cal* i . oleo . *cal* i . apio . ius *cal* i . per triduo bibat.

2.1.9 Item marrubio *fascl* iii . apio foliis et radicibus . leuestico radice . costo radices . sclareia . serpullum . ruta . sauina . senetionem . uuismalua . satureia italica . ysopo . betonica . agrimonia . caulo crispo . plantagine . ueruena . artemisia . elna . ane<t>o . tanaceta . feniculi radice . brusalzinatia . saluia . nepta . ambrosia . coliandro . a<b>satureia . uino uetere *s* iii . mel . libram i . butiro libram i . oleo *cocler* iii . coque <usque> ad medietatem colas . exinde . tepid<e> accipiat *coclr* i . in as balneo . mane . et uespere . s<au>res permiserint . Postea facis . calidum . ex cenamo . costo . gariofilo . spico piper . bagas lauri . gingiber . cum uino et melle calide bibat.

2.2 *Contra artetricos*, f. 2v

2.2.1 Contra **artetricos** . peretro . pens\an/t . *dnr* . ii . saluia tenerrima . *manplm* . i . ieiunus bibe.

2.2.2 Item alia eiusdem . diptamno radice . *m* . i . centaurea folio . *m.* i . basilisca . similiter . frasica . iua . artemisia . ambrosia . caprifolio \similiter folio/ calcatrippa radice . lupopectino radice . caprahulso . similiter radice . plantagine folio similiter . edere terrestre . grossa urtica . saluia similiter . piper grana . ccc . uinum staupos . l . quos debes bibere per dies . l.

3 *Lat. 11218*

3.1 *Inplastrum Afrodites*, ff. 45v–46r

3.1.1 **Inplastrum afrodites** . facit ad capitis dolorem et temporum uel fronte in aluta inductum et inpostum statim curat et recte dentis capitis plagas . aui . rupturas cum cruorem adpositum sine fibolas glutinant aurium uerum uulnenera emitentis resoluis medicamen in oleo roseo . et tepefactum adicies in auriter in diem istatim curat facit ad scouolas . ad panocolas et ad apostimas et ad duricias et ad ordiola in cilia et ad neruorem dolores . sed contraccionis . aut incisionem et ad ignis agro et ad fluxum sanguis stagnan . uiris . aut feminis et ad stuporem neruorum facit ad epaticis . et ad spleneticus et ad stomachum debile . et balneom uel terso inductum inponis hoc tercius credas quia omnia super memoratas passionis non surgant nisi curarent facit et ad tumorem et ad inflamacionem stomachi . et ad uulnus curat eum cancrum et fistolas humurosas . et percussus scorpionis et ad morsum humanum et ad canis rapidi morsum uel ad cuiuslibet morsum serpencium tolitum in eiusdem inplastrum inuenies ad magnitudinem auelane mortifero uenino inde tersum superinponis . facit ad omnem mammillorum dolorem et ad nescia et ad renium dolorem et ad articulorum dolorem et ad steroni percussum superinpositum sed ad sterpe et producit foras et ad ragadias et ad si . qua ibi aliena tisunt facit et ad podacrius mirifice . et ad ceparcius cum oleo mirtino conficis sic litargiro ~ ii . đ ii galbano ~ ii đ ii . eruginem ~ ii . amoniaco nittido ~ x . mirra ~ i . cera pontica ~ x . colofania *lb* i *s* . oleo dulce uetere mittis per statem *lb* i . et per hieme *lb* . ii . conficis autem sic primo oleo cum tebidauerit mittis litargiro et moues . et quoqus lento ignem ad pauorem et semper agitas quousque ad molentem fiat . et digito . non quo in qui nentur postea cera et amoniaco . et risina deinde mirra postea galbano cumtundis cum parte cera macera birbene et in tebido mittis similiter et eruginem et agitas dum refrigidant mandalionis.

3.1.2 **Item de afroditis . ad ipsas passionis** . Galbano ~ . i . spuma argenti ~ . i . et dinarius vi . et dimedio . erugine cupria ~. i . amoniago ~ iiii . mirra dinarius . vii . cera pomica dinarius . xiiii . colofania ~ . i . oleo uetere dulce quod sufficit.

3.2 *Item catapodias Eufimie*, ff. 46r–46v

Item catapodias eufimie qui facit ad tussem qui de presenti mitigant causa storaci ~ . i . mirra ~ i . croco ~ i . opio ~ i gabbano ~ . nuce pineus purgatus ~ i . teris omnia galbano uero relequauis et miscis facis catapodias ad magnitudinem proue in ouo aut cum uino ieiuno <e>t post cena binas aut ternas dabis.

3.3 *De capite dicit*, ff. 50r–50v

De capite dicit . cum ad capite morbus oretur solet capites dolor timtare supercilia grauantur . Tempo erapsallunt aures sonant uel molestantur . Oculi mane lacrimantur uel ad somno et caligenantur . Naris obcluduntur . et odorem non senciunt.

De cura dicit . cum his aliquid accederit . oportit capitis purgacionem adhibere isopi coma uel poleie . tur . igane macerato in dulce disri de mensura . emina . et acito tantum . tepefacto gargaridiatur expedit ab homine ieiuno . aut colerato senape . in mulsa tepida similiter ieiuno <s>upinato capite ad sole caledo calefacto cerebro gargaridiare et naribus infundere sucus radicis bitarum p[.]artes duas . mellis . parte una . in se mixtum ut dixi tepidum naribus infundere . quare conuenit iam humor hominis qui in capite consistit . ut ieratur et cycli cura . adibeat . uel ciborum . quam qui se negliunt . Cade ante pyforis . oculorum . et tragomata . palpebrorum et emigranium aurium . dolores et erupciones . interdum et pariotidas . post aures . et glandolas fiunt uel iscrofe et uicia circum fauces . et ceruicis doloris . ori se solent . et strumas . et in facia scabies . et distillacionum faucium tumoris . uel grauido interdum ulcera in capite nascuntur eciam et capilli difluunt et dencium doloris et adiutacionem et in cerebro uertiginis . et suffocaciones in guttere.

3.4 *Antidotum qui dicitur acharistus*, ff. 57v–58r

Antidotum qui dicitur acharistus . Facit ad tipus ante ora accessionis ex mulsa aut ex uino facit et ad desenthericos . mirrae croci casiae spica nardi (.) singulas . cinamomum . ~ . i . aut casiae duplum . piperis longi piperis albi . castoreum galbani . costi .

opii . storacis . ~ . singulas . mel dispumatum quod sufficit . dabis in modo faue ita ut in singulis pocionibus aque et mellis coclearius . iii . adas et aceti boni digito guttas xii.

3.5 *Ad oris uicia*, ff. 89r–89v

3.5.1 **Ad oris uicia** . apii radix cum mel cocta ulcera oris caelerius sanat.

3.5.2 **Item** lapacium in uino coctam gargalidias umorem dencium dolorem tollit raucam uocem et tussiculas purgat.

3.5.3 **Item** ficus nigra sicca adque conbusta cum tot eadem <t>enerem solsorem capitibus in uas fictile conbustis et in puluerem redactis in melle collectis uulneribus ex quacumquae causa infantibus in ore natis et peruersantibus sanati.

3.5.4 **Item** alumen iscisum . *sem* . *un* . i . mirra trocliten penso . *sem un* . cupe *drag* . una trita puluere spars<o> ceri dencium sanat.

3.5.5 **Item** oliastri uiridi . cimas . lauri folias . iii . inflamatas . aprotani uiridi cimas . iii . piper grana . xvii . carofoli . granas . iii . lasari gemma . i . bettuminis pars una . sardinarum capita . iii . mastice granas . iii . teris in acito emina . i.

3.5.6 **Item** ad gingiuas qui reumatizant . id est lenteum nouum in melle modefactum conburis et pulueris ipsas gingibas . adponis.

3.5.7 **Item** folia oliastri lentisci et alaterni mastice folium piper factis simul unum testum conbustum cardi radicis ustum omni aequaliter teris et ponis prius tamen de uino optimo os labit cancrum sanat.

3.5.8 **Item** ad omnia oris uicia uel rane siue uulnera rossiricum *un* . ii . gallas *drag* . ii . alumen scisum *drag* . i . factis pulueribus inponis.

3.5.9 **Item** ad cironico uel cicatricem . expertum ferruginem ferri qui de includi ne cadit . tritum cum melle et acito inpone.

3.6 *Ad scabule dolorem*, f. 96v

Ad scabule dolorem . herba sanguinaria et uerbina tunsa in coc<l>us menu<...> faua farisa cocta in uino infusa et exungia uetus contundis unum corpore facis in panno et ponis calido.

3.7 *Ad costas fractas*, f. 97r

Ad costas fractas . uitro pice acito resoluis in patena bene adiuuat.

3.8 *Ad puncta que in lateribus superuenit*, f. 97r

Ad puncta que in lateribus superuenit hoc est defecciones se in febre acute superuenit . abrotanum in aqua tritum et euaporacione ne adhibeatur propere omnia et agriamen uetandum est.

3.9 *Antidotum ad sthomachum frigidum qui dicitur climax*, ff. 98v–99r

Antidotum . ad sthomachum frigidum . qui dicitur climax . Recepit ec enula ~ . v . fenuculi semen . ~ . iii . piper ~ ii . gingiber ~ . i . mel attico crudo . *lib* . ii . aut qualem inuenis dispumato . eruci semen ~ . i . si eruci non habes mitte senape semen ~ . i .

sicionus siriacus hoc est nigella ~ ii . sili . ~ i . apii . ~ i . petrosilino ~ i . in omnibus enim melior uisum est magnificus et in multis rebus . ad inflacionibus stomachi et indegescione pacientibus sic in mulieribus minstrua . perducit . et ad modicus mirabiliter operatus est . facit ruptus suauis datus et ad omnem tussem . et quibus est capite in torace reuma fluit et ad omnes pectoris dolores . mirabiliter effectus est.

3.10 *Pocio mirabilis contra omnes infirmitates*, f. 99r

Pocio mirabilis contra omnes infirmitates . gariofilo grana . xxx . piper grana . xl . gingiber peciolas iiii . spico iuxta consideracione myrra *drg* . i . amoniaco *drg* . ʃ galanga tercia parte de dinario cynamo *dir* . ii . capparo *dir* . i . agarico *dir* . ʃ . saluia manipulo . i . abrotano . *manp* . i . quinquefolia . *manp* . i . triscalamo . *manp* . i . gamendrea *manp* . i uermiculosa *manp* . i . et parum saturegia hec omnia tere cum mel dispumatum . parum et cum uino uetus . staupus viiii.

3.11 *Pucione ad ebrugine*, f. 102r

<P>**ucione ad ebrugine** herba ebula . college radices . iiii . <.>ribus ante sole leuante in contra oriente ipsas college . feno<g>rego grana . v . lauro folia . iii . piper grana . xxx . cum ceruisa leuan<t>e facias staupo pleno . et dabis ei bibere . et cum ipso bibet abeat <.>no ouo fricto dabis ei ad comedendum et in lecto . sic coperes <.a>ledo usque ad uesperum.

3.12 *Antidotum sotirie*, ff. 113v–114v

Antidotum . sotirie qui interpretatur saluatrix tocius corporis qui omnes . causas pagat qui sunt . intrinsecus constitute capitis anticum dolorem soluet . escotomatecus et epelempticus . et post accessionem aurium dolores cessat . oculorum . impetus cessat . dencium dolorem sanat . tussem antiquam . et recentem tollet . pleorisem et perepleomonia pectorum . et eparis tensionem desoluit siccat enim et pulmonum humorum sic cum mul<..> aut calida aqua . bibatur . ad sanguinem ex<c>re<an>tibus . cum oximelle dabis . singultum tollet et qui cibum non continent . degescionem parat et uomitum constringet . et omnem uentositatem istomachi uel aquali . coli dissoluit ictericus et habundancia fellis ruffi dissoluit et ad pristinam colorem reuocat melenconia isplenus . graui dolores . releuat fleoma per interiora reduc<it> reniculorum causas sanat sablonis de uisica ad exitum deducit quiliacus uero . grande adiutorium prestat brachiorum solucionem uel dor et coxarum ad pristinam sanitatem reducit . feminarum . uero . causas uel omnes . matricis molestis sanat . et eos qui per dolorem . somnium \non/ capiunt . membra uero . resoluta suo calore ad pristina sanitatem reducit necessarium uero est podagricis . et contra omne uenena et serpencium morsum mirifice prodest . ut non solum cum mulsa . donetur . sed ut antidotum morsibus apponatur ad tipus ante ora uel duas oras . accessionis cum aqua calida dabis . et quartanariis hoc propter longinquas infirmitatis hutilem est . nam si quis sanus frequencius cum mulsa bibatur numquuam infirmi<tates> das antidutum istum iuxta uiris . uel etatis dabis <i>n modo abila\i/ne . **Recipit** . hec mirra troclite *drs* . xviii . castoreo . *drs* . viiii . opio . *drs* . xviiii <pet>rosilino . *drs* . xviiii . aniso . *drs* . xii . apii . semen . *drs* . xx . isquinoantus . *drs* . xv . piper . *drs* . xv . senenus *drs* . xv . cenamo . *drs* . xii . costo . *drs* . xviii . ispica *drs* . xiii asaro . *drs* . vii . croco maucma . *drs* . vi . seselleus . *dr* . vi . cassia *dr* vi . istorace *dr* . vi . croco . *dr* xvi . piper albo *dr* . xii . amonio *dr* . iiii . piper longo iscriptulum . i *s* . mel discumato . quod sufficit.

3.13 *Ad prugine qui uocatur morbus regio*, ff. 115v–116r

Ad prugine qui uocatur morbus regio . In primis cum illam infirmitatem cognoueris statim fleugumare debis de uena epatica qui subtus brachio iacet . et minimas ei sanguinem usque libras . iii . et post tercio uero die aut iiii . in assu balneo faceas ducere et ibi fortiter sudet et antequam sudare ceperit das ei bibere sucum de rafani cum oleo mixto dimedio . staupo et postea egressus de balneo duces eum in lecto et fortiter cooperis illum ut et ibidem sudet et exterges illam sudorem et mittis in uas et inuenies ipsam eruginem supernatantem In alia die ducis eum in balneo et antequam sudare aperit das ei plenam cocleariam de rasuram eburnei cum mel et uino staupo pleno . tercio uero die duces eum in balneo et antequam sudare ceperit das ei bibere liuestico radices cum apio et piper mel et uino staupo pleno . quarta uero die ducis eum in balneo et antequam sudare ceperit das ei bibere sauinam et adriplicem cum uino et mel et piper *stau* . i . v uero die ducis eum in balneo et antequam sudare ceperit das ei bibere centauream et cardonem cum uino et mel et piper *stau* . i . vi . uero die ducis eum in balneo et antequam sudare ceperit das ei bibere rutam saluaticam et camitriam et liuestico saluatico cum uino et mel et piper *stau* . i . vii . uero die ducis eum in balneo et antequam sudare ceperit das ei bibere . radices et folia de erba apollonia et sarpullo minore cum uino et mel et piper . viii . uero die ducis eum in balneo et antequam sudare ceperit das ei manducare . radicis de \<c>/rud[.]i nape in melle co<nsectas> viiii uero ducis eum in balneo et antequam sudare ceperit das ei bibere sucum de celedonia cum uino et melle et piper staupo . i . ista aut ad<iuto>ria ad presens sunt . et cib<i> eorum talis erit uetus lardum manducet et bucc<in>am carnem aut multon<inam> et pisces et oleo et aceto et panem <tenerum> et abstineat se de oua de lacte de casio et de omnia a<g[r]en>ti se abstineat appio et liuestico et ruta campana et faciat metus et istas erbas ibidem mittat bullire et das ei bibere.

3.14 *Ad dentes stringendas uel si dolent uel putrescunt*, f. 122r

Ad dentes stringendas . uel si dolent uel putrescunt . uini austero *ff* . i . porrorum sucus ~ i . usque ad medias decoquis et tepido diu in ore <teneat>.

3.15 *Ad ueretrum suscitandum*, f. 122v

3.15.1 **Ad ueretrum suscitandum** . Tincum in cute fricet et destellatam gut<tam> bibat cum uino et quando iterum uolueris <et non> dare refriga ipsum tincum in aqua modice aut in metus et bibat.

3.15.2 **Item ad ipsum suscitandum** . de persicis nucleos viiii . in medus aut in melle tinctos comedat ante altare et deum omnipotentem precare debet qui omnes sementes et corporibus . et hominibus et herbis dedit ut ei det semen bonum ad uoluntate dei <f>acit.

3.16 [Title faded and no longer legible], f. 124v

petrosile . [....] liuesti pastenace . bitonica . pipenella agrimonia milfolia . apio saluia poleio . ruta millo saluatice . galanga . auerio . lasari . ortica flores . bagas edere . bagas lauri bagas iuniperi piper elebyro grano mastice pulpodia casia fistula.

4 *Lat. 11219*

4.1 *Puluera ad epaticos*,[1] f. 221vb

Puluera ad epaticos recipit haec .
piper ∻ i .
cinamomo ∻ i .
spico ∻ i .
costo ∻ i .
gingiber ∻ i .
galinga ∻ i .
reopontico ∻ ii .
aloen ∻ i .
granomastice ∻ i .
gariofilo ∻ i .
peretrum ∻ i .
bagas lauri ∻ i .
genciana ∻ i .
apio ∻ i .
satureia ∻ i .
absentio ∻ i .
centaurea ∻ i .
marrubio ∻ i .
nepta ∻ i .
feniculo ∻ i .
polipodia ∻ i .
anetum ∻ i .
ermodactulo ∻ i .

1 This recipe is recorded as a list with each ingredient on a new line, so I have replicated the structure in my transcription.

aristolicia rotunda ∻ i .
lupino ∻ i .
fenogreco ∻ i .
Haec omnia puluera facis dabis ex <bibere> <eu>ndi dormitum *denr* iii <pensante>.

4.2 *Potio ad carbunculum*, ff. 223va–223vb

Potio ad carbunculum quod clao uocatur et omnia uenenata potione siue ictus serpentium uel bestiarum morso probatissimum est id est zedoar cum aqua trita bibat . utilis et ualedissimum adiutorium est.

4.3 *Puluis ad implere plagas et si ossa habet minuata discutit*, p. 225ra

Puluis ad implere plagas . et si ossa habet minuata discutit . id est . irius . aristologia longa . panacus regius ana *unc* . i . manna turis *un* iiii . puluerem facis et uteris.

4.4 *Puluis uera ad faucium tumorem et omnis oris uitia siue sordicia*, f. 225ra

Puluis uera ad faucium tumorem et omnis oris uitia siue sordicia . Id est irius alumen . scise . myrre . ana *un* . *s* . puluerem facis . addis mel et uino sufficienter conmiscis et uteris.

4.5 *Puluis ad uuam leuandam uel oris ulcera*, f. 225rb

Puluis ad uuam leuandam uel oris ulcera galla non forata *drag* iii . costo . croco . irius . myrra . alumen scisse . cortice i malagranate . strucio ana *drag* ii teris cernis et uteris.

4.6 *Ad eos qui urinam facere non possunt*, f. 225va

Ad eos qui urinam facere non possunt petrosilino semen ∻ i apii semen ∻ i fenicoli semen ∻ i olisandri ∻ i saxifrica ∠ galinga ∻ i reopontico ∠ piper grana xx . uino staupos iiii . per quattuor dies bibere dabis in balneo.

4.7 *Potio contra paralesin* ff. 226va–226vb

Potio contra paralesin ad confectum faciendum . debet habere myrra *lib* . i . \bacas *lib* i/ petrisilino macedonico similiter . centaurea similiter . nasturci semen similiter Istas v . causas denominatas siccas unamquamque ex parte in mortario tribulare faciat . et postea ad unam pensam coaequare debet . et cum melle mundo misce dare debet usque perducat ad confectum . et postea quando ipsum confectum accipere debet per diem cotidie . non amplius accipiat nisi quantum unus mancosus pensat . et multitudine eum tribulare faciat . et quando ipsum debet accipere . debet habere plenum staupum de aqua calida . et sic ipsum distemperat uel tepidum bibat . et aliam causam cum istis mittere non presumat . et si ista omnia impleuerat . pro certo sciat . quia de ipsa infirmitate sanus erit.

4.8 *Timiama*, f. 227v

Timiama . Cotsumber *lib* i . *unc* i . Cumfiti *unci iii* . *dr* v . Aloa *unc* iiii . Cinamo *unc* ii . Ambar *dr* ii *s* . Storace *unc* i . Tus *dr* xv . Gariofilo *unc* i . Muscho *unc* i . *dr* ii . Cafora . *unc* i . *dr* i.

4.9 *Tymiamam*, f. 227va

Tymiamam . guzuber ℥ . v . đ . ii . aloa . *unc* . ii . et đ . xviii . cinamomum . per iii ℥ . i . et *dr* . xviiii . thus per . đ . iii . *sol* . i . gariofile . per đ . ii . *sol* . i.

4.10 *Item alia*, f. 227va

Cotsuber ℥ . ii . tus . *s* . cynamo . *dr* . vi storace . ℥ i . gariofile *dr* . iiii . aloa ℥ i et *s* . gumfiti similiter musco . đ . iii . caffora . đ . ii.

4.11 *Alia*, f. 227va

Cotsuber . đ . x . tus . *der* . *s* . spica *dr* . *s* . Aloa . *dr* . v . gunfiti *dr* . iii . musco *dr* . i . caffora *dr* . *s* . storace calamitei . *dr* . ii.

4.12 *Confectio timiamatis adgragantum*, f. 227va

Confectio timiamatis adgragantum cozzuber . *unc* . v . *den* . ii . aloa . *unc* . iiii . storace calamite . *unc* . ii . cinamo . *unc* . ii . tus . solidum . i . gariophile . *sol* . i . gumfiti . *unc* . i . spico . *sol* . <i> . cafora *den* . ii . amber . *den* . ii . musco . đ . ii<ii>.

4.13 [untitled recipe], f. 227va

Cozzuber . *unc* . ii . tus . *dim* . *unc* . cinamo . đ . vi . gariophile . đ . iiii . aloa . *unc* . i . gumfiti . similiter . storace calamite . similiter . cafora đ . ii . musco . đ . iii.

4.14 [untitled recipe], f. 227va

Cozzuber . đ . x . tus . đ . ii . cinamo . đ . ii . gariophile . đ . i . *s* . spico . đ . i . *s* . aloa . đ . v . gumfiti . đ . iii . storace calamite . đ . ii . cafora . đ . i . *s* . musco . đ . ii.

4.15 *Confectio timiamatis*, f. 227vb

Confectio timiamatis . cotzuber *lib* vi . storace calamite ℥ viiii . gumfiti ℥ xviii . cariofile ℥ iii cinamo ℥ v<i> ciperum ℥ v . tus ℥ v . myrra ℥ iii . mastice ℥ ii . spica ℥ vii croco ℥ i aloa ℥ vii . cafora ℥ ii et *denr* ii . musco *denr* xviii ambar *dr* iiii.

4.16 *Item*, f. 227vb

Item Timiamatis confecis . cotzumber *lib* i storacem calamitem ℥ i cariofile *sol* . ii . cinamomum ℥ i tus (.) gunfiti ℥ iiii spico ℥ i amber *sol* i aloa ℥ iiii cafora *sol* i . musco *sol* . i.

4.17 *Item*, f. 227vb

Item Aloa ÷ ii gunfiti ÷ ii . croco duas partes *denr* . cafora similiter . musco similiter . spico *denr* . it us . duas partes de *denr* et *dim* storace . calamite similiter gariofile similiter . cotsumber <÷> vi.

4.18 *Item*, f. 227vb

Item . gumfiti . aloa . tus lucidissimum . musco . ambar.

4.19 *Confectio timiama*, f. 227vb

Confectio Timiama . [g]cotzuber ÷ vi . aloa . ÷ ii . gumfiti ÷ ii . cenamo ÷ i tus . ÷ *s* . storace ÷ *s* gariofilo ÷ *s* . caffora ÷ *s*.

Stiftsbibliothek St. Gallen

5 *Cod. sang. 44*

5.1 *Antidotum sotira*, pp. 234–6:

Antidotum Sotira antidotum quod dictum est saluatio . conficitur . sic . murra . ʒ[2] . xviii . croco ʒ . xv . opio . ʒ . xviii . anisu . ʒ . xii . squinantu . ʒ . xvii . piper longo ʒ . xiiii . sinonus ʒ . xi . amomu ʒ iiii . nardo statio ʒ xiii . castoreo ʒ viiii . petrosilino ʒ xv . semen appii ʒ xx . cassia ʒ iiii . piper nigrum ʒ xv . storace ʒ vi . ydrococumaum ʒ vi . cinnamomum ʒ iiii . quod sufficit mel . facit autem his causis ad omnem corpus cum mulsa bibantur caput dolentibus soluit stomaticis epilenticis . et accessiones mania compescit insomnietas ad somnum perducit . et freneticis somnum prestat . et aurium dolores soluit . et nimium dolorem in pessimum oculorum et reuma constringit . et paracintidiatos sine dolore punctum soluit dentium dolore compescit anelitum nimium pausare facit et omnem causam corporis extinguit tussem antiquam peripleomonia . et uiscerum tensiones et partes omnes causas reuelat dessicat de pulmonem uomicationem flecma uel saluia cito reiectare facit . cum mulsa bibat . si aliquem sanguinem resceat cum oximelle dabitur aut sucu policoni ad mensura egrotantis siue addere stomachi est magnum adiutorium lesum constringit . et non delectantes cibum uomica stomachi et uentris tollit acciditas indigestionem et uiscerum morsus soluit epaticis punctiones

2 The symbol in this recipe fluctuates but appears to reflect variations on the same character. While it does not quite fit the 'ʒ' symbol, it looks closest to this; there is, however, some uncertainty given that it is glossed with *dr* in the preceding recipe. In Sigerist's transcription, 'Z' is used to represent the symbol in question, a symbol/unit he does not address in his comments on weights and measures; see *Studien und Texte*, ed. Sigerist, 80–81 (*Antidotum sotira*) and 175 (weights and measures).

et dolores mitigat et in morbum regium colera refusa in corpore in bonum colorem et naturalem perducit et prouocat . et malencoba multum cogitantes et asperitatem eorum pulmonis tollit grauitudinem . et colorem malum in antiquum reuocat reuma uel colera per stentinas ponit mediocrem febrem per stentinas . et urinam prouocat . et statim in rene sanat facit per [...] diureticus perducit in uissicam constrictiones uel lumbi renum et uisi[c]cę purget disuriam malam \in/ iunctam etiam in naturam uirorum paralisis eius curat . et reuocat in usum uenerium . Quando iam et tentica nihil profecerit ciliacę causę [i] uehementer curat uentositatem tollit et uentrem stercus . et humorem eorum soluit torquimina mitigat te[r.]nsione intestinorum et spasmum finit paralisis brachiorum et femorum tollit silentium facit . non oppressionem sed exponit naturalem somnum . Illis autem qui per hos non possunt bibere per clisterem datur . cum succo fenogreci matricis omnem causam et dolorem et insomnietatem eorum soluit et tentionem eorum uel duritiam commalaxat sanguinis fluxum uel humorem si bibat constringit . et cum uino calido inculpidiata constringit . Dabis autem matricis podacricis sciaticis in doloribus magnis uirtutem huius medicamenti non solum per os soluat . sed et illi[s] faciens lixopiritum . est autem in maioribus . febribus . et in tipicis modum abellane ante hora accessionis dabis . Quartanis autem plus dabis medicamentum et in tres potiones dabis . haec autem omnia in nomine domini.

5.2 *Antidotum pigra Gallieni optimum*, p. 238

Incipit antidotum pigra Gallieni optimum Qui facit stomaicis epilenticis melancolicis freneticis epaticis spleneticis podacricis uertigines caligines typus subito metus saltus membrorum neruorum contractiones perfrictiones . et quod liber stupor uel mulieris uitia . et ad omnes causas quę subito ueniunt emendant . Recipit hęc . aloen *lib* . i . costo amomu axentio rosa ficca . ana ~ v . xilobalsamo cinnamomum . spica mastice . croco cassia fistola squinuantus ameu ~ ana . v . exinde puluere fac addis mel quod sufficit . da exinde . ∠ i . si febr[u]\i/erit cum mulsa si non febrierit cum uino ad pullorum cantus.

5.3 *Antidotum filantropum*, p. 238

Incipit antidotum filantropum Facit tissicis dipnoicis cefalargicis stomaticis ad toraces limosotis dissolutis epaticis spleneticis colicis . aliis doloribus nefreticis podacricis . recipit hęc petrosilino ʒ ii . cipero squino\antum/ indico [cesaro] \asarum/ eufurbio ana ʒ i . dispumatum mel dabis cum aqua frida.

5.4 *Inplastrum apostolicon*, pp. 238–9

Incipiunt emplastra singularia infirmis in primo[m] inplastrum apostolicon. Apostolicon facit ad omnes causas . et ad omnia uulnera antiqua siue recentia ad pleumones ad neruos pręcisos ad musculos et omnes plagas quę a ferro inciditur siue utres siue uitro siue canna sagittas educendas infixas corpori uel ad morsum et ad punctus anima uenerorum terrena et maritima et uenena trahendo foras quę in alto sunt oculta facit etiam apostematicis ad cancros ad ignis agr[a]um ad ceruicis dolorem nimium ad sacrofas rumpendas et per modico foramine omnia trahit et sanat ut catrix non pereat et qui inter costas apostemas habent in epate in splene a foris inponis et intus rumpitur per egestione et cyros in splenis soluit et sanat . facit autem arteriacis ad percussuras uel cironia quę in genua uel in pedes et meliceridas rumpit et sanat . facit autem ad reuma uel quacumque dolore et tumore coxas genua et ad talos descendit ut ad cataplasmas inponas . facit etiam ad fistolas . Recipit autem hęc . Ligargi\r/o . *lib* . i . et ~ i . *s* . galbano ~ i . *dr* . i . gutta ammoniaci . ~ iiii *dr* . i . cera ~ vi . mirra ~ . erugine campano ~ i *dr* . i . bdellio ~ i . et *s* et manna turis ~ i . et *s* opopanace ~ i . aristologia quale uolueris . ~ i . oleo uetere *lib* . i . et *s* . quę tuenda sunt cribellas . deinde cera colofonia et oleo solues in foco et miscis litargirum . et postea miscis residuas species et tamdiu coques dum mutet colorem.

5.5 *Emplastrum qui sine ferro rumpit uulnera et scrofas et aperit*, p. 243

Emplastrum qui sine ferro rumpit uulnera et scrofas et aperit salis ammoniaci *lib* . i . mollibdine *lib* i . oleo *lib* . i . cineris sarmentorum *lib* . i . femus columbino ~ iii . conficis et uteris.

5.6 *Oxira crucira emplastrum*, pp. 243–4

Oxira crucira emplastrum qui facit epaticis spleneticis ad ipocondria tensione nefretici . et omnes neruorum passiones . pleuretici peripleomonici artitici podacrici sciatici neruorum contractiones ad luxu ad fracturas et incisus neruus soluet ad serpentem ad canes rapidi morsum ad omnia recipit hęc . pice sicca *lib* . ii . cera *lib* . i . amoniaco . *lib* . i . arisenum galbano ana ~ iiii . croco ~ ii . aceto fortiter *ser* . iii . teris ammoniaco et libano cum aceto ad mellis cocti pinguedinem et teris <cum> pice autem . mittis in cacaposteo . et supermittis aceto et coquis agitando semper . postea mittis galbum et cum fuerit solutum mittis et effundis in altero mortario et conficis manibus.

5.7 *Confectio timiame*, p. 247

Confectio timiame . cozumbrio *lib* . i . storace ~ ii . et *dr* . ii . confiti . ~ iii . et *dr* vi . thus ~ i *dr* . ii mirra *dr* vi mastice ~ *s* spica ~ i et *dr* vi croco *dr* . ii . alo[e]\a/ ~ i et *dr* . vi . cafora ~ i et *dr* i . musco *dr* iiii . ambar *dr* . i.

5.8 *Dentisfritium bonum et salubrem*, p. 248

Dentisfritium bonum et salubrem qui recipit multas species costu ad bonum odorem cipero ad fauces linendo cardamo ad [h]oris uulnera bratheum et piper et pro pessimum humorem illirica ad dolorem iusquiami ad prurigine scisti ad uuam . bacas lauri ad frigorem . samsucu ad suauitatem thus ad ginguia tumida piretrum et stafidagria ad humorem sicandum . de hęc omnia ana ʒ i et perbelle[3] utis.

5.9 *Dentisfritium ad gingiuas confortandas et dissicandas*, p. 248

Dentisfritium ad gingiuas confortandas et dissicandas . mastice ~ i . stipteria scut[4] ~ i . yreus iliricis ~ i . perfoliu ~ i . salis frixus ~ i *s* cornus ceruunus ∠ iiii.

5.10 *Catarticum artriticis et idropicis*, p. 250

Catarticum artriticis et idropicis . lacteridia ʒ ii . ermodactilo . ~ iiii . gingiber ℈ viii cimino etiopicum . piper ana ℈ viii . teris et cernis piper album ℈ viii . mittis et reponis et cum opus fuerit tollis de puluere . ss[5] pensum *sol* i . et ℈ iiii . et admiscis diacridium sub ora tritum ʒ i . dabis sera eunti dormito tamen ipso calice ubi sunt pigmenta soluta in calida aqua deponas donec tepefiat . sed hoc ieiuno dabis . expertum est.

5.11 *Oleo roseo*, pp. 256–7

Oleo roseo uirtutem habet scipticam reprimit et refricdat et potatus soluet stomachum et causos stringet . est autem ulcerum nutritor et cectica uulnera tegat et capitis dolorem tollit . et ad dentium dolorem in os missus facit et ad palpebras duras ut mollis fiat intestinarum dolores et matricis sanat in inchoatione . Conficitur autem sic . rosa rubea exungulata et in umbra exsucata die et nocte mittis . ~ iii oleo umfacium italicum . *ses* . ii . mittis in ampulla uitrea . et ligas diligenter linteo et desuper pellem cooperis propter pluuiam aut solem et ponis ad solem diebus xl . et postea tollis et ponis sub tectum in locum temperatum . Alii non ponuntur ad solem . sed in puteum aut in fontana mittunt diebus . xl . et postea sic reponunt . sed prima confectio qui ad sol<em> ponunt . omni cura expediens est subtilios . et miticantium . frigidiorem est ex aqua et spissior . de terra autem grauior est . ergo his qui ad solem ponuntur facit ex capitis dolore qui ex nimia febre fuerint exsiccati aut solis ardore accensus et pro aliis causis mitigat dolorem et somnum adducit . Qui autem in aqua conponitur ad nimium sudorem capiti uel ardorem potest adhiberi ad omnia nimia ardentia adhibitum mitigat ad ardorem in uisceribus quod per de coleribus accenditur potatur cum aqua calida aut frigida refrigerat et dolorem stomachi tollit etiam si cum nimia modacitate fiat

3 The abbreviation 'pbl' remains puzzling and is entirely absent from Sigerist's transcription (see *Studien und Texte*, ed. Sigerist, 89); my thanks to Conan Doyle for suggesting *perbelle* as a possible way to expand this.

4 It is unclear what 'scut' is abbreviating (mark of abbreviation over 'u'); with *stipteria* meaning 'alum', I suggest that it possibly was intended to mean a word such as *schistum* or *scissum* that are often descriptors of another word for 'alum', *alumen*.

5 It is unclear what 'ss' is abbreviating; given the measuresments that follow, it appears to be an ingredient (rather than an alternate abbreviation of *sextarius*), but there are a variety of possible ingredients that could work with this abbreviation (e.g., *samsucus, sisimbrium, solsequia*, etc.).

. ad lumbricos similiter datur . colum laborantibus ita datur et sanat . ad omnia calida adhibendus est interius et exterius.

5.12 *Oleo lentisscinum*, p. 258

Oleo \lentis/scinum fit de semen lentisci . cum autem maturauerit . facis sicut de lauri bacas . facit autem ad omnes matricis dolorem uirtutem habet calefacturiam et stipticam malaxaturiam facit ad omnem duritiam stomachi et ad ciliacum et disentericus . et ad oris uitia . et de facię omnia purgat et colorem bonum et furfures et ordeola capitis facit.

5.13 *Ad podacra*, p. 260

Ad podacra aristologia rotunda centauria agatia puluis ęquali pondere cum succu ciclaminis distemperas et superpone proficit.

5.14 *Confectio saponi Constantini*, p. 282

Confectio saponi constantini recipit hęc . blaustia . rodon . cerussa . nitru mastice . thus aloen . mirta amoniaco . pumix stafidacria . gariofilo . spica indica . folio sarcocla . croco . licio . calcantu . alumen . scissum . alumen rotundum . ossa sipię . et ostrię costo amomu ana ~ i . *s* . ca\r/pobalsami confiti . xilobalsami . squinoantus afronitro dracantu sandaraca nardo celtico ana ~ i . balsamo . ~ *s* musco *dr* iii *s* ouarum uetella . ii . albumen . iii . sapone gallico . *lib* elixatura lupini quod suficit . optimum est nimis.

5.15 *Potio maniacis siue gutta catiua*, p. 285

Potio maniacis siue gutta catiua lasar . stupio . opopanace . castoreo . amiantu . pionica lucia . fel ursinum fel taurinum . byro martira . canta psalmo nono . et missa super et lege passionem domini . tres cime elene . iii . cime de rubo . iii . cime ortica . iii . cime de fusago . iii.

5.16 *Ut infantibus dentes sine dolore exeant*, p. 304

Ut infantibus dentes sine dolore exeant cerebrum leporis coctum gingiuas fricas.

5.17 *Ad fagidinica*, pp. 330–1

5.17.1 Ad fagidinica ad amantium ad diuturnas quę dificile cicatricant uulnera . bulbus scillis quod mollis est in oleo ʒ is mittis coquis donec ad tertias reuertatur et de hoc oleo uteris perunguis ulcus cum pinna absque mutario haec purgat carnem nutrit et cicatricem ducit uide ne morcare redeat super ulcus ex hoc in noto.

5.17.2 Item aliud ad fagidinica ulcera . pastinace folia trita cum mel superpone . melior enim est pastinace siluestris folia quam domestice . si non inuenis agrestem domesticam uteris.

5.18 *Potio ad nescia*, p. 345

5.18.1 **Potio . ad nescia** Sauina . *manip* . iii . piper grana . xviii teris cum uino et mel . qui patitur dolorem in balneo bibat . postea super ipsa coxa que dolet iaceat et in ipsa potione tres staupos uini mittat . ut per triduum hoc bibat.

5.18.2 **Item ad ipsum** . Ebolo qui solus nascit radicem ipsius tere in acetum . cum nouella ceruisia bibat . et ambulet . ut sudet.

5.18.3 **Item ad ipsum** . Azaro . libra . i . piper . grana . xv . in uino . aut in ceruisia nouella bibat.

5.18.4 **Item ad ipsum** . Brasia . et agrimonia . et caballopeia teris . in nouella ceruisia maneat cooperta . et crastinum bibat . sanus erit.

5.18.5 **Item ad ipsum** . Fenuculi semen quantum in tres digitas . leuas . bibat . sanat.

5.19 *Ad renum dolorem uel coxarum*, p. 345

Ad renum dolorem uel coxarum . Flos feni in aqua coquis . tepefactum superliga et dulce potione bibat . sanat.

5.20 *Ad luxatura*, p. 348

Ad luxatura . Agrimonia tusa superponis . et uena incidere debes sanat.

5.21 *Item ad ipsum potio bibenda contra ipsos uermes eiciendos*, p. 350

5.21.1 **Item ad ipsum** . Potio bibenda contra ipsos uermes eiciendos . aut quacumque maleficio in se habuerit Herba basilerica quae nascitur per montes . in loca arida ubi petras minutas sunt . folia simili porro . radix eius crispa . et fistolas . colligis eam mense septembre luna decurrente die martis aut iouis . aut sabbati . herba ipsa teris diligenter . miscis cum nouella ceruisia calice pleno das ei ieiuno bibere . et ante die abstineat se a cibo die iouis luna uetere debet bibere . si uermes ipsa die iactauerit . priusquam manducet calido bibat aut exouera.

5.21.2 Ranas et craxantos . haec potio expellere solet . et si de ha[n]c potione . non exierint . bibat . alia potione . ad occidendos . ius de mora campestria teris et exprimis . et teris folia cannapi manu plena . et si folia non fuerint semen ipsius dabis ei potione calice pleno . et si ius more non habuerint aut cannapo inuenire non potuerit . lacte caprino calido bibat . mortuos uermes proiciet.

5.22 *Ad flegma curandum*, p. 351

Ad flegma curandum . Marrubii sucum . Mente sucum . Matresilue sucum . Azari sucum . Agrimoniae sucum . Betonicę sucum . [Agrimonię sucum] aequali mensura . de aceto . et aloen . et apii semen . de uino calice pleno . piper grana . c haec omnia simul miscis . et in olla noua coquis . ad tertias . sic per tres mane . ieiunus bibat . sanat.

5.23 *Ad glandolas siccandas*, p. 353

Ad glandolas . siccandas . celidonia radice . manipulo . i . bladonna . radice . manipulo . i . Rodenapo radice . manipulo . i . polipodia . similiter . ebolo similiter . mater herbarum similiter frafolio . similiter . azaro . similiter . betonica . similiter . agrimonia similiter uermiculo folia similiter . plantagine similiter . edera siluester similiter . pico lingua similiter . gamandrea similiter . quinquefolia similiter . herba benedicta similiter . piper grana . xxxiii . haec omnia simul teris et in sex staupos de ceruisa distemperas et das bibere . sanat.

5.24 *Ad dentem cauum*, p. 360

5.24.1 **Ad dentem . cauum** . Stercus corbino . ibidem inponis . dentem rumpit . et dolorem tollit.

5.24.2 **Item** . Plantagin[e]\is/ radix commasticetur . dolorem tollit.

5.24.3 **Item** . Farina de negella . intus in dentem cauum mitte sanat.

5.25 *Ad exasperatione gingiuarum*, p. 361

5.25.1 **Ad exasperatione gingiuarum** . Folia rose . teris cum mel diligenter . inde gingiuas inunguis . et oleo crudo . non manducet nec nullum agramen . sed salsamenta . manducet.

5.25.2 **Item** . Oleo uetere . naribus infundatur . frequenter.

5.25.3 **Item** . Quinquefolia radices gargarizet sucum cum aqua.

5.26 *Ad ulcera oris uel quicquid in labia fuerint*, p. 361

Ad ulcera oris . uel quicquid in labia . fuerint Rumice . et pampinis folia . tenenter[er] ad tertias in uino decoquis . et ipsum uinum . ore teneatur.

5.27 *Ad scapularum dolorem*, pp. 361–2

5.27.1 **Ad scapularum dolorem** . Betonica scripulos . iiii . cum mulsa . ciatos . iiii . dabis bibere.

5.27.2 **Item** . herba berbena . et faua fresa . coquis in uino cum axungia contundis inducis in linteo . et calido superpone.

5.27.3 **Item** . uino uetus . cum axungia ferue simul . quousque soluatur . Postea lana succida carpinata intinguis . et exprimis fortiter . ut omne sucus dimittat . sic ipsa lana ponis super ubi dolet.

5.28 *Ad serpentes uel alios uermes de homine expellendos*, p. 364

5.28.1 **Ad serpentes** . uel alios uermes . de homine . expellendos . Potio probata . ius de cocurbita saluatica . nuce plena cum nouella ceruisia ieiuno dabis bibere luna decurrente.

5.28.2 **Item** . Medulla ceruina . aut de osso . aut de corno ipsius . cum lacte caprino bibat.

5.28.3 **Item** . Ius de mora campestra exprimis . et teris folia canapi miscis simul et bibat calice pleno . semen mitte s\i/ mora non est . lacte caprino calidum mittis . haec potio . herbas uel omnia maleficia . et omnia uermes proiciet.

5.28.4 **Item** . Ad uermes de infantes eiciendos pingue de lardo porcino *cocla* . iii . ieiunus bibat.

5.29 *Ad punctas qui in latere superueniunt*, pp. 364–5

5.29.1 **Ad punctas qui in latere superueniunt** . Abrotano trito in aqua colato medio calice . tepidum bibat . admiscis modicum sal.

5.29.2 **Item** . herba . antola manipulo . i . teris cum uino . calice . i . ieiuno das bibere . superiaceat ubi dolet.

5.29.3 **Item** . Amoniaco . *sol* . pensum . oleo . aceto . et sal . singulo cocleario insimul teris . et ieiunus bibat . et tamdiu super ipso latus iaceat . usque . dum sudet.

5.30 *Ad uentris dolorem uel tumores stintinarum*, p. 366

5.30.1 **Ad ventris dolorem** . uel tumores stintinarum . Sementis bete decocta ex aq<ua> fomentas uent<.....> . et tumorem tollit si per triduum hoc feceris.

5.30.2 **Item** . Herba quinquefolii sucu[s]m dabis bibere . *cocl* . ii . sine mora dolorem tollit.

5.30.3 **Item** . Si tumor fuerit . Herba plantagine sucum eius tepefactum fomentando dolorem tollit . et ipsa tunsa . et inposita dolorem tollit . et sucum eius bibitum et toracem . et uentrem sanat.

5.30.4 **Item** . Betonica . *drag* . i . in aqua calida . ciatos . ii . bibat . his autem apta erit fomentando . dolorem tollit . ipsa tusa . et inposita tumorem tollit . ius eius bibitum . et toracem . et uentrem sanat.

5.30.5 **Item . Ad intestinarum dolorem** . Herba nepta cum uino bibat . sanat.

5.30.6 **Item . Ad duritiam uentris** . Lino semen cum mel tritum . in ceruisa . ieiunus bibat mirum . est.

5.31 *Ad lumborum dolores*, pp. 367

5.31.1 <**Ad**> **lumborum dolores** . Betonica *drag* . iii . uino rubeo . ciatos iii piper grana xviii tritum et calefactum ieiunus bibat.

5.31.2 **Item ad lumborum** uel coxarum dolorem . Betonica *drag* . ii . ex mulsa dabis bibere.

5.31.3 **Item** . Herba senicion per se trita potui data mirum prodest.

5.31.4 **Item** . Alium non mundatum . cum axungia contusum in panno superposito mire sanat.

6 *Cod. sang. 217*

6.1 *Ad capitis*, pp. 257a–258b

6.1.1 **Ad capitis** . Oportet diu permanere capitis . dolore precipuae . sine febri matheriam . detrahere per nares . uel per os . quaeres . etiam aures . uel dentem diutius dolentibus . prode est . brasice sucus naribus . infusus . capud expurgat dolorem mitigat.

6.1.2 **Item** . Bete nigre radicis sucus minus quam dimidium et mellis . mixtum in nares infundes ita ut palatum non transeat . pituita omnes . defluit et cum his cessare oleum in os accipiat.

6.1.3 **Item** . caerefolium in aqua decoctum . et \e/ aqua potui data . pituitas extrahis.

6.1.4 **Item** [R] Sinapis . ∻ i . rape seminis . ∻ i . piper . grana . xx . nasturcii semen ∻ i . erucae origani . ∻ i . apii . seminis . ∻ i . tantumdem ex aceto et melle . colligis . et ex ea . aqua calida . per dies vii . gargarizauit.

6.1.5 **Item** . origani . comam . uel ysopi herbam conelam in mellitissima mulsa triduo macerabis . De hinc coqui facies . et sereno . celo tepidum ieiunus per triduum gargarigaes.

6.1.6 **Item** . Senapis . cocleario . ii . et aque mulsa cyatum . i . miscebis . calefacias.

6.1.7 **Item** . malue semen . ex uino nigro . contrito . gargarizato . tepidum . pituitas . capitis . extrahis.

6.1.8 **Item** . mellis . semina sape . aemina . aceti acerimi [m] . ff . i . sinapis triti . ∻ i . ysopi . tusi et creti . ∻ i . origani tusi . et cribrati ∻ i simul omnia coquis . ita ut pinguinem . aquatioris melli . asum<.>t . et colatum diligiter . gargarizet . ad solem quamdiu potest.

6.1.9 **Item** . ysopi ∻ i . origani . ∻ i . timi . ∻ i . istafidosagrias . ∻ i . pulei . ∻ i . sape optime ff i . aceti acerimi aemina omnia infusa tertia die coques carbonibus lentis donec . una parte decocta dua remaneant hinc quartam . partem contra solem hora tertia . gargarizet . postea . recentem in ore teneat ut humoris abuncia restringatur et ieiun<a> usque hora viii.

6.1.10 **Item** . ad dolorem . capitis et insaniam . quamquam plurime sint . cause . dolorem capitis . tamen si sol acerimus . celebrum. percusserit . subito mens . auferetur . et uelut insanus . differtur homo aliena . loquens . et nullum agnuscens . hoc cum uideris statim eum in obscuro loco et conlocari . et conprimi faties . uinum autem . uel poscam nęc ipse odoretur hec . quia ei . ministrant bibant . post hec . faties ex quo qui anetum . in aqua et ex ipsa calida capud ei fouebis . septies in die . et iter in nocte . lumen uero nec diei . uideat . nec ignis . ad hubi ceperit resipiscere . offeres ei lumen . lucernam postea oleum . roseum calidum . inpones ęi in cerebrum cum lana . et ligas . hoc die . et nocte sepius mutabis . cum iam ceperit . conualescere tunc ęum producis ad lumen et dilotum . uinum bibat ante rodomeli in aqua calida . accipiat . post rosatum . et sic uinum hoc modo quasi de morte suscitabis hominem . res est enim saluberis na experimentata.

6.2 *Antidotus Atrianus*, p. 262

Antidotus atrianus . faciens . . ad multas . passiones colocis dabis . in calda quam agdutinis . hebis . aepatiois . in ino melle similiter . epilemticis . epistotonicis . calda aqua . pleureticis . in mulsa . stomaticis . in pusca . quiatiter . ex c<rudi>ditate<m> conpelluntur . humoris . in aqua frigida . quiatos tres . n<on> freneticis in aqua calida . ad prefocationis . matricis . tisicis . ac nocte datur . et qui frigus . patiuntur . curat autem

. et dolorem dent<i>um . et pausat . inpositum in dentum . et orto non o[c]cisi tubat datum in pusca . sciaticis . cum uino . dulce . quiatos . iii . est lexopiritur . Recipit hec . amomu budro id est dracmas . iii . costu đ ii . euforuiu . đ i . opiu tiuaicu . đ xii . grocu . đ . v. foliu đ i . murra . troclide đ i spica nardi đ i . ruta sicca . đ i aloę epatite . đ i . maratre semen . đ iiii . piper . albo . granas . xx . apii . semen . đ i . Iosquiamum . semen đ xx . piretru . đ . i . dauco semen . đ i . cassia . đ. i . petrosilino . đ ii . rosa sicca đ . i . cassamu đ iii . mel . dispumato . quod sufficit.

6.3 *Antidotum Theodosion*, pp. 263b–264b

Antidotum theodosion . faciens . ad multas . pasiones . accipitur . uernum . et autumnum . qui facit . ad dolorem . et ad uertiginem . capitis . et epilemticis . et ad c\u/aleri nigra . et ad pectoris . siue laterum . dolorem . a digescionem . ciperum quibus . accessit . ad dolorem . uentris . siue . sthomaci . et longa egritudinem lauorant . et minime conualiscunt . auriginosis . uero . ydropicis . tisicis . et ad neruorum dolorem et ad colum et ad eos qui corpus grauem habent extrasordinariis uel longas egritudinis sudores incongruos et incipiaentes dolores podagricos et mulierum . uitia stomaci . aciscentis sub haec autem uentris sine molestiam que intus sunt producunt non autem presentis sed future preuenit necessitatis . Recepit hec aloae *dr* iiii groco Э xii reuponticu Э xii mastice Э xii . cenamum Э xii . agaricu ∻ ii . scamonia Э xii xilobalsamum . Э vii piper . albo . Э viii piper nigro . Э vi piper longo . Э vi meu . Э vi squinuantos Э vi . gingiber . Э vi gentiana . Э vi amomu . Э vi interiones coloquintidos Э xii costu Э vi acoru Э vi asaru Э . xii spica nardi Э vi cassia . Э . vi . camedrios . Э xxxvii mel dispumatum quantum sufficit.

6.4 *Ad dolorem aemigranii*, pp. 266–7

6.4.1 **Ad d**olorem aemigranii . stercus . suricis . cum aceto . inpone.

6.4.2 **Item** corni cerbini . cinis . aceto et roseo . mixtos fronti inpositus . magnifice . uitia . emundat.

6.4.3 **Item** sucum de radice bete purpareae mittis . cum modico . lasa\i/ris . et in modum trium guttarum . mittis in narem . ex ea parte que dolet . et statim sedabitur.

6.4.4 **Item** lasar cum lacte mulieris . resolutum . et in alteram partem auris . infusum . tepefactum . sine que dolet . agittans mandubula cubet . emigranii dolorem careuit.

6.4.5 **Item** opii . Э . dimidium . groci . Э dimidium murre . *ro* dimidium . iosquiami erbe . sucum . apii seminis . Э . i . aneti . seminis Э dimidium . grocum seorsum . tundes . et in mortario . simul conteris . diutissime . ex aceto . optimo . conspargis . et formabis colliria . cum uero opus fuerit . in cute . ex aceto conteris . et spissum fronti \uel/ . temporibus inducis.

6.4.6 **Item** . iii . grana . alei . et viii . grana piperis . trita fronti inlines uel in ea . parte qua dolet.

6.4.7 **Item** . iii . \a/ grana alei . tundes ex quorum sucus infundes lana et utraque aures claudis.

6.4.8 **Item** . ut spiritus . uel cerebri . mundas aleum et teris diligenter et facis pastillos . ex eo et pones in cerebro siue in migranio et desuperligabis . donec ustulet . uessicam faciet . quam decoperies ut hude currat.

6.4.9 **Item** bace lauris puluerem et senapis puluerem . cum aceto acro . temperabis . et linis . partem que dolet.

6.4.10 **Item** agacie puluerem cum oui album . permisces et uteris.

6.4.11 **Item ad** emigranium . seu ad dentium dolorem croci . Э vi . maligran<...> cortices . ∻ vi . yreos . Э . xi . aluminis scissi Э vi has omnes . spe<...> cum uino uetere . in unum permisces . et in mel temperabis . ut colliria si de<ntes> dolent . uel mouentur . in melle resolues . et inde gingiuas tangis si emigraneum est . qui celestis . cesterne in cuticula . resolues et fr<on>tem linis . effectum miraueris.

6.4.12 **Item** fisicum . ad emigraneum . p<...> yreos et stercus columbinum in oleo et melle decoctum fronti inposi<tum> conpescit . dolorem . fisicum est.

6.4.13 **Item** fisicum ad emigraneum . farina lolii cum amoniaco . equaliter . aceto mixto . anacollema facta . emigranio in de<...>.

6.5 *Ad dolorem auricule uel aque ingressu*, p. 267

6.5.1 **Ad dolorem . auricule uel aque ingressu** coriandri sucum lacte mulieris mixtus et auricule infusus dolorem efficaciter . tolet.

6.5.2 **Item**. ad auris doloris siue quae uermes hab<ent> sucum calamente . permixtus cum cedria . et infusus prodest.

6.5.3 **Item** lasaris . granum modicum . aurem inicies . statim dolorem paus<at>.

6.5.4 **Item** cardamomi sucus . auribus instillatis dolorem aurium et moli<a>riorum . dentium sedat.

6.5.5 **Item** porri uirginis sucum . sanat.

6.5.6 **Item** adeps . galinaceus . ad ora solutus . tepidus . auri infusus plurimum prodest.

6.5.7 **Item** rute sucus . si mittas . curabitur.

6.5.8 **Item** si aqua in aurem introierit . et dolorem fecerit . solus sucus coriandri . in aure expressus sine dubitatione liberat . ac sanat.

6.6 *Ad uitium oris*, p. 273

6.6.1 **Ad uitium oris** . Sepiarum ossa in cinere redacta . et ori sparsa uitia emendat.

6.6.2 **Item** coclearum uacuarum cinis cum murra tritus adsparsus uicia emendat.

6.7 *Ad uulnera oris siue tumores gingiuarum*, p. 273

6.7.1 **Ad uulnera . oris siue tumores gingiuarum** . aprotanum uiridem . teris diligiter . cum melle misces . tangis loca deintus que dolent . et deforis ubi tumor est . apponis et mirabilater curat.

6.7.2 **Item** ad oris uulnera . uel gingiuarum . in mustum dulcem recens . mittens malum granatum siccum plenum et alterum uiridem cum cortice . et coques . in stagnato ad carbones ut spissitudinem mel adsumat . et leuas de foco et addis murre et stiptiriae . scistis puluerem . tenuissimum conmisces et ex eo uulnera linis.

6.8 *Ad fetorem oris*, p. 274

6.8.1 **Ad fetorem oris** . Puleium et serpillum siccum commanducatum benefacit.

6.8.2 **Item** uades dormitum acetum bonum os labet.

6.8.3 **Item** mastice commaesticet et uino suauios colluat.

6.8.4 **Item** mur<i>nus cinis cum mel dentibus infregatu<r>.

6.8.5 **Item** foliam myrte et lentisci pari pondere et galle siriac<em> dimid<i..> *pond* simul tere . et asparsa uino uetusto matutin[o]\i/s mand<...>.

6.8.6 **Item** si alitus f<..>et cum dormitu uadit aceti boni ciatum per partes sorb<.nt> hoc et in coctionem faciat . et mane sero inde sorbe . prodest quod si spleneticis hoc dederis in paucis diebus sanus erit.

6.8.7 **Item** hedere uace cum casia et myrra pari pondere ex uino.

6.8.8 **Item** s<...> herba que gallice lauria dicitur ieiunus commanducet et gl<...>.

6.8.9 **Item** ad eos quibus subitus humor fetorem facit siue putridinem gingiuas ita ut dentes cadunt quod grece helpe dicitur . hiu ∻ i cum <mel> ∻ vi coquis bene tritum et curabis.

6.9 *Item ad dentium dolorem*, p. 335

6.9.1 **Item ad dentium . dolorem** . aspar<a>gis siluaticis radix in uino decoquet et in ore tenitus et dolor<.> sedat . sucus eius similiter facit.

6.9.2 **Item** hedere . radicem coques in uin<.> puro quod in ore tenes et transit dolor.

6.9.3 **Item** brasica . coma<s>tica dolorem statim sedat.

6.9.4 **Item** . secum hedere cum aceto et paru<.> sale in diuersam narem mittis.

6.9.5 **Item** timum et piretrum . pare pondere . tusum denti adices.

6.9.6 **Item** piretri radix . et posca . et melle gargarizetur et tenetur in ea parte . qua qua dolet.

6.9.7 **Item** ciperi puluerem dentes et gingiuas rep<...>.

6.9.8 **Item** . pentafilon . cum radice sua . in aceto . aut uino . decocta in ore continetur.

6.9.9 **Item** . adicies in olla acetum satureia<m> et sale in uno feruentem et maxilla continebis.

6.9.10 **Item** fen<.>culum uiridem . masticet . et sucum contineat.

6.9.11 **Item** . tus et uace lauri . in uino deferueant . et in ore deteneat quamdiu potuerit.

6.9.12 **Item** uiolam si\c/cam ex uino coques et calidum ori continebis.

6.9.13 **Item** . uinum et piper misces et tepidum ori continebis.

6.9.14 **Item** urtices [e] minores . radices . commasticet . s<.>cum eius . in aceto . ore continebit aut gargarizet.

6.10 *Ad dentes molares*, p. 336

6.10.1 <A>**d dentes molares** uel ad omnes . ut sint . incorrupti . et inpassibiles inmouiles . que magnum remedium uitis albe burionis sucum cotilis duabus mori radices . cortices coques ad tercias . et in ore teneat ac diluat per dies . vii . numquam dentes dolebit.

6.10.2 **Item** inuiolati prestantur . dentes . in si quis cotidie . mane ieiunus . habeat sub lingua salis granum donec linquiscat.

6.11 *Ad uuam distillantem et ad fauces tumentes*, p. 337

6.11.1 Ad uuam . distillantem . et ad fauces tumentes . corium de nuce u<...>de tundes et expremis hinc mittis ∻ vi . et mellis ∻ i . coques do<...> spissetur ex eo *cocl* . i . ieiunus gargarizet.

6.11.2 **Item** . cimas . de oliua <...> coques in aqua fontana ad medietatem . et gargarizet.

6.11.3 **Item . ad** <u...> reprimendam . et gingiuas <t>umentes . betonica ex aceto . decoqu<..> et ore conteneat . diu que calido . gargarizet.

6.11.4 **Item** ad uam iacentem uel distillantem . sucum herbe absentii . subleuas.

6.11.5 **Item** . cinis testa<r..> ostrearum . addito melle inlinitur.

6.11.6 **Item** . gari optimi *cl* subici<t..>.

6.11.7 **Item** senapem . gargarizetur cum aceto . et melle.

6.11.8 **Item** . ad uuam n<.> molesta sit . brasice folium . crudum liuisime terito . ex eo suco . uuam tangito . continuo silit.

6.11.9 **Item** ad ubam reprimendam pruni silu<.>tici . folia decoques . ex uino . austeri et subinde gargarizas.

6.11.10 **Item** confeccio . antere . pulueris . ad ubam subleuandam . qui ad o<m>nes reuma facit . ciperum . ∻ iiii . murrae ∻ ii . aluminis scisi . <...> sandaraca . ∻ iiii . grocu . Э vi . hec omnia trita . et cribrata in unum puluerem . rediges.

6.12 *Ad synances*, p. 338

6.12.1 <A>**d synances** . costu alumen . scisu . spica nardi . grocu . <fl>os rose . et gallam . equis po\n/deribus . in puluerem mollisimum . redigis . et cum <m>el dispumato . uteris . Si autem uulnera . intra os quasi alba nata fuerint <..>imum de uinum foueas et sic puluerem inponis.

6.12.2 **Item** . apii semen . stafidasagrias <...> numero xii . lasar primum piper. spungie. noue . in cacauo rudi conbusti . omnia contri<..> miscentur melle et pinna uel digito inducis.

6.12.3 **Item** . lupinorum crudorum . fari<..m> . similiter . et costi . admixto suco . nasturcii . teris in modum mellis . et uteris.

6.12.4 <I>**tem** . murra . et casia sulfor . uiuum . et melle et menta uiridem . comisces omnia <i>nsimul puluerem facta murra et casia . et sulfor . et postea . commiscis . et fri<.>atum ore faucium . et humidum . dentes constringit.

6.12.5 **Item** . sal frixum cum aceto <o>leo et mel . utere.

7 *Cod. sang. 397*

7.1 *Si tertiana aut cottidiana febris hominem tangit*, p. 22

Si tertiana aut cottidiana febris hominem tangit colligat de ueruena manipulum . i . quae alio modo isarnina uocatur et viiii grana de pipero . et cum uino mixtam componat . et ante accessionem inde bibat staupum . i.

7.2 *De fico emendando*, p. 22

De fico emendando . Accipe plantaginem et herbam acerem quae alio nomine gundereba nominatur . et seuum de multone . hoc est unslit . et ista tria tundantur in mortario . et fricantur in patella et sic ieiunus comedat cum pane . Ceruisam et medum nec aquam bibat . antequam sanetur.

8 *Cod. sang. 550*

8.1 *Istam causa facias contra morbum qui dicitur nesse*, p. 54

Istam causa facias contra morbum qui dicitur nesse . tollat unum modium de amar bene uersum et faciat eum in bracium duas ebdomadas et faciat illud ad ceruisam et tollat de uuisto sicut inter duos manus posses capere et pluet illud et tollat de illo ceruisa . xii . stoupas et uuistun miscit et simul et illud scias quando castum fuerit descendit intus adfetes et tollat viiii . stoupas et lxxxx piperes cortices et minuet usque ad puluerem et discuciet inter duos uasculos et viiii manes bibet illud antequam quicquam custasset et si <titiu> nihil bibet nisi quod superfuit de ceruisa illa et non manducet ane<tam nec augam> nec crudum carnem nullum nisi de ouibus nec alem nec barbum nec <vinum> rufum et de illis abstineat se u<...> unum annum.

9 *Cod. sang. 751*

9.1 *Ad ilii dolorem*, pp. 304–6

9.1.1 **Ad ilii dolorem** urinam ircinam singulas potiones per triduo ieiunus bibat . femum ircinum primo die pilolas . iii . tritas ex uino bibat . alia dię v bibat . tertia die . viii . ieiunus bibat.

9.1.2 **Item ad ilii dolorem** Saxifraga *unc* . ii . uettonica *unc* . i . ispica nardi . *unc* . vi . casia *un* vi . piper . *unc* . i . piper albo *unc* . i . zinziber . *unc* . i . costo *unc* . i . isopo *unc* . i . uinci radices . *unc* . i . timu *unc* . i . apii semen *unc* . i . asaro uncia . i . triblas et dabis bibere ieiuno.

9.1.3 **Item ad ilii dolorem** Et ad cauculosis et istraguiriam patientibus et corum urina retinetur piper . *iscrip* . vi . lauri bacas . *iscrip* . iii . uisicularia *unc* . ii . erba istrumus sucus haec omnia teris in uino uetere et obtimo calices viiii . admiscis mel quantum extimas in modum conditi facies et ieiunus tepefacto bibat calice pleno et suspendis eiusdem cibos graues et alius usque ad ora tertia.

9.1.4 **Item ad ilii dolorem** uel uesicae et difficultatem urinae nucleus pineus purgatus . xxx . amendolas . xx . tracant . *unc* . i . dactulus . xiiii . teris in mortario quomodo medulla nucleus pineus . et amendolas extra et tracanto infundis si mutae in mellę et in mortario teres et admisces cum illas alias et dabis de ipsum medicamen quantum medium cocliare in careno aut in medus bibere.

9.1.5 **Item ad ilii dolorem** apii radices coquis cum dulce apiato aut condito qui lapides habent lini semen bene tritum quantum solidus pensat et addis de condito . et ceres ipsa farina bene et facis potione et dabis bibere.

9.1.6 **Item ad ilii dolorem** anetum siccum et uiridem et ruta equaliter teres et colas cum uno et das bibere una cum oleo bono cocliarem unum prendis paritales uiuos et mittis in ulla rudę et coperis illa ulla cum coperculo et lotas et potiones in foco et tandiu quoquis ut perustulent illi passares toti ut cinis fiant et de ipso puluere dabis bibere qui patitur.

9.1.7 **Item ad ilii dolorem** Erba c[i]\a/pilli ueneris et papauer et nitru teres omnia equaliter pensas et cum aqua aut uino calido dabis bibere.

9.1.8 **Item ad ilii dolorem** Remedium bonum leporem uiuum prendis et laterem de luto facis . unde fabricant domus siccus facis in medio fassam et ponis super tripede ut calefiat quomodo caletilli lateris occidis leporem . et ibi fundis sanguinem ipsius super ipso latere in ipsa fossa ita ut pedes ipsius . ad retro sursum teneat ut sanguis illi bene decurrat super illum lateris fossam . et cum bene colauerit leuas illum laterem de foco et ponis usque quę refrigerit bene et sic tollis illum sanguinem coagolatum.

9.1.9 Item pellem illius decorias et ustulas super latere usque bene ustulet ut fiat puluer et de ambas res ęquali pensas et teres diligenter et das ad illum qui laborat cocliare pleno cum uino calido bona . et si uis expermenta rem . istam rem mittis in calice de ipsas pulueres cocliarium unum . et petra . i . aut duas in modum fabę aut cicer et mittis aqua tepida ut copenas bene et alia die requires et inuenias solutum lapidem.

9.1.10 **Item ad ilii dolorem** Saxifrage radicęs petrosileno radices . isparagi radices elene radices . libistici radices [isparagi radices] fenugreco apii radices aneto cento capitis radices bacas lauri . *unc* . iii . orticę semen *unc* . iii . trita da bibere in uino.

9.1.11 **Item ad ilii dolorem** origano hoc est illaris saxifragia poleio apio petrosileno tere cum uino bono da bibere.

9.2 *Unguentum acupo galastico ad omnem dolorem uel tumorem tam podagricis quam artetricis*, p. 319

Unguentum acupo galastico ad omnem dolorem uel tumorem tam podagricis quam artetricis . axungia purcina uetere . *unc* . i . cera *unc* . ii . sapone *unc* . ii . oleo laurino *unc* . i . conficis et uteris quia utilis . est.

9.3 *Unguentum artitricis uel geniculorum dolorem*, p. 320

Unguentum artitricis uel geniculorum dolorem terebentina . (.) i . amoniaco . ş . iiii . mastice . (.) ii seuo arietum . (.) vi . lardo elexum . (.) \v/iii . cera alba . (.) iiii . conficis et uteris expertissimam habet medicinam.

9.4 *Item trociscus Eraclio*, p. 364

Item trocis\c/us Eraclio Ad auris uitia ad gengiuas ad fistolas ad uulnera uerandarum digitorum ad usquiones ad igni agrum ad uulnera canciriosa superponis ad uitiorum iniurias frontem lenis melagranatę . *unc* . iii . aristolicia ciatos . v . murra troclitus *dr* . iii . sisti et facis trociscum dabis quando opus . est.

9.5 *Qui facit ad tibias putridas et ad omnes plagas sanandas*, pp. 367–8

In christi nomine qu<i m... c..... et p...> qui facit ad tibias putridas et ad omnes plagas sanandas . Picae carsetane<a> *lib* . iiii . amoniaco *lib* . i . sinopido *unc* . iii . uitro uirgine . *s* iii . cera uirgine . *lib* . i litio bonum . i . croco . *unc* . i . tus masculi . *s* . iiii . masticae . *s* . vi . aloę . *s* . ii . rasina molle . *lib* . ii . smirra . *s* . iii . spuma argentea . *s* . iii . sabo orientale . vi . haec omnia mittis in buccola requoquis et postea maceras et omnes plagas sanat.

9.6 *Ad osso fracto*, p. 378

Ad osso fracto Solfor bibat per die . viiii . terciam partem dinarium pinsantem ieiunus cum uino et aqua.

9.7 *De mandragora*, p. 392

De mandragora . Dicitur ipsa mandragora habet similitudinem hominem iacentem .

9.7.1 Ipsa radice teris et dequoquis cum oleo et super plaga pone mirum sanat.

9.7.2 Ipsa teris cum uino albo et mel dabis bibere matricis uel cauculorum dolorem tollit et ad mulieres qui partum uolit habere ipsa radicina ad mulie ipsa poma dabis biberere concepit.

9.7.3 Ipsa trita cum garo dabis bibere profluuium sanat.

9.7.4 Ipsa trita cum ficos edropicos curat.

9.7.5 Ipsa trita epelenticos et lunaticos dabis bibere remedium est diodis probauit.

9.8 *Si homo de arbore uel de equo ceciderit*, p. 395

9.8.1 **Si <homo de arbore uel de equo> \ceciderit/** Recipis illa pastera sumen de illam aut de ebisteris cum aceto et albumen oua in linteo superpone.

9.8.2 Item sulfor bibat et mater erbarum bibat.

9.9 *Si spina in pede uel in alico membro fuerit*, p. 396

Si spina in pede uel in alico membro fuerit unctum leporis superinpone.

9.10 *Ad luxum*, p. 400

Ad luxum Ad luxum uel quolibet casum si percussum fuerit ut liuorem faciat . calce uiua et sinopitę cum mel conspargis et ad locum lesum ponis miraueris effectum.

9.11 *Ad uicia articulorum*, p. 404

Ad uici\a/ . articulorum . Erba quinquefolia tunsa cum exungia ueteri sine sale inposita sanabitur.

9.12 *Ad luxum*, p. 405

Ad luxum . Erba agrimonia contrita et opposita mirae doloribus et tumoribus ex luxo tollit.

9.13 *Ad capitis fractura*, pp. 405–6

Ad capitis fractura In primo battę lardo et [……] de lino simul inpone et muta mane et sero si uideris ossa fractam diu inpone usque quod fractum fuerit eicias inde foris postea mittis mel aput carpia ad curandum deinde ad sanandum facias medicamen de cera et oleo et mel pauco resina de pino grano masticae et colofonia simul in unum misces et quoq\u/is uno corpore drapicello mundo inledas et in plaga inpone.

9.14 *Ad capitis fractura*, p. 408

Ad capitis fractura Verba uittonica contusa in capitę in plaga inpositam rase celeritate gluttinatur.

9.15 *Ad dentium uitiae*, p. 409

Ad dentium uit<iae> Herba uittonica cum uino uetere aut aceto ad tertias decoctae gargarizata . dolorem dentium tollit.

9.16 *Ad fico*, p. 413

9.16.1 Ad fico que dicitur quiliacus d<m>ittis in lapidia ouo . i . cum uitello suo et alio tanto de oleo et tertio de mel tepęfactum das ei bibere et sanabitur.

9.16.2 Item cucurbita saluatica nuce plena cum molle ceruisa dabis diebus supra dictis.

9.17 *Potio ad oua colobrina*, p. 413

Potio ad oua colobrina . Collegis radices de erba dosinatia et de ipsis radicis inuenis nudiculus quasi nuces auillania si satis infirmus <a lasu sunt> fuerit usque tria grana dabis bibere in nouello medus per dies septem et intermittis die . i . ipsa potio probata ad uermis qui in stomaco iacient . uel ad omnia maleficia intra hominem ad expellendos.

9.18 *Pocio ad podalo uermo occidere*, p. 416

Pocio . ad podalo uermo occidere . accipe radicinas de callilada . iii . et tres staupus de aceto uehementi et mitte in olla noua et coquis illas . ii . partes ut ad unum staupum . ueniat et tunc mitte piper grana . viiii . et bibat tantum qui hac infirmitate patitur et bibat in luna decurrente.

9.19 *Ad pulmones curandum*, p. 417

Ad pulmones curandum ius de marubio albo staupo pleno aceto staupus duos . mel staupo . i . qui omnia bulliat in unum corpus ita ut sit spissum sicut mel et per singulos dies singula cocliaria accipiat et curat pulmones.

9.20 *Sales ieraticas qui faciunt ad acies oculorum usque senectutę et flegma impetum deducit et suspirium relaxat et dentes putresce non sinit*, p. 418

Sales ieraticas qui faciunt ad acies oculorum usque senectutę et flegma impetum . deducit et suspirium . relaxat et dentes putresce non sinit ameos . ∻ i *s* cimino thebaico . ∻ *s* poleiu . ∻ i . *s* . ysopi semen . ∻ iiii . sales frixas . ∻ xx . dabis supra.

9.21 *Sales catarticos*, p. 418

Sales catarticos qui faciunt podagricis in omni feruore et artitricis . et asmaticis . gingiber . *dr* . iii . petrusilenu . *dr* . iiii . epitemu . *dr* . iiii . silfiu . *dra* . iiii . ameos . *dr* . iiii . apii semen . *dr* . iiii . ciminu . *dr* . iiii . liuestico . *dr* iiii . piper *dr* . iiii . dacridiu *dr* . iiii . sales amoniacus . ∻ vii . dabis dose *sold* . i . semis secundum uires unius pullis in oua uel in idrogarum aut in calida aqua.

9.22 *Oxira podagricis*, p. 419

Oxira podagricis ad omnem dolorem picae bitria libras . ii . cera *lib* . i . amoniaco . ∻ \iii/ tormenella . ∻ ii . libano . ∻ i . galbano . ∻ i . aceto *dr* . i . et dimidia.

9.23 *Ad serpentes uel alios uerme de omine expellendum potio probata*, p. 423

9.23.1 **Ad serpentes uel alios uerme de ominem expellendum potio probata** Ius de cocurbita siluatica nucae plena cum nouella ceruisa ieiuno bibere dabis luna decurrente.

9.23.2 Item de medulla ceruuna aut de osso aut de corno ipsius cum lacte capruno bibat.

9.23.3 Item ius de mura campestria expremis et teris foli\a/ de canepa miscis sim\u/l et dabis bibere calicę pleno si folia non habes semen mitte ipsum ualet uel.

9.24 *Emplastrum apostolicon*, pp. 423–4

Emplastrum . apostolicon qui facit ad omnes causas et ad omnia uulnera antiqua siue recentia ad pleomones ad neruia precisa ad musculos et omnes plagas quae a ferro incidetur siue de uitru carne sagittas educendas infixas corporis uel ad morsum . et pugtus anima uenenorum terrena et maritimas et uenena trahenda facis et qui in altum occulta sunt facit etiam apostematicis ad cancros ad igne agrum . ad ceruicę dolore nimium ad iscrofarum penda et per modico foramine omnia traet sanat . et cicatrix non pereat et qui intercosta apostema habent in epatę et in splene a foris inponis . et intro rumpe egestione et sciros in splenis soluet et sanat . Facit autem arteriaces ad percussuras uel cirronias que in genua uel in pedes et meliciridas rumpes et sanat . facit autem ad reumam quecumque dolore et tumore et coxas a genuas et ad talos descendit ut captaplasma inponet facit etiam . ad fistolas litargirum *dr* . g . viii . galbanum *dr* . viiii . gutta amoniaci . *dr* . xxvii . cera . *dr* . lvi . panum dicitur[6] . viiii . bidellium *dr* . xii . manna turi . *dr* xii . opopanace *dr* . viii . aristolocia quale uolueris . *dr* viii . oleo uetere *lib* . i . que tundenda sunt criuellas deinde cera colofonia et oleo solues in foco et miscis litargirum et postea inmisces . residuas species et tamdiu coques quam mutet colore.

9.25 *Ad ossa si fuerint fracta in testa*, p. 432

Ad ossa si fuerint fracta in testa de pipinella [s]puluis facis super teola exsiccas et super puluere ponis si ret[e]\i/colus fuerit ruptus . lana de pap[a.r]\i/ro super reticulo ponis et [a]\i/nde aceto et mel lauabis.

9.26 *Ad ulcera quae in ore nascuntur*, p. 435

Ad ulcera quae in ore nascuntur mentastri sucu in uino inmixto collectione hore frequentium facta.

9.27 *Ad uitia oris*, p. 435

9.27.1 Ad uitia oris apii . radidicis \cum/ mel dequoquis olla . ore sanat.

9.27.2 Item lafasio ex uino decoctum gargarizet ore sanat.

9.28 *Ossa in capite si fracta fuerint*, p. 437

Ossa in capite si fracta fuerint erba agrimonia contusa cum exungia ueteri fractis oponis solidat.

---

6 It looks like a *dr* abbreviation for *denarius* was misinterpreted as *dicitur* at some stage in the transmission of this recipe.

9.29 *Ad luxum*, p. 440

Ad luxum erba agrimonia contusa et inposita super legata sanati fermentum cum acito lenissimo trito . inposito sanat.

9.30 *Antidotum podacricum ad pedis dolorem sedatur*, p. 444

Antidotum podacricum ad pedis dolorem sedatur piper album . ℈ viiii . filo armatico . viiii cimino ℈ viii . gingiber . ℈ viii . hermodictalus . ℈ viiii . isui id est eoforbio ℈ viii . tundis cribras et reponis cum opus fuerit dabis cum aqua calida aut cum uino . ℈ vii.

9.31 *Potione ad ebrugine*, p. 447

Potione ad ebrugine erba qui dicitur ebulae college radices ante sole leuante in contra oriente ipsas colleges fenogreco grana . v . lauro folia . iii . piper grana xxx . cum ceruesa leuante facias staupo pleno et dabis ei bibere et cum ipso bibes habeas uno ouo fricto dabis ei ad comedendum et in lecto sic coperes calido et usque ad uesperum ipse custodiat.

9.32 *Antidotum ad stomaco frigido qui dicitur climax*, p. 448

Antidotum ad stomaco frigido qui dicitur climax recepit haec euulo . ∻ v . fenuculi semen . ∻ iii . piper . ∻ iii . gingiber . v . mel atico croco . *lib* . i . aut qualem inuenis dispumato . erucae semen . ∻ i . si erucae non fuerit . senapi semen . ∻ i . siciopurciri . hoc est nigella . ∻ ii . sili . ∻ ii . apio ∻ i . petrosilino ∻ . i . in omnibus melior uisus . est . magnificus et in multis rebus ad inflationibus stomaci et indegentio pacientibus sic in mulieribus menstrua producet ad madicus mirabiliter operatus . est . facit a ruptus suauis dattus . et ad omni tussę . et quibus capite in toracę reuma fluit . ad omnis pectoris doloris mirabiliter effectus . est.

9.33 *Ad dolorem ceruicis*, p. 457

9.33.1 Ad dolorem ceruicis artimissia contundus et sucum eius expremis et adis oleo quantum sucus est pones cera et facis cerotum simplice . haec permiscae et unguę dolorem.

9.33.2 Item si escapulas doluerint ruta in aceto coquis et in linteo infunde et pedum inpone.

9.33.3 Item uinum uetus oleo aut exungia uetere ita ut solu[a]etur bulliat . et postea lana sucida carpenata intinguis et expremis fortiter ita ut omnem sua cumque acciperat emittat quantum fiere potest et sic lana ipsa inponis in aqua cumque parte dolor . est . mirificae sanat.

9.33.4 Item si tormentos post aurem natus fuerit rutae sucum cum oleo miscis et cocliare in aure mittis et iaceat in ipsa.

9.34 *Purgaturium capitis*, p. 457

Purgaturium . capitis porcia ad uipus mamentum capitis dolore precipuerit sine febri materia detrahere per mane res uel per hos que res uel dentibus diucius dolentibus prodest.

9.35 *Ad laterum dolore*, p. 461

9.35.1 Ad laterum dolore artemisia cum uino bibat.

9.35.2 Item caulae cumbustae cum exungia lateribus uel coxis et lumbis adpositus mire sanat.

9.36 *Ad dentes ne cadent neque putriscant*, p. 472

9.36.1 Ad dentes ne cadent neque putriscant sal granis ieiunus sublingua opponatur donec liquiscat.

9.36.2 Item ad dentes confirmandos et dolorem cessat et dentes confirmat.

9.36.3 Item ad dentem cauam piper in ipsa partę conmastica.

9.36.4 Item ad dente cum dolore erba centauria ieiunus masticem dentes firmat.

9.36.5 Item rosmarino masticet et inter dentes teneat.

9.36.6 Item ad dentes qui mouentur cornum ceruinum conbustum dentesfricium utatur confirmat.

9.36.7 Item ad dentium dolore erba simphoniaca radix cocta in uino austeri teneat in dente qui dolit mox sanatur.

9.37 *Ad gengiuas plenas sanguinem*, p. 473

9.37.1 Ad gengiuas plenas sanguinem murae agrestae sucus sextarias tres croco uncia . i . \a/lumen optimum \∻ i/ mel sestario . i . in suam orę mel admiscis et lento ignis coquis donec ad spissitudinem mellis ueniat et si cum croto et \a/lumen mittis et sic diu igita non solum gengiuas cumtetiris utile est . sed a dentes . et faucis et uuam . oportum est.

9.37.2 Item ad siccandas gengiuas et stringendos dentes alumen liquendum in carta nuda inuoluis et carbonibus conburis tundis adquę triuelas uncias tres sal tostata et trito uncias sex et sic diustissimę in mortario mortario paretur tere donec tenuissimae estinguae.

9.37.3 Item ad hoc et ad renas qui sub lingua nascuntur alumen ci barbarica . et piper omnia quod sufficiat tere pariter misee et sic abundantur omnem intrinsecus os et paletum et ubicumque puteris cum digito tangere etiam ipsam uuam perfricabis.

9.37.4 Item ad pinnolas quę iusta uuam nascuntur que aliquando electum intrare aut egere de re non sinunt super dicta medicina et hec eas delent si frequenter perfrecentur cum digito alon triton . cum mel mixtum prodest probatum.

9.37.5 Item ad exasperationem gengiuarum . folia de rosa tritum cum mel diligenter et inde gengiuas tanges adsta uero gengiuarum exasperationem alium crudum non expedit manducare nec alia agraminas et salsidumen debet usare.

9.37.6 Item ad gengiuas si ipsa carnes super dentes creuerit anguistia paciuntur ut cibum glutire non possunt adsiduę ruptantur dolore in dorso uel in scabolas et renibus patiuntur his uirtus non de est fleotomandi sunt et post hoc fomento ei sunt talem facis oleo in quo infusum est mellilotum . et absentio masticę et castoreo dequoquis et ut super diximus stomacum foues aut mellido stomacum ungues et aspargis desuper pu[c]\l/uerem talem masticae trito ale<m> . et piper uetella et desuper pagella inponis calida aut lane sucidum floaum et fecit desuper et epitemacium post expoliarcion aut diespermatum aut [a]sapaptaenos aut milion . absentio pontico in calda infuso.

9.38 *Antidotum podagricum*, pp. 489–90

Antidotum podagricum quod dicitur calipodium . quod ego terentius eoticianus accepi post annos sex dolui . fortiter quod in aetate in uani annorum xxxvi . Cum uino lenter fuissem adflictus ista potionem usus sum per dies . ccclxvi . Ad omnem aut podagram facit potio haec quem podagrae sunt septem . id est tarda cidata frigidalida contractiosa uulnerosa et lapidosa sic lapidosa curant . ita ut a uiciis p<o>dagrae sit recessum lapides pedis postea nascuntur et exeunt et mureor lapidum orum loca medici quomodo non uulnerant non morbo podagreado est [a] quo est haec potionem liberatus . Uirtus autem podagricae pontionis talis . est . ut cum moueat sic nimietatem per ipsam orina inmittat cuius confectio talis . est . et qualiter sit utendum uel a quibus rebus sit abstinendum quousque conpleantur numerum ccclxvi . dierum . Id est ergo aristolocium rotundum *lib* . i . mirra troclitae *lib* . i . bacas lauri *lib* . i . centauria *lib* . i . tundis et cribellas postea mittis mellis atici uel distillatio dispumati quantum sufficiat . confectio seruabis in doleo uitreo dabis ex eo uno *sol* pondus diurnam in aqua calida uatis tribus.

10 *Cod. sang. 752*

10.1 *De melancolicis ad fel nigrum deponendum purgatorium quod deponit umores frigidos et siccos*, p. 5

De melancolicis ad fel nigrum deponendu<m> <purga>torium quod deponit . umores frigidos et <siccos> epitimo . đ . x . menta sicca . *lib* . x . Ə ii . piper ∻ . i . hęc conteres subtilissime et dabis exinde int<egra> potione . Ə . x . et media potione Ə v . cum uino uetere medio calice . faciat hoc frequenter . utilissimum est.

10.2 *Ad paralisin*, p. 5

Ad paralis<in> . sucum erbę salu<[u]\i/>e . đ vi . sucum <sauine> . đ . iiii . mel dispumatum đ . ii . uino ∻ i . ieiunus bibat <mirifice> sanat.

10.3 *Thymiama Paltgrimi*, p. 82

Thymiama Paltgrimi . Gozumbri – iii . Gumfiti . – i . Aloa *den* vi . Musci *den* . ii . Cafforę *den* . ii . Haec omnia terendo miscentur.

10.4 *De fico emendando*, p. 158

De fico emendando . Accipe plantaginem . et herbam acerem . quae alio nomine gundereba nominatur . et seuum de multone . hoc est unslit . et ista tria tundantur . in mortaliolo . et fricantur in patella . et sic ieiunus comedat cum pane . ceruisam et medum . nec aquam bibat antequam sanetur.

10.5 *Si tertiana aut cottidiana febris hominem tangit*, p. 158

Si tertiana . aut cottidiana febris hominem tangit . colligat de ueruena manipulum . i . quae alio modo isarnina uocatur . et viiii . grana de pipero . et cum uino mixtam componat . et ante accessionem inde bibat staupum unum.

10.6 *Quibus cibis abstinere debeant quem paralysin tangit*, pp. 158–9

Quibus cibis abstinere debeant . quem paralysin tangit A pane hordeatio et omni pane azimo . A carne boum et porcina et caprina . Ab omni aue aquatili . Ab omni pisce squammam non habente . Ab omni legumine pręter lentem . et foenumgrecum . Ab omni olere crudo . Ab omni fungo . Ab omni potione quae inebriat pręter uinum album tenue . et medum tenue et ceruisam tenuam ac leuem . Utatur autem in cibis . panem de speltu . et frumento bene leuato . Carnem birbicinam . ceruinam . edat et omne genus uenationis . omnem auem domesticam . et agrestem . et siluestrem . praeter aquatiles . Omnes pisces squamam habentes excepto sal[o]mone . De legumine lenticulam et foenumgręcum . De oleribus porrum coctum . et omnia olera cocta . et oua sorbilia . Bibat uinum album et tenue . Medum leue . et ceruisam leuem . Crebro sanguinem minuet . In stuba non lauet . et saluiam assidue bibat gagarismum sumat . Piretrum masticet . et saliuam proiciat . sternutamentum sibi moueat.

11 *Cod. sang. 759*

11.1 *Anteditum Teodoritum*, p. 2

Anteditum teodoritum ad omnia ut celissimo purgaturio qui facit ad dolorem capititis stomaticis epilemticis melancolicis maniaticis ad pectoris ad lateris dolorem ad malus humoris coniectus quibus esca acedis contra in estomacho ad tisecus ad eos qui reumaticas passionis patiuntur et ad eos qui in magrosia ueniunt hoc est in longa egritudinem ad hictericus ad itropicus ad neufriticus et qui graue corpus habent ad colum per hunc anteditum repletus et sane fiunt ad pedes plurimum dolentes ad incipientem dolore podagricis et mulieris aborsum et ad eos corruptillam uentris patiuntur uel stomacho ad epaticus ad spleniticus soluit autem uentrem sine molestia acipiendum est uernum et autumnum uel statem simel aut bis non solum presentibus curat egritudines sunt et futuris aduenientis infirmitates repellit Si quis autem sanus usitauerit numquam infirmatur cuius confecis hec est aloe patiti ∻ i croco *s*∻ reupontico *s*∻ mastice *s*∻ cenamo *s*∻ scamonia *s*∻ \epitemo *s*∻/ asaro *s*∻ pionie radices *s*∻ interionis *s*∻ <er>ingio hoc est cardo pane ∻ i polipodia ∻ i escolopendrio ∻ i camitrius ∻ i *s* exilobalsemo ∻ ii *s* piper albo ∻ ii *s* piper nig[e]\i/r\o/ ∻ ii *s* meu ∻ i . brateus ∻ ii scinoentos ∻ ii . gingiber ∻ ii . gentiana ∻ ii . amonto ∻ ii costo ∻ ii . aguro ∻ ii . capare ∻ i mel quod sufficit.

11.2 *Ad uulnera in ore*, p. 5

Ad uulnera in ore <n>ata costo tundis et criblas ulceribus quae in ore sunt fretas sanant.

11.3 *Ad dentis laxos*, p. 5

Ad dentis laxos galla sulpor iudaico carta usta equale mensura \in/ puluerem redigis et ex ea dentis fricas et gingibas.

11.4 *Ad dentes dolorem trociscus*, p. 48

11.4.1 Ad dentes dolorem trociscus murra teris et in dentis ponis.

11.4.2 Item nitrum teris ex uino aceto in pultario deferueat tepefactum dentibus teneat.

11.5 *Infussio ad capud et ad colera*, p. 51

Infussio ad capud et ad colera agrimonia uitonica frafolio benedicta gamendrea absentio edera terestria cardone radices menta sisimbrium ortolanum apii folia petrosileno ruta celedonia iouis barba caulo sauina nepta cerifolia tanacita saluia sal nigro pugnata aceto tertia parte de staupo oleo tertia parte de *lib* califactum et super capud inponis edera nigra cum oleo roseo et cum sucu eius mixtum cum uino tempera et freta in fronte.

11.6 *Ad fracturas ossorum*, p. 52

11.6.1 Ad fracturas ossorum margile alba puluis *lib* . i . sal *lib* . ii . conmiscis cum aceto et album ouarum ponis super non soluis usque vii . dies et bibat uiola cum uino et piper et sal uiola.

11.6.2 Item farina de faua miscis cum aceto et albumen de ouas et bolo et superponis dies . vii . et ipsa pocione.

11.7 *Catarticum artreticis ydropicis*, p. 58

Catarticum artreticis ydropicis lacteredas . ÷ ii . ermodactulo ÷ ii . cum oximelle datum miro est.

11.8 *Potio ad podagra*, p. 60

Potio ad podagra qui dicitur calapodia qu[a]/e\m ego terentianus accipi et post annus ex dolui cum in etate iuuenile annorum xxxvi . essem in omne aut podogra[s] facit quem podagri sunt . vii . id est tarda citata frigida et calida constrictiua uulnerosa et lapidosa ista potio curat omnes podagras omnem enim morbum per urinas deponit post mens uel iiii . urina ualde adsidue mouet per mensis . ii . bibatur ergo ista potio per ccclxvi dies et si propter aliqua necessitate numerus de ipso anno dierum non fuerit conpletus in alterum annum conpleatur et tamen anno absteneat se a bubula caprina ueruicina ceruina lactuca beta rafano [cum] curbita cucumere et mellone alio cybas et de porrus crudos aceto crudo senape piper et si potest fieri a mulieri si non uel rarius curabus stomachum conficis autem sic aristolocia rotunda cardamom[a]\o/ petrosileno macedonico murra tr[i]\o/clite bagas lauri centauria ana *lib* . i . omnes tricoci<na.> mellatico quod sufficit reponis in dolio dosis ÷ i . in aqua ciatus iiii.

11.9 *Gyma artreticis*, p. 61

Gyma artreticis radices euoli subtilioris *lib s* . mel *lib* . i . aqua *ff* iii . cimino ÷ i . bullis in aqua usque ad tertias reddatur et dabis bibere die intermisso.

11.10 *Puluis qui facit ad implire placas etiam et si ossa minuta habuerit excutit*, p. 61

Pul[7] qui facit ad implire placas etiam et si ossa minuta habuerit excutit yrius ÷ i . aristolotia longa ÷ i . panacus rigius ÷ i . mannis ÷ iiii . omnia in puluere redacta sic uteris.

11.11 *Malagma aduersus dolores uel fracturas et podagra ad luxum*, p. 63

Malagma aduersus dolores uel fracturas et podagra ad luxum pice *lib* . i . colofonia *lib* i . cera *lib* i . sulfol uiuo *lib* . i . nitro *lib* . i . pice liquida ÷ vi . fenogreci puluere ÷ iiii.

11.12 *Confectio ydromellis*, p. 66

Confectio ydromellis malorum cidoniorum suci *ff* v . mellis optimi *lib* xx aqua pluuialis *ff* xv omnia misci diligenter et in sole esse pondere dies xl postea in uaso recondis.

---

7 There is no mark of abbreviation around *pul*, but it can be assumed that *puluis* was meant, hence the edited title I have used.

11.13 *Medicamen mirabile ad placas ad sagita percusso*, p. 67

Medicamen mirabile ad placas ad sagita percusso oleo roseo et cera et ouarum mediolus coctus insimul conmiscis cera uero ante remitis et facis medicamen et uteris.

11.14 *Remedium ad punctas*, p. 68

Remedium ad punctas lias de ceruisa recentis colas n<..tri> das et alio tando buter simul miscis et bibe dabis statim sanabitur.

11.15 *Ad talorem dolorem quis luxauerit ut dolor pausit*, p. 72

Ad talorem dolorem quis luxauerit ut dolor pausit uirgas de rubo haec rumice facis cinus et oleo conmiscis bene et ubi dolet inponis.

11.16 *Ad dentes ut numquam doleant*, p. 73

11.16.1 Ad dentes ut numquam doleant rasumus de corium ceruinum in olla rude ad tertias quoquis et ipsa aqua in ore tenis una iactas alia mitis sanat mox.

11.16.2 Item spina nigra fodis cum oratione dominica scorcia mediana de ipsa radice *man* . iii et *col* . iii . de uino decoquis ad tertias in olla rude et ipso uino in ore tenis una iactas et alia mitis mox sanat.

11.17 *Unguentum ad fractura uel luxatura*, p. 75

Unguentum ad fractura uel luxatura buterum berbicino *lib* i . cera ÷ ii . oleo uetus *lib* . i . oleo laurino *lib* . i . lini semen sucus ÷ i miscis omnia et inungues mire adiuuat.

11.18 *Ad dentium dolorem*, pp. 75–6

11.18.1 Ad dentium dolorem plantagine radices turnelle radices manipula singula coquis in uino ff i . ad tertias et gargalicit ad solem aut ad foco subinde usquedum sanat.

11.18.2 Item milfolio bucco mellis lupopectine scorcia de nogario ana insimul teris et cum modice ceruisa mis[cus]\cis/ colas mitis ubi dentes dolent apud hoc dormiat si potit tempore uiesue dentes numquam dolent.

11.19 *Confectio ydromellis*, pp. 88–9

Confectio ydromellis hoc et pro uino usui essę potest \mellis optimi/ aqua fontis . *p* . xl . utrumque [mellis optimi dispumato . *p* xx .] miscebis diligenter in uas fictili tenue et petito recondis et claudis et mitis ad sole sub tecto diebus xlv . hoc est ex die kalendae iulio in . ii . o id est agusto Ita ut inter quinque dies uas conuertas ut partis que quinque diebus <ini>e fuerint superioris fiant . hoc genus poculi ut uinum uetustati melius reditur et nescientes si bibant putant se uino obtimo bibere.

11.20 *Conpositio thymiamatis*, p. 89

Conpositio thymiamatis myrrae ∻ ii . bidellio ∻ ii . casia fistola ∻ vii . storacis ∻ vi . ladane . ∻ ii . yrinilirici ∻ ii croci ∻ vi . ungiculas marinas . iii . amomi ∻ vi . uino ueteris ƒƒ . i . mellis optimi ƒƒ i . hec omnia miscebis pastillus ex eo facias quos in umbra siccabis.

11.21 *Tymiama simplex*, p. 91

Tymiama si[n]/m\plex . storace ∻ ii . mastice ∻ ii myrnę ∻ i . onecus <id est> ungellas ∻ ii . rose uiridis ∻ i . het omnia minute tundis et miscebis et facies pastellus.

11.22 *Ad dentes stringendos uel si dolent uel putriscunt aut sanguinant*, p. 92

11.22.1 **Ad dentes** stri\n/gendos uel si dolent uel putriscunt aut sanguinant uino auster\o <. i> porri sucum . ∻ i . usque ./ ad medias decoquis et tepido in ore <diu \t/enis>.

11.22.2 **Item ad dentis** dolorem ad ea parte que dolunt de summa auricula <sang>uinem auferis cum fleotimum hoc probatum a multis hominibus.

11.23 *Ad ycterícus*, p. 93

11.23.1 **Ad yctericus** collegis atriplicis satis et in enio mittis ut . diutissime bulliant postea in tina mittis et quomodo refrigerat ibidem balneare debit et antequam ibidem intret de ipsa aqua pleno staupo bibere debit facis hoc per triduum et in quarto die bibat garo staupo dimedio et postea fleotomas.

11.23.2 **Item add** ictericus ut inter triduum sanus sit croco ∻ i *s* . nardo ∻ x . cassia fistola ∻ x . scinuantus ∻ v . amomum ∻ v . piper longo ∻ viii . interionis ∻ viii . cucumeris similis ∻ i *s* . murra ∻ xii . ex melle actico conficis et das cum aqua mulsa in modum auellane maioris.

12 *Cod. sang. 761*

12.1 *Ad incontinentiam hurinae*, pp. 55–6

12.1.1 Ad incontinentiam hurinae ungularum apri . uel suis cinis potione spargitur.

12.1.2 Item leporis cerebrum in uino bibitur . et eiusdem testiculi cocti eduntur.

12.1.3 Item anserum trium linguae asse in cibo sumuntur.

12.1.4 Item cocleae africanę cum sua carnę conburuntur . cinis que earum ex uino signino bibitur.

12.1.5 Item uisica suis sterelis cinere redacta ex uino bibitur.

12.1.6 Item uisica capraeę assata manducatur.

12.1.7 Item ciminum quantum tribus digitis leuatur conterito . et adiectis uini quiatis . duabus totidem que aque ieiunus bibito.

12.1.8 Item olei nardi . *lib* . i . terbentina . *lib* . i . cera ÷ viii . piper ÷ i . aut si piper nolueris . nitri . ÷ ii . mittis et facto cerotario uteris supra pectinem quamdiu sentias beneficium.

12.2 *Oxyra crocira*, pp. 59–60

Oxyra crocira facit epaticis . spleneticis . et ad ypocondriae tensiones . nefreneticis . et ad omnes neruorum passiones . pleureticis . peripleumonicis . sciaticis . et ad luxus . ad fracturas et incisos neruos sanat . soluit autem et omnem duritiam . et ad serpentium morsum . uel ad morsum canis rapidi . extrahit spinas . aut quecumque infixa fuerint corpori . expurgat ulcera malitiora . pice sicca brutia . *lib* ii . cera *lib* . i . amoniacum timiamatum ÷ iiii . libanum arrinum ÷ iiii . galbanum ÷ iiii . croco . ÷ ii . acetum acerrimum *ss* . iii . teris amoniacum . libanum cum aceto ad mellis cocti pinguidinem et in alio mortario teris c\r/ocum . picem autem mittis in cacabo testeo non in aereo et supermittis quod superauerit acetum et coquis agitas frequenter . et cum acetus fuerit consumptus . supermittis amoni\ac/um et libanum . agitas frequenter ne foras exeat . et postea mittis crocum effundis in mortario bene et uteris.

12.3 *Emplastrum somato filax*, pp. 62–3

Emplastrum somato filax qui facit ad canis morsum . curat etiam si sit rabidus uulnera uetera sanat sciradas parotidas furunculas et omnia apostema curat oculorum rupturas uel percussuras sanat . Neruis prodest . podagricos paragorizat dolorem aurium leuat . si ex hoc emplastrum inponatur . condilomata et omnia soluit . et quicquid circa caput uicii nasci potest . qui cauculum patiuntur si ex hoc [pa] emplastrum accipiat ab umbilico pub<is> tenus per urinam lapides exyre compellit . oris uitia curat . si buccis fuerit inpositum syringia sanat . tussientibus et tisicis adiuuat . in stomacho uitia omnia mala curat . conficis sic . lupini uiridis sucum . ÷ ii . maratri sucum ÷ ii . nepite sucum ÷ ii . lapatii sucum ÷ ii . arnoglose sucum ÷ ii . iusquiami sucum ÷ ii . prassii sucum ÷ ii . medullae ceruunae . ÷ viii . resina pituina ÷ v . seu taurino *lib* v . gipsu speclaris *ff* i . omnia cum fuerint diligenter soluta mitte sucos et agita diutissime ut totum misceatur et postea mittis gypsum et ad ea quę suprascripta sunt utere.

12.4 *Emplastrum apostolicum*, pp. 65–6

Emplastrum . apostolicum qui facit ad omnes causas et ad omnia uulnera antiqua siue recentia ad flegmonas . ad neruos pretiosos . ad musculos . et ad omnes plagas ferro incisas . siue sordidas . uitro canna sagittas educendas infixas corpori . uel ad morsus et punctas animantium uenenosorum [neruorum] terrenorum uel maritimorum et ad uenena extrahenda foris que . in alto occulta sunt . facit etiam apostematicis ad cancros ad ignem acrum . ad ceruicis dolorem nimium ad scrofas rumpendas . et per modicum feramen omnia adtrahit . sanat ut cicatrix non appareat . et qui intercostas apostemas habent in epate et in splene a foris et intus rumpuntur . per gestionem et scirosin splenis soluit et sanat . facit artriticis . facit ad percussuras uel cironia quae in genibus uel in pedibus et meliceridas rumpit et sanat . facit autem ad reumam quecumque cum dolore et tumore ad coxas ad genua uel ad talos discendit ut cataplasma inposita . facit etiam ad fistolas . litargirum . *lib* i *s* . galbano ∠ viiii . gutta moniaci ∠ xxvi . cera ∠ vi . colofonia ∠ lvi . myrra ∠ viii . eruginis campane ∠ viii . bidellui ∠ xii . manna turis ∠ xii . opopanace ∠ viii . iii ∻ i . aristolocia ∠ viii . oleo uetere *lib* ii . quae tundendas uel cribellas . et deinde colofoniam ceram et oleum soluis in foco . et miscis lytargirum et postea miscis residuas species . et tamdiu coquis quamdiu mittitur colorem.

12.5 *Thimiama*, p. 66

Thimiama . cozzunbar ∻ iii . aloa arbor *den* iii . confitum . cafora *den* . i . musico *den* . i.

13 *Cod. sang. 878*

13.1 *Ad fracturam uel uulnera ferri*,[8] p. 333

Ad fracturam uel uulnera ferri . Farina *melo*/ ordeacia *hirstan*/ . Adeps *smero*/ aprinus uel uerrinus . urtica minor *nezzela*/.

13.2 [Recipes for incense],[9] p. 334

13.2.1 [Untitled recipe]

Cotzubri . *lib* . vi .
Storace calamite . *unc* . viii .
Gumfiti . *unc* . xviii .
Aloa . *unc* . xviii .
Cafora . *unc* . ii .
Musco . *denar* . xviii .
Amber . *denar* . iiii.

13.2.2 **Item aliter**

Cotzubri . *lib* . vi .
Storacis ysaurici . *unc* . viiii .
Confiti . *unc* . xviii .
Cariofili . *unc* . iii .
Cinnamomi . *unc* . vi .
Ciperi . *unc* . vi .
Turis . *unc* . v .

---

8 Inserted, italicised words are interlinear glosses in Old High German that were added by a later scribe.

9 These recipes are recorded as lists with each ingredient on a new line, so I have replicated this structure in my transcriptions.

Myrrae . *unc* . iii *s*
Masticis . *unc* . ii *s*
Spici . *unc* . vi .
Croci . *unc* . i *s*
Aloa . *unc* . xvii .
Cafora . *unc* . ii . *den* . v .
Musco . *den* . xviii .
Ambar . *den* . iiii.

14 *Cod. sang. 899*

14.1 *Si tertiana aut cottidiana febris hominem tangit*, p. 131

Si tertiana aut cottidiana febris hominem ta\n/git colligat de ueruena manipulum . i . quę alio modo isarnina uocatur . et viiii grana de pipero et cum uino mixtam componat . et ante accessionem inde bibat staupum . i.

14.2 *De fico emendando*, p. 131

De fico emendando . Accipe plantaginem et herbam acerem que alio nomine gundereba nominatur et seuum de multone hoc est unslit et ista tria tundantur in mortariolo . et fricantur in patella et sic ieiunus comedat . cum pane . ceruisam et medum nec aquam bibat antequam sanetur . De libro Grimaldi tuli.

14.3 *Confectio timiamatis*, p. 137

14.3.1 **Confectio timiamatis** . Cotsumber . *lib* vi . rasina stiru\a/x stora\c/ę calamite ∻ viiii . gumfiti ∻ xviii . gariofile *unc* iii . cinamo ∻ vi . ciferus ciperum *unc* v . thus *unc* v . mirra iii . mastic ∻ ii . spica ∻ vii . croco ∻ . i . aloa ∻ vi . cafora ∻ ii et *din* ii . musico *din* xviii . ambar *dinr* iiii.

14.3.2 **Item alia** . Timiamatis confectio cotsumber *lib* . i . stora\cę/ calamite ∻ i . gariofile *sol* ii . cinamum ∻ i . tus ∠ gumfiti ∻ iiii . spica *unc* i <ca> *sol* i . aloa ∻ iiii . cafora *sol* i . musico *sol* i.

14.3.3 **Item alia** . Aloa (.) ii . gumfiti (.) ii . croco duas partes de *dr* . caphora similiter . musico similiter . spico *din* i . tus duas partes de *dr* . cynamo *dir* i *s* . stora\cę/ calamite similiter cariofilo similiter cotsumber (.) vi.

14.4 *Cataplasma ad tumorem brachii que ex fleubotomo contingit*, p. 141

Cataplasma ad tumorem brachii que ex fleubotomo contingit . farina tritici cum ouo et lacte conpastas et superpone per triduum.

14.5 *Cataplasma ad tumorem*, p. 141

14.5.1 Cataplasma ad tumorem . stercus caprinum cum aceto teris inpone sub nocte sanat.

14.5.2 Item ad tumores liuores . contusiones lenticula cum aceto et mel coquis . et sic cataplasma.

14.5.3 Item ad liuorem tollendum absinthium tere cum mel et fac cataplasma in linteo inducis et inponis.

14.6 *Ne cadant dentes neque putrescant*, p. 141

Ne cadant dentes neque putrescant . salis granum sub lingua ieiunus oppone donec liquiscat . confirmat dentes nec putrescant sinit.

15 *Cod. sang. 1396*

15.1 *Ad dentes molares*, p. 19

Ad <dentes> molares uel ad omnes <..e........nupi/t... n.. pasib..um in uino uiles qui m..g..m nome d..........is albe burionis suco cotilis duabus in oc...ul..s... cordices coquis ad ter...s et...ore ....dil...t per dies vii num...de....ol.....>.

15.2 *Ad luxum uel contussim*, p. 20

Ad luxum uel <con>tussim origanum cum aceto et oleo cum lana sucida superponitur.

Biblioteca Apostolica Vaticana

16 *Pal. lat. 1088*

16.1 *Medicamentum ad maculas oculorum et ad caliginem*, p. 34v

Medicamentum \a/d maculas oculorum et ad caliginem . licio . ∠ i aloe . ∠ i . caffora . ∠ ii . teris cum uino uetere albo . licio . et aloe . insimul teris caffora uero . puluera facta postea . super ipsum . medicamentum . adiungis . et miscis insimul . et repones in uas uitreo . aut in ęreo et cum opus fuerit . mittas in oculo guttas ii . mane et uespere.

16.2 *Ad dentium dolorem*,[10] ff. 35r–35v

16.2.1 Ad dentium dolorem radices fraxini uino calices . iii . decoquis ad tertias et sic inde in os dentis qui dolet diu ibidem teneat . frequenter faciat et mitigat dolorem.

16.2.2 **Item** herba ueruena radices ex uino uetere decoquis et exinde frequentius dentes lauet qui dolorem infra biduum tollit.

16.2.3 **Item** alium cum aceto in dentes qui dolet intus teneat frequenter.

---

10 The inserted, italicised word in 16.2.5 is an interlinear gloss in Old High German that was added by a later scribe.

16.2.4 **Item** herba millefolia ieiunus frequenter masticet.

16.2.5 **Item** he\r/ba simphoniace \<*oss…zunge*>/ in uino fortissimo cocta et sic ipsum ius in os mittit et teneat diutius super dentes qui dolet et sanabitur.

16.2.6 **Item** uittonica ex uino uetus et aceto a tertias decocta gargarizata dolorem dentium discutit.

16.2.7 **Item** ad dentem cauum stercus coruinus ibidem inponis dentem rumpit et dolorem tollit.

16.2.8 **Item** plantaginem radice masticetur.

16.2.9 **Item** farina de nocella in cauum dentem mittat sanabitur.

16.2.10 **Item** larice in dentem mittis super noctem sanat.

16.3 *Ad experatione gingiuarum*, f. 35v

16.3.1 Ad experatione gingiuarum olia rosę teres cum mel diligenter inde tangis gingiuas et oleo cru<dum> non manducet nec ullum agrumen sed menta manducet . et sanus fit.

16.3.2 **Item** oleo uetus nares infundat frequenter.

16.3.3 **Item** qui\n/quefolia radices sucus cum aqua gargarizetur.

16.4 *Ad ulcera oris uel quidquid intra labiis fuerit*,[11] f. 35v

16.4.1 Ad ulcera oris uel quidquid intra labiis fuerit rumicis \<*ebeohowe*>/ et pampinis folia tenere a tertias . in uino reteneat.

16.4.2 **Item** plantaginis sucum in ore teneat.

16.4.3 **Item** porri folia sine pane manducat.

16.4.4 **Item** ad asperitudinem lingue sucum mente cum mel mixtum mistificat.

16.5 *Ad serpentes uel aliorum uermes de homine expellendum potio probata*, ff. 37r–37v

16.5.1 Ad serpentes uel aliorum uermes de \h/omine expellendum potio probata sucum de cucurbita siluatica . nuce plena cum nouella ceruisa ieiuno dabis bibere . luna decursa.

16.5.2 **Item** medulla ceruina aut de ossum aut de cornu ipsius cum lacte caprino bibat.

16.5.3 **Item** ius de mora campestria exprimis et teris folia de cannabe miscis simul et dabis bibere calice pleno et si folia non habes semen mitte ipsum ualet si mora non est lacte caprino calidum facis . Haec potio herba uel omnia malefitia aut uermes omnes prohicit.

16.5.4 **Item** Ad uermes de infantes prohiciendos pingue de lardo porcino cocleares . iii . ieiunus bibat.

---

11 The inserted, italicised word in 16.4.1 is an interlinear gloss in Old High German that was added by a later scribe.

16.6 *Ad punctas que lateribus superueniunt*, ff. 39v–40r

16.6.1 Ad punctas que lateribus superueniunt aprotano trito in aqua colatum medium calicem tepidum bibat admiscis modicum sal.

16.6.2 Item herba candula manipulum . i . teres cum uino calice . i . dabis bibere ieiuno et sic iaceat super dolorem.

16.6.3 Item gutta ammoniaci siue pannace . *sold* . pensante aloę aceto sale singula coclearia omnia insimul teres et dabis bibere ieiuno et tamdiu . super ipsum latus iaceat quousque sudat.

16.6.4 Item sanapidos distemperas cum aqua frigida mirum est.

16.6.5 Item flores de cardos qui dicitur caletrepa siue radices eius cum tres nucleos de persico diliter teris et cum aqua dabis bibere et iaceat super ipsum latus probatum est.

16.7 *Ad uentris dolorem uel tumores uel intestinarum*, f. 40v

16.7.1 Ad uentris dolorem uel t[o]\u/mores uel intestinarum sementis uitae decoctum ex aqua fumentabis uentrem dolores et tumores tollit si per triduum hoc feceris.

16.7.2 Item erba quinquefolia sucum dabis bibere cocleare ii . sine mora dolor tollitur et ipsa tunsa inposita dolorem tollit et sucum eius bibat et toracem et uentrem sanat.

16.7.3 Item uittonica . ʒ . i . in aqua calida ciatos . ii . bibat . his autem <a\p/ta\r/[i]> potio si non cruditate ciborum intestinarum quiebunt.

16.7.4 Item ad testinarum dolorem herba nepita sucum bibat et sanat.

16.7.5 Item ad duritiam uentris lini semen cum mel tritum in ceruisia ieiunus bibat mirum est.

16.8 *Ad lumborum dolores*, ff. 41r–41v

16.8.1 Ad lumborum dolores uittonica . ʒ . iii . uino rubeo ciatos iii . piper grana . xvii tritum et calefactum ieiunus bibat.

16.8.2 Item ad lumborum uel coxarum dolores . herba sinicionem per se trita potui data.

16.8.3 Item alium non mundatum cum axungia contusso in panno superposit[o]\um/ resanat.

16.9 *De simplices uulneribus ad capitis fracturam*, f. 44v

De simplices uulneribus ad capitis fracturam uittonica contussa et super uulnus inposita mira celeritate gluttinat . eo quide sanabis si tertio quoque die recentiorem frequentius inposueris donec sanescat etiam et ossa fractura extrahit.

16.10 *Ad alia uulnera uel plagas ubicumque a ferro aut quolibet*, f. 44v

16.10.1 Ad alia uulnera uel plagas ubicumque a ferro aut quolibet facta menta per se inposita uulnera recentia glutinat.

16.10.2 Item herba plantago tunsa cum axungia uetere sine sale inponitur.

16.10.3 Item herba millefolium cum axungia pistata inponis.

16.10.4 Item ad plaga recente porri folia in quantum super terra esse uidetur . pista et exprimis sucum . et iterum pistas coque usque non habeat sucum et ponis ipso pistato super plagam et die tertio soluis et inuenies eum sanum probatum est.

16.10.5 Item potiones ad ipsas plagas sanandas uel fistulas uel quecumque uulnera ubicumque uittonica . agrimonia fragisfolia consoldas minores . ii . maiores . iii . ptron\i/ola siue fastidiosa tribulos . ii . haec omnia manipulos xxii mel coclearia . ii . et si uelis addis grano mastice . facis potionem dabis bibere cum necesse fuerit probatum est.

16.11 *Ad neruos incisos*, f. 45r

16.11.1 Ad neruos incisos lumbricos terrenos combures teres leniter cum mel permiscis et inponis superconglutinat.

16.11.2 Item et ipsos uiuos cum mel superponis.

16.11.3 Item saluiae folia tunsa sucum eius exprȩssum desuper stillatum et quod remanet ponis super.

16.11.4 Item cocleas uiuas cum testa sua combustas et tonsas adiecto libano pari pondere inponis praecisos neruos sanat.

16.12 *Ad contussione uel luxatura de praesenti*, f. 45v

16.12.1 Ad contussione uel luxatura de praesenti cineres et sale ponis in bo<c>colare calefac et cum aceto bono fermentabis et ligas super.

16.12.2 Item ad luxaturas aut talorum dolorem stercus caprinus in aceto solutum coquis ut cataplasma . inponis.

16.12.3 Item herba origanum cum aceto et cum sucida lana inponis.

16.12.4 Item agrimonia contussa superponis sanat.

16.12.5 Item lili folia tunsa et superposita sanat et tumorem tollit.

16.12.6 Item femus uituli recente calidum adpositum sanat.

16.13 *Ad eos qui cum toxicata sagittasi sunt*, ff. 46v–47r

Ad eos qui cum toxicata sagittasi sunt beta domestica et saturegia aequaliter teres et cum uino dabis bibere et in ipsa plaga mittis sale et sputas.

16.14 *Puluis ad dentium commotionem*, f. 50r

Puluis ad dentium commotionem . costu . gallas . piper uaca cipressi in furno coctas corticem panis ordeacii combusti . yris ylirica foliu sale scammoniacu aequis ponderibus.

16.15 *Dentifricium ad dentium splendorem*, f. 50r

dentificium . ad dentium splendorem ordeum et sal commixto mel dispumatum donec sibi cohibeant . mitte omnia in linteolum conbures terito hoc dentifricium usus nigros dentes ad candorem rediis et oris graue molestiam corrigis.

16.16 *Dentifricium odoris fetorem*, f. 50r

Dentifricium odoris fetorem speculare coctu . piper puleiu contere cribella et in unum commisces et utere . Usu ergo cottidiano dentes confirmat gingiuas essiccat . uuam loco suo reuocat oris fetorem tollit . Uim pridiani . uel acriitio . iiii . odorem aufert . quamdiu quo usus fuerit . nullum dentes perdent . conficitur ergo huius dentifritii . siue medicaminis sic costum ad bonum odorem ciperum ad fauces deliniendas . cardamomum ad oris uulnera . erba sabina propter elefantiam yris illirica ad dentium . yusquiamum ad pruriginem . alumen scisum ad uuam bacas lauri . ad frigdorem . piretrum et stafidoagria propter umorem capitis exsiccandos . mastice propter suauitatem tus ad gingi.

16.17 *Dentifritium qui omnem humorem exsiccat*, ff. 50r–50v

Dentifritium qui omnem humorem exsiccat . ad omnia quae in ore sunt passiones . quod obtime curat dentes nigros candidos facit . agitantes solidat . dolentes saluat . reumaticos densat humestos constringit . uulneratos soluit . putrida expurget . uuam reumaticam siccat . Sed odorem bonum dat ori . cum melle uteris ad uulnera sordida . Recipit haec sales cammoniacos . *lib* . i . sales communes . *lib* . i . pumice combusta . ∻ vi . corni cerbini combusti . ∻ vi . specularia uirgine ∻ vi . testa ostreae . ∻ vi . sippie testas . ∻ iii . amomu . ∻ ii . piper . ∻ ii . radices arga ∻ ii . galba . ∻ ii . yreos yllirice . ∻ iii acoru . ∻ iii . lentisci folia . ∻ iii . iunci radices . ∻ iii . alumen scissum . ∻ iii . spicana nardi . ∻ iii . flores rose . ∻ iii . cassia fistula . ∻ ii . masticae . ∻ ii . myrra . ∻ ii . foliu . ∻ ii . costu . ∻ ii . semen balsami . ∻ . i . corallu . ∻ . ii . haec omnia separatim combusta miscebis ea . quae combusta sunt . cum his quae contundis cribellas et uteris ad omnia suprascripta.

16.18 *Puluera ad plagam assucandam et stringendam et celerius sanandam et carnem mortuam manducat*, f. 50v

Puluera ad plagam assucandam et stringendam et celerius sanandam et carnem mortuam manducat . et confectio eius haec est mirra . \li/banum masticae colofonia pice nigra . Auropigmentum . bolorminum . galla . aloę . gipsu cornu ceruinu incensu . Aristolocia rotunda . Omnia aequis ponderibus trita cribata puluerem factum et cum opus fuerit uteris ad supra scriptas causas.

16.19 *Antidotum Adrianum*, f. 52v–53r

16.19.1 **Antidotum adrianum cuius uirtus est** ammirabilis fatigatis aduersus uires dabis omnibus tamen in modum fabe aegiptiae . facit autem ad has causas aepaticis in uino et mel . frebricitantibus in hidromelle . epilenticis similiter opistotonicis in mulsa tepida pleureticis in hydromelli . ciatis . iii . stomachum dolentibus in pusca ciatis . iii . Eis qui de fluxu uentris laborant id est . eis qui de fluxu corporis laborant in frigida ciatis . iii . Ad renum dolorem cum calida . cauculosis id est ad morbum regium cum ydromelli ydropicis cum mulsa eis qui perfrictionem patiuntur ieiunis periodicis . typicis ante a\cc/essionem . Ad dentium dolorem in gargarismo uel modice exinde in ipsum dentem adpositum . et orem apertum habeat ut omnis umor de capite in terram decurrat . Eis qui sanguinem uoment in pusca . disintericis cum pusca . s[.]ciatis cum mulsa speneticis cum pusca paraliticis cum mulsa . Eis qui precordia in feruore habent uel inflantur . aut ex dolore conpunguntur . et ad secundas mulierum cum ydromelli uel cum sucum fenigreci purgat uero apostoma in interiora laborantibus Tisicis ad noctem in ydromelli . eis qui tussem patiuntur addito mel cum idromelli . Eis qui a serpente mordentur cum mel eis \qui/ a spallangione mordentur id est qui a mure cecum mordentur cum pusca . Eis qui uenenum acceperint cum suco tipsane uel oleo cuius antidoti uirtutem si cognosceris includis gallum et serpentem uenenosum serpis uero occidet gallum postea ponis de antido\to/ huius granum in ore uel in aure galli et mox reuiuescet de quo antidoto nihil dubites quia ex ultima morte reducit homines [d]ad pristinam sanitatem . quia frequenter probatus est in omnibus passionibus Recipit hęc calamum arromaticum . ʒ . vi costu . ʒ vi daucu . \id est semen pastinace/ ʒ ii . castoreu . ʒ . ii . siseleos ʒ xii . cardamomum . ʒ . iii . ameos . ʒ iii . carpobalsamu . ʒ vi . sagapinu . ʒ iii . piper albu ʒ iii piretru . ʒ iii . crocu . ʒ xliiii . ciperu \id est iunco triangolo radix ./ . ʒ vi . e\u/forbiu . ʒ. iii . amomum . ʒ iii . spica nardi . ʒ . iii . rute ag\r/este semen . ʒ . iii . mirra . ʒ . viii . opiu . ʒ xxx . cassia . ʒ viii . appii semen . ʒ iii . y[o]\u/squiami semen \id est canilata/ . ʒ xxxiii . rosa sicca . ʒ . iii . petrosilinu . ʒ vi opobalsamo . ʒ viii . gentiane radices . ʒ iiii . gamedreos . ʒ ii . aristolotia ʒ ii . bacas lauri . ʒ ii . mel acticum sufficienter . uteris ad omnes causas supra scripta nihil dubites.

16.19.2 Item adrianum ad eadem quod supra . Recipit haec . opiu . ʒ x . piper album ʒ xx . crocu . ʒ v . amomum . ʒ . i . piretru . ʒ . i . foliu . ʒ . i daucu . ʒ . i . cassia . ʒ . i . petrosilenum . ʒ . ii . sagapinu . ʒ ii . ciperu . ʒ ii costu . ʒ ii . yosquiamu . ʒ xx eu\for/biu . ʒ . i . spica nardi . ʒ . i . \ruta/ piganu . ʒ i . apii semen . ʒ i . castoreu . ʒ i rosa sicca ʒ ii . anissu . ʒ i . ci\n/namomu . ∠ . xilobalsamu \lignum ipsum/ . ʒ ii . nitru . opobalsam[o]\u/ ana . ʒ ii . mel dispumatu quod sufficiat.

16.20 *Antidotum panchristum*, ff. 53r–53v

Antidotum panchristum qui ad omnes aegritudines necessarium est qui sic accipitur in similitudine fabe aegiptiae colligis in aqua calida pensu *sold* . i . in ciatis . iii . epaticis cum uino calido . epilempticis caducis cum aqua calida ipsa mensura . stomaticis cum pusca calida . renes dolentibus cum aqua calida ictericis cum uino obtimo . febricitantibus cum aqua calida cauculosis et stranguiriosis similiter dabis et qui tipum patiuntur . cum ydromelle quartani siue tertianis ea hora sanantur . dentes dolentibus caraxatis de ferro exinde fricentur et aperto ore umor decurrat . sanguinem excreantibus cum pusca frigida ipsa mensura desintericis catapotias per nocte accipiant cum uino aut cum calda aqua aut cum cond<it>o detur . Tortiones iuxta uires cum aqua calida detur inflationes habentur ut supra datur menstrua mulieribus prouoca\n/t\tes/ cum idromelle aut cum suco fenigrece et cum omni celeritate parebunt . Ad morsum serpentis cum melle bibatur et de ipso medicamine in plaga inponis . et ad uenenum mirifice prodest . cum suco gentiane . Recipit haec calamu aromatico cardamomum costu . ana . ʒ v . castoreu ae\u/forbiu amomu piretrum spica nardi . dauci cretici semen . rute agresti\s/ semen . cassia rosa sicca fenuculi semen . ana . ʒ iiii . siseleos . ʒ xii . opiu . ʒ xxx crocu . ʒ . xv . zimziber ʒ iiii . apii semen yosquiamu ana . ʒ iiii petroselinum dragmas . v . opobalsamo ʒ vii carpobalsamo . ʒ v . sagapinu . ʒ iiii . meu piper albu . ana . ʒ iiii . mel acticum quantum opus fuerit misces haec omnia simul tritas diligentissime et sic ammiscis postea mel.

16.21 *Antidotum gera Galieni fortissima*, ff. 55v–56r

Antidotum gera galieni fortissima quae facit cefalargicis . scotomaticis epilempticis colericis melancolicis fleumaticis quartanariis . stomacis emitritaicis ydropicis pleureticis . diaforeticis elefantiacis podagricis artriticis siadicis disintericis ciriacis apoplecticis paraliticis et qui maniam patiuntur . ydrofobicis hictericis colicis epaticis spleniticis ambliopiasis litargicis nefreticis facit et ad oculorum passiones . id est semosin extenuat oculis uisum cerebro medetur auribus auditum prebet fauces et arteria purgat dentium dolorem conpescit renibus est ammirabilis mulieribus salubris uocem claram restituet asmaticis et suspiriosis medetur et longinquas aegritudines sine mora curat . strumaticos sanat febres omnes auertit omnes malos dolores curat . lepras omnes permundat cancros curat et si quis uenenum biberit omnia curat quae confectio prima est omnibus Recipit haec aloę . ∻ iii . petrosilinum absintium piper nigrum ana . ∻ iiii coloquintidos \cucumera agrestis/ interioris squilla cocta in pane agaricu \bollidus larice/ ammoniaco . diagridium \scamonia/ gariofiri . ipericu \. triscalamo ./ . ana . ∻ x . epithimum polipodius siccu bdelliu camedreos prassius siccu cassia ana ∻ viii . smirna \mirra/ sagapinu aristolotia longa p\i/per album piper longum cinnamomum opopanace . castoreum ana ∻ iiii . mel quod sufficit . dosis est . ∠ dabis cum mulsa et addis salis tri\ti/ coclearium . i . est autem potio haec \ni/mis admirabilis dabis ad omnia supra scripta nihil dubites.

16.22 *Antidotum sotira*, ff. 59r–59v

Antidotum sotira facit ad omnes causas inuisibiles post autem cum aqua calida bibitum capitis dolorem soluit stomachi umorem desiccat in accessionibus et diebus aneticis uigilias in somnum perducere ad frenetico dolorem oculi mitigat et reumatismum oculorum constringit superinuntum cum lac mulieris dentium dolore conpescere anelitum nimium pausare facit omnem causam corporis extinguit . tussienti quam et pleuresim p[l]eripleumonia et uiscerum tensionem aepaticis et omnem causam releuat desiccat etiam de pulmone umectationem flegmam uel saliuam pinguem cito reiactare facit si cum mulsa detur . et emoptoicis cum suco poligoni et aceto datur . uel arnoglosse suco uirtutem aegrotanti praestat non delectantibus cibos manducare facit . uomitum stringit hictericos sanat melancolia et qui multum cogitant . et uigilias in somnum reuocat . pulmonis grauitudinem sanat . colorem bonum facit . flecma de corpore per intestina deponit . urina prouocat et poros ureticos perducit conscriptiones uel trobos renum et uesice purgat . dissinteria sanat . paraliticis medetur . maxime si in ueretrum fuerit . ciliacos firmiter curat . spa\s/mos sanat . paralisin omnibus curat . illis autem qui non possunt per os accipere per clistere iniciatur . Adiecto suco fenigreci . matricis impetus soluit . sanguinis fluxum . uel humorum uicia constringit . enconpilmauis ad artriticis . podagricis . sciati\ci/s in doloribus magnam uirtutem ostendit . non solum per os saluat . sed in illis locis inunctus lixoperitu autem est . In maioribus febribus dabis ad omnem tipus quartanis plus dabis . me uero de quartana febre in tres potiones liberauit . Recipit hec murra ∻ ii . ∠ . i . anissum ∻ i . ∠ i castoreu ∻ i . ∠ i . opiu . ∻ ii . ∠ . ii . cassia . fistula ş . petrosilini . ∻ ii . apii semen ∻ ii ∠ ii . piper longum . ş . piper nigru ∻ ii sinonu suriac<ci> ∻ i ş . cinnamomum ş . storace ∠ . vi . siseleos . ş . idiocrocomagmatos . ∠ . vi . amomum ş . squinantu ∻ i . ş . costu . ∠ . vi asaru . ∠ . vi spica indica ∻ i . ∠ . v . crocu . ∻ ii . mel dispumatum quod sufficit . datis . ut supra dictum est . et miraberis.

16.23 *Oxira crocira*, f. 60r

Oxira crocira facit epaticis spleneticis ad [i]ypocondria tensiones nefreticis ad omnem neruorum tensiones . pleureticis peripleumonicis artriticis sciaticis et omnem neruorum contractiones . et luxas et fracturas et incisos neruos soluit autem et omnes duritias et ad serpentium morsus et canis rabii morsum . Recipit hec . pi[s]ce sicca brittia *lib* . ii . cera *lib* . i . ammoniacam ∻ iiii . galbanum ∻ iiii . libanu ∻ iiii . crocu ∻ ii . acetum fortem sextarios . iii . teris ammoniacam et libanum cum aceto . ad mellis spissitudinem cocti . et in alio mortario teris crocum . pice autem mittis . et quod superauit acetum in cacabo et coques et agitas frequenter . et cum acetum fuerit consumatum . supermittis ceram . et cum se soluerit supermittis ammoniacam . et libanum et agitas frequenter adtende ne foris exeat de olla et posthec mittis . galbanum . et cum fuerit resolutum et ammolentum sic supermittis crocum et fundes in mortario et miscis bene et fac magdaliones et uteris.

16.24 *Unguentum ad febrientes*, ff. 62r–62v

16.24.1 Unguentum ad febrientes . nepte suco partes . ii . oleo partem . i . commisces calidum . a cubitis usque ad summitatem digitorum perunges . similiter a genibus usque ad summum articulorum . et modicum in uertice capit[e]\i/s id est coclearia . inungues . et miraberis uirtutem eius.

16.24.2 Item . unguentum absinthio sext[e]\a/rium . i . oleo *sex* . i . aceto *sex* . i . commisces et coques donec ad mensuram olei ueniat . addes ceram facies cerotum . in li\n/teum induces . super stomachum impones . cum sudare ceperit tolles.

16.24.3 Item unguentum . ius ueruenę . et oleo roseo ana mensura misces . et quamlibet febrem inunges expertum est.

16.24.4 Item unguentum rasura de \cu/curbita exprimis sucum eius . cum oleo roseo admisces ana mensura frigidum totum corpus perungues . et si hiems fuerit calidum appones certum est.

16.24.5 Item unguentum iusquiami radices tritis *lib* . i . nepte suco bibat . ii . oleo *lib* i . medulla ceruina *unc* . iii . cęra *unc* . i . mittes in ollam rude[s]m . coques lento igne semper agitando donec ad medium ueniat . et sic calidum per linte[o]\u/m excolabis . et cum refrigerauerit . quod super est induratum mitte in mortario cum modico aceto . bene conteres et repones in buxta et uteris.

16.24.6 Item artemisię suco cum oleo perungues mirum est.

16.25 *Potio contra artreticam siue nesciam uel podagram*, f. 65v

Potio contra artreticam . siue nesciam uel podagram . Aloę *dr* . iii . pensante . Centauria . *manps* . iii . Absintio . *manps* . ii . Aqua calices . vi . quoquis in olla rude usque ad quatuor uenies et sic utere.

16.26 *Antidotum gira deacoloquintidis*, f. 90r

Antidotum . gira . deacoloquintidis . facit . ad uertiginem . et dolorem capitis . epilenticis qui subito angustia incurrit ad dolorem . pectoris et qui de nigra colera laborant pleoreticis et ad malas humores indegestibiles stomaticis . epaticis . et uentris dolorem colicis et qui longam egritudinem habent . eruginosis . et qui malam colorem habent neufreticis . et qui grauitudine corporum habent . idropicis et qui subito grauantur . tisicis . podagricis . incipientis mulieribus uitia . et corruptela uentris intrinsecas rupturas curat . sine molestia soluit . omni tempore . accipienda est . non solum presentes infirmitates curat . sed futuras egritudines defendit . Recipit hęc . eringio radices . polopodię radices . sirobalsamo amomo . piper longum . meu . gingiber . gentiana . brathea . costo . spico . \casia ./ agarico . agaro . interiones . ana . dragmas . ii . scolopendria . camitrius . cafora . ana untia . i . et dimidia . aloę . croco . reopontico . masticę . cinamo . diagridiu . epithimo . asaro . pionia . ana *unt* . i . omnia pulueraem facis adde mel dispumatum quod sufficit . terendo commiscis in buxtea reponis . da exinde prima die cum aqua calida scripulos . iii . alia die . *scrbl* . ii . tertia die *scrpl* i . si uelis uentrem bene purgare da exinde dragma . i . scamunia *scrpl* . i . ista gira . est aloetica . et est maior et melior et suauior in omnibus utilior quia per hanc antidotum omnes egritudines minuantur.

16.27 *Potio ad nesciam*, f. 90r

Potio ad nesciam . Ueruena . manipulum . i . artemisia . manipulum . i . Bledonne . radices rotellas nouem . Lupopectine radices . similiter . piper . grana . viiii.

17 *Reg. lat. 598*

17.1 *Antidotum sancti Paulini*, f. 124r

Antidotum sancti paulini Quod facit [ad] ydropic[o]\i/s . dissentericis tisicis . febribus . melancolicis . spleneticis . epaticis . tussientibus . sciaticis . humorem bonum nutrit . colorem bonum facit . fastidientibus uomitum . et distemperantiam distringit . facit ad omnem dolorem corporis . urinam prouocat dęmoniacis bonum . facit ad os fetidum . ad albulas oculorum . super tempora imponis . et in tercio die sanabit . si super carbunculo<ri> aut nascentia mala impositum fuerit . rumpit dolorem et tumorem tollit et sanat . Et sanat plagam mirifice absque uicio . super epar aut splen impositum . sanat . Intussuram et tumorem mitigat . dentium dolorem tollit si inter [posueris] \miseris/ aut si super pulsum qui iuxta auriculam . posueris . Quid dicam . medicamen melius non inuenies . potes ex ipso omni tepefacit quo uoleris accipere . quia multum calefacit et calorem detergit . colera . satis minuit . cardiacam passionem de quarta . aut de . quinta . potione curat et sanat . dabis cardiacis . et ad dolorem siue ad tussem ad dissinteriam . tisicis . ydropicis . cum mulsa calida . aut cum melle ciato . dęmoniacis cum uino caldo . sine febribus mire sanat . Recipit hęc . Aloe . ∻ v . Mirram . Amo<ni>acum . Terebintinam . Galbanum . ana . ∻ iii . Serapino . Opopanace . Crocum . Corallum . ana . ∻ ii . Libanum . Mastice . Bdellium . Storace . Agaricum . anacard[ce]ium . Costum . Yreos . Opium . ana . ∻ i . Balsamum . Folium . ana . *z* . i<iii> . hęc omnia teris cribras . Opium solue in mortario ad carbones cum terebintina . et galbano . et balsamo modice tepefacto . Et si non habueris balsamum . m<itte> oleum laurinum . et postea cum tepida . misce et conficis diligenter . et sic reponis . Quando uolueris fac catapocias in mo<d>um piperis . et exinde dabis . vii . ad dolorem . ad cardiacos uel uitium pectoris . ad ultera in stomacho potes dare cum melle . et miraberis eius effectum.

18 *Reg. lat. 1143*

18.1 *Anthidotus Teodori*, ff. 81r–82r

Anthidotus teodori qui facit ad omnes doloris capitis et his qui pectoris doloris patiuntur pleureticis et quibus indegestio escarum preuenit et qui suspirium patiuntur epaticis uel spleniticis et quibus dolor uentris aut stomachi et eis qui de post longa egritudine uix reparantur et malum colorem habentes et eis qui morbo regio <...>is et per totum corpus se <..fu...t> et soluta membra habentes et ad renum dolorem et podagricis dandum sed priusquam eis dolor accedat mirabiliter occurat . **Incipit eiusdem confec\tio/** Aloe . *scip* . x . agaricu *scrip* . xxxvi . crocu . *scrip* . viiii mastice . scripulos . viii . cassia fistula *scrip* . viii . cinamomum . *scrip* . viii . sed qui a cinamomum non inuenis mittis cassia . *scrip* . xviii . absque illos *scrip* . viiii . iam quod pensatum ligno balsamis . *scrip* . vii . costus *scrip* . xii . anacardia *scrip* . xii . mellis quod sufficiat omnes supra dictas species redigis mercis cum melle et das cum uino cuius aduersus faba egiptiaga . uel abellane qui uult ante <acciper.. rarum> quae egrotant nec dolores patiuntur accipiant semel in septimana aut in quindecim dies semel . si enim uolueris ut purget adauges in una dolose hoc est grana fabae aegiptiace aut abellane diacridius siliquas . viii . et purgat quomodo catharricus si enim uolueris in tota confectionem anthethiti . adicies dicridiu ∻ una que est habet *scrip* . xxiiii . ita est accipiendum ueris semel si necessitas non ex\i/gerit sin uero quod absit causa poposcerit sepe accipies sicut scriptura continet autumno . frequenter usque ad initium hyemis.

18.2 *Ad emigranium siue dentium dolorem*, f. 99r

18.2.1 Ad emigranium siue dentium dolorem laseris gemmam in aqua soluta in aurem et partem quam dolet tres guttas de digito expremis ipsa quidem hora grauauitur sed in perpetuum sanus erit.

18.2.2 Item gulbano semuntia inducis in carta et inponis in ea parte qua dolet remediabitur.

18.2.3 Item balsamum guttas quinque in aurem stillat prodest.

18.3 *Ad cadiuo homine*, f. 109r

Ad cadiuo homine potionem probatam aut in pectus sit . aut in caput . uertiginem mittit . tus . myrra . et opio . et gingiuer . et euforbio . et reupontico . et spaltro . et custo . et piper et cynamo . et gariofoli . et timiama . et petroselino . saxifica cassia sigilada . pulegio . non fumicato . rosmarino . uetonica et agrimonia . et saturegia . et luuestici . et apio . haec omnia puluerem facis et cummiscis cum uino . potui dabis bibere et ad sanitatem perducat mirifice prodest.

18.4 *Apostolicon*, ff. 133r–134r

Apostolicon qui facit ad omnes causas et ad omnia uulnera antiqua siue rentia ad fleumones ad nerbia praecisa ad mysculos et omnes plagas quae a ferro inciditur siue sudes uitro cannas sagittas educendas infixis corpori et punctus anima uenenorum frena et maritima et uenena trahenda quae in alto foris occulta sunt facit etiam apostomaticis ad cancros ad igne sacrum ad ceruicis dolorem nimium ad scrufas rumpendas et permodico foramine omnia trahet sanat ut cicatrix non pareat et qui inter costas apostemas habet in epate in splene in foris inponis et intus rumpuntur per egestionem et sciros in \s/plenis soluit et sanat facit autem arteria ad percussuras uelitronia quae in ienua uel in pedes et melicedas rumpet . et sanat autem facit ad reuma quaecumque dolore et tumore a coxas ad genuas et ad talos discendes et cataplasma inponet facit etiam ad fistulas recipit li\tar/girum . *dr* cviiii galbanum *dr* viii gutta ammoniaci *dr* xxvii cera *dr* lxi colofania *dr* lvi . myrra *dr* viii . erugine campane *dr* viii \be/dellium *dr* xii manna turis *dr* xi opopanece *dr* viii aristologia *dr* viii . oleo uetere *lib* ii . quae tundenda sunt cribellas deinde cera colof[a]\o/nia et oleo solues in foco et miscis litargirum et postea inmiscis re\si/duas et tamdiu coques quam mutet colorem.

18.5 *Ad dentes laxos*, f. 148v

Ad dentes laxos id est lupini xii . castaneas siccas ueteres cum scortia non tres incendis ut fiant carbones et facis exinde puluere subtilis et mittis modicum sale bedica mittis in aceto faciens fiolas tres ut ferueat et tertiam et posteum facis puluerem de pipe grana uiginti et . vii . mittis in ipso aceto et quomodo potest durare mittis in os et per totos dentes diffundes et facis per tres dies in aere sereno aut in balneo aut in caminata.

18.6 *Antidotus polichristus*, ff. 161v–162v

Antidotus policristus a marcello accepta melius operatur . quam illa quae ex multis migmatibus conficitur uel illa mitridatica croci *sc* . v . opii *sc* ii eurforbii *sc* . i . piperis ∻ i pyretri *sc* . i . spicae nardi . *sc* . i dauci *sc* i . petroselini *sc* ii yosciami *sc* ii opobalsami *sc* . ii cassiae fistulae *sc* ii . omnia tunsa creta melli optimo admiscentur et bene malaxantur et ex hoc fabe magnitudine singulis passionibus ministratur ad colum cum aque cyathis tribus epaticis cum uino mulso frebricitanti cum aqua . lateris dolori cum aqua mulsa sthoma\ci/cis cum posca indigestis similiter . Disintericis cum aquae frigidae cyatis duobus renibus laborantibus ante hora accessionis si ex eo gluttiant releuabuntur . Dolorem dentium conpescit si loco dolenti inponatur . Sanguinem uomentibus cum posca frigida ministrabis cyatis tribus . Coxas dolentibus cum passo cretico praebebis . paraliticis similiter in passo dormitum euntibus iuxta uires dabis . Tumores praecordiorum uel qui tortiones patiuntur ut supra dabis secunda seducit si cum aqua mulsa bibatur et uulnera quae intra torace nasci possunt si cum uino bibatur ptisicis prodest si cum melicrato sumatur . morsibus serpentium resistit si cum uini cyatis tribus bibatur . et ipsum uulnus medicamine more emplastri contegatur.

18.7 *Unguentum ad artiticus*, f. 169r

Unguentum ad artiticus Eoforuio ∻ i . gitter ∻ i . sinape ∻ i anithino aut commune oleo quod sufficit.

18.8 *Oxyra grocira*, ff. 172r–172v

18.8.1 Oxyra grocira . facii epaticis pleneticis ad ipocondrias tensiones nefreticis et ad omnes neruorum passione pleureticis peripneumonicis artriticis sciaticis et ad neruorum contritiones et luxus et fracturas et incisus nerouus soluit autem et omnem duritiam et serpentem morsus et ad canis rabidi morsum . pice sicca brutia £ . [li .] cera £ . i . amoniaco ∻ iiii liuano ∻ iiii . galuana . ∻ iiii . crogo ∻ ii . aceto agro ſt . iii teris amoniaco liuano cum aceto ad mellis cocti pinguidinem et in alio mortario teris c\r/oco picem autem mittis in caccabo testeo non in ereo et supermittis quod sup[er]erauit acetum et coquis agittas frequenter et cum acetus fuerit consumm\at/us supermittis cera et cum resolserit supermittis samoniaco et liuano agitas frequenter et atende ne foras exeat de ulla et posthaec mittis galuana . et cum fuerit resoluta et cum lentum fit supermittis crocum effundis in mortario miscis bene et uteris.

18.8.2 Item oxyra qui facit podacricis artriticis et ad omnem dolorem et luxatis pice brutia £ . ii . cera £ . i . amoniaco ∻ iii . tereuentina ∻ ii aceto . *s* . i . i *s*.

18.8.3 Item aliuo oxyra afrodesi . amoniaco ∻ iiii . colofonia ∻ ii . boellius ∻ vi . medulla ceruina ∻ ii . tereuentina ∻ iii senopedem . *s* ii . resina pitoina pensante ŏ ii . mannis ∻ i . confecis et uteris.

18.9 *Potionem probata ad ilica passio*, ff. 185r–185v

Potionem probata ad ilica passio agrimonia radices prinde manipulos tres mitte in ulla noua et addis ibidem uinum staupos nouem et coquatur usque ad tertiam partem et bibit quando oporte fuerit radicem de rusco radicem de tribulo radicem de sparago radicem de olisatro radicem appio radicem de petroselino puleio siccum allii capitinas . iii . semen de malua sicca uncia una porros iiii . cum radicinas suas bettonica cum radice sua siue sicca siue uiride radicem de uiola nasturtium ruta siluatica et si non domestica coriandrum anetum oleum quod sufficit. Haec omnia coques insimul et bulliat usque ad tertium postea mitte ciminum et fricas panem et bibe cum uino ieiunos.

18.10 *Ciraturiu artriticus opotatricus aparlasensis*, ff. 187r–187v

Ciraturiu artriticus opotatricus A<p>arlasensis . Recipit haec teruentina . *unc* . ii . colfonia ∻ iii . galbano ∻ iii bedelio ∻ i . amoniacu ∻ iii . agatio ∻ i aloae ∻ iii . thus . ∻ iii . mirra ∻ iii mastice ∻ iii . croco ∻ i spicu ∻ i sal<ui>ola ∻ i gingiber . ∻ iii cariofola ∻ iii cynamo ∻ iii . piper ∻ i . steteria ∻ i cerosa ∻ i . litazero ∻ iii . sarampinon ∻ i reopontico ∻ i . opio ∻ i . traganto fistriolo ∻ i . staratio calamitis i baca lores ∻ iii rastelogo rotundo ∻ iii elebro albo ∻ ii . elebro nigro ∻ iii gentiano ∻ iii . coconidio ∻ iii . aspaltro *unc* . iii . sarcocola ∻ iii . licio ∻ iii . cozumbra . ∻ iii . opopanice ∻ ii adarcio . *unc* . i . uisco malba *lib* iii . pastinacu *lib* iii olmo scortia mediana *lib* . iii . malba ortensa *lib* i . medulla ceruina ∻ ii uino uetus sexterios . iii . uncto portino *lib* ii . seuo *lib* ii . butero *lib* ii . cera *lib* ii . oleo *lib* i . simul quoquis Lupino ∻ iii . fenogreco . ∻ iii . aniso ∻ ii ameu ∻ iii . taridio ∻ iii . gipto ∻ ii pastinaces semen . ∻ iii . caulas semen ∻ iii . anetu ∻ iii . ratoregia ∻ iii leuestice ∻ ii . olesera ∻ iii . anito ∻ iii . ruta . ∻ ii . micon ∻ iii . fenoculo ∻ iii.

19 *Vat. lat. 5951*

19.1 *Potio muscata ad omne infirmum*, f. 1r

Potio <m>uscata ad omne infirmum . Recipit . muscu <ʒ i> libanu ma<… m>ittes modicas . ʒ . viii . cinnamomum ʒ . iii . mel et uinum uetus quod sufficit.

Bibliography

List of Manuscripts

Note: the following is a list of all manuscripts mentioned in the text; see Appendix 1 for more information on the primary manuscripts involved in this study.

Bamberg

Staatsbibliothek

Msc. Med. 1

Digital facsimile: http://digital.bib-bvb.de/view/bvb_mets/viewer.0.6.5.jsp?-folder_id=0&dvs=1708862996938~573&pid=4685473&locale=en_US&usePid1=true&usePid2=true.

Bern

Burgerbibliothek

Cod. A 91.7

Digital facsimile: http://www.e-codices.ch/en/list/one/bbb/A0091-07.

Cambridge

Corpus Christi College

MS 223

Digital facsimile: https://parker.stanford.edu/parker/catalog/th953kw1763.

Glasgow

University Library (UL)

Hunter 96 (*olim* T.4.13)

A digital facsimile is not currently available online.

Karlsruhe

Badische Landesbibliothek

Aug. perg. 120

Digital facsimile: https://digital.blb-karlsruhe.de/blbhs/Handschriften/content/titleinfo/64141.

Laon

Bibliothèque Municipale

MS 199

Digital facsimile: https://initiale.irht.cnrs.fr/codex/12831.

London

British Library (BL)

Harley MS 585

A digital facsimile is not currently available due to the cyber attack; previously, it was accessible at: http://www.bl.uk/manuscripts/FullDisplay.aspx?ref=Harley_MS_585&index=1.

Modena

Archivio Capitolare

O.I.11

Digital facsimile: https://archiviodiocesano.mo.it/opere-digitalizzate/cat/15-o-i-11-sancti-isidori-episcopi-chronicon.

Paris

Bibliothèque nationale de France (BnF)

lat. 2849A

Digital facsimile: https://gallica.bnf.fr/ark:/12148/btv1b9067647m/f4.image.

lat. 2858

Digital facsimile: https://gallica.bnf.fr/ark:/12148/btv1b10318625w.r=%22Latin%202858%22?rk=21459;2.

lat. 5543

Digital facsimile: https://gallica.bnf.fr/ark:/12148/btv1b10502052p/f5.image.r=calendarium.

lat. 6882A

Digital facsimile: https://gallica.bnf.fr/ark:/12148/btv1b90767579/f1.image.

lat. 7021

Digital facsimile: https://gallica.bnf.fr/ark:/12148/btv1b10035236o/f1.image.

lat. 9332

Digital facsimile: https://gallica.bnf.fr/ark:/12148/btv1b60004321/f2.image.

lat. 11218

Digital facsimile: https://gallica.bnf.fr/ark:/12148/btv1b9066936j/f1.image.

lat. 11219

Digital facsimile: https://gallica.bnf.fr/ark:/12148/btv1b8438662j.r=lat.%2011219%20lat.%2011219?rk=21459;2.

lat. 13955

Digital facsimile: https://gallica.bnf.fr/ark:/12148/btv1b9066978w?rk=21459;2.

St Gall

Stiftsbibliothek St. Gallen

cod. sang. 44

Digital facsimile: https://www.e-codices.unifr.ch/de/list/one/csg/0044.

cod. sang. 217

Digital facsimile: https://www.e-codices.unifr.ch/de/list/one/csg/0217.

cod. sang. 397

Digital facsimile: https://www.e-codices.unifr.ch/en/list/one/csg/0397.

cod. sang. 550

Digital facsimile: https://www.e-codices.unifr.ch/en/list/one/csg/0550.

cod. sang. 751

Digital facsimile: https://www.e-codices.unifr.ch/de/list/one/csg/0751.

cod. sang. 752

Digital facsimile: https://www.e-codices.unifr.ch/de/list/one/csg/0752.

cod. sang. 759

Digital facsimile: https://www.e-codices.unifr.ch/de/list/one/csg/0759.

cod. sang. 761

Digital facsimile: https://www.e-codices.unifr.ch/de/list/one/csg/0761.

cod. sang. 878

Digital facsimile: https://www.e-codices.unifr.ch/de/list/one/csg/0878.

cod. sang. 899

Digital facsimile: https://www.e-codices.unifr.ch/en/list/one/csg/0899.

cod. sang. 1092

Digital facsimile: https://www.e-codices.unifr.ch/de/list/one/csg/1092.

cod. sang. 1396

A digital facsimile is not currently available online.

Vatican City

Biblioteca Apostolica Vaticana (BAV)

pal. lat. 187

Digital facsimile: https://digi.vatlib.it/view/bav_pal_lat_187.

pal. lat. 1088

Digital facsimile: https://digi.vatlib.it/view/MSS_Pal.lat.1088.

reg. lat. 421

Digital facsimile: https://digi.vatlib.it/view/MSS_Reg.lat.421.

reg. lat. 598

Digital facsimile: https://digi.vatlib.it/view/MSS_Reg.lat.598.

reg. lat. 1143

Digital facsimile: https://digi.vatlib.it/view/MSS_Reg.lat.1143.

vat. lat. 5951

Digital facsimile: https://digi.vatlib.it/view/MSS_Vat.lat.5951.

Vienna

Österreichische Nationalbibliothek (ÖNB)

Med. gr. 1

A digital facsimile is not currently available online.

Printed Sources

Abū al-Qāsim Khalaf ibn ʿAbbās al-Zahrāwī. *Albucasis* On Surgery and Instruments*: A Definitive Edition of the Arabic Text With English Translation and Commentary*. Translated by M. S. Spink and G. L. Lewis. Berkeley, CA: University of California Press, 1973.

Admonitio generalis. Edited by Alfred Boretius, MGH *Capit.* 1, no. 22. Hanover: Hahn, 1883.

Agnellus of Ravenna. *Lectures on Galen's 'De sectis'*. Translated by 'Seminar Classics 609', State University of New York at Buffalo. Buffalo, NY: Department of Classics, State University of New York at Buffalo (Arethusa Monographs), 1981.

Alcuin of York. *Carmina*. Edited by Ernst Dümmler. MGH *Poet.* 1. Berlin: Weidmann, 1881.

Alcuin of York. *Epistola*. Edited by Ernst Dümmler. MGH *Epp. kar. aevi* 2. Berlin: Weidmann, 1895.

Alexander of Tralles. *Alexandri Tralliani Latini Liber tertius: De febribus singulis. Introduction, Edition, Translation, Notes, Indices*. Edited and translated by David R. Langslow. Santiago de Compostela: Andavira Editora, 2020.

The Alphabet of Galen*: Pharmacy from Antiquity to the Middle Ages*. Edited and translated by Nicholas Everett. Toronto: University of Toronto Press, 2012.

Alphita. Edited by Alejandro García González. Florence: SISMEL Edizioni del Galluzzo, 2007.

Angelbert. *The Battle of Fontenoy*. In *Poetry of the Carolingian Renaissance*, translated by Peter Godman. London: Duckworth, 1985.

Angelbert. *Versus de bella quae fuit acta Fontaneto*. Edited by Ernst Dümmler. MGH *Poet.* 2. Berlin: Weidmann, 1884.

Annales Bertiniani. Edited by G. Waitz. MGH SS *Rer. Germ.* 5. Hanover: Hahn, 1883.

Annales regni Francorum inde ab a. 741 usque ad a. 829 qui dicuntur Annales laurissenses maiores et Einhardi. Edited by Friedrich Kurze. MGH SS *Rer. Germ.* 6. Hanover: Hahn, 1895.

The Annals of St-Bertin. Translated by Janet L. Nelson. Manchester: Manchester University Press, 1991.

Anthimus. *De observatione ciborum ad Theodoricum regem Francorum epistula*. Edited and translated by Eduard Liechtenhan. CML 8. Berlin: Akademie-Verlag, 1963.

Anthimus. *On the Observance of Foods*. Edited and translated by Mark Grant. 2nd ed. Totnes: Prospect, 2007.

Antonii Musae De herba vettonica liber. Pseudoapulei Herbarius. Anonymi De taxone liber. Sexti Placiti Liber medicinae ex animalibus etc., edited by Ernst Howald and Henry E. Sigerist. CML 4. Leipzig: Teubner, 1927.

Ars medicinalis de animalibus: Estudio introductorio, edición crítica y traducción. Edited and translated by Arsenio Ferraces Rodríguez. Santiago de Compostela: Andavira Editora, 2016.

Die Briefe des heiligen Bonifatius und Lullus. Edited by Michael Tangl. MGH *Epistulae selectae* 1. Berlin: Weidmann, 1916.

Caelius Aurelianus. *On Acute Diseases and On Chronic Diseases*. Edited and translated by Israel Edward Drabkin. Chicago: University of Chicago Press, 1950.

Caelius Aurelianus. *Celerum Passionum Libri III. Tardarum Passionum Libri V*. Edited by Gerhard Bendz. Translated by Ingeborg Pape. CML 6, 2 vols. Berlin: Akademie-Verlag, 1990–93.

Caelius Aurelianus. *Caelii Aureliani operum omnium quae exstant Concordantiae*. Edited by Brigitte Maire and Olivier Bianchi. 4 vols. Hildesheim: Olms-Weidmann, 2003.

Caesarius of Arles. *Sermons*. Translated by Mary Magdeleine Mueller. 3 vols. Washington, D.C.: Catholic University of America Press, 1956.

Capitula a sacerdotibus proposita. Edited by Alfred Boretius, MGH *Capit.* 1, no. 36. Hanover: Hahn, 1883.

Capitula de causis cum episcopis et abbatibus tractandis. Edited by Alfred Boretius, MGH *Capit.* 1, no. 72. Hanover: Hahn, 1883.

Capitulare de villis. Edited by Alfred Boretius, MGH *Capit.* 1, no. 32. Hanover: Hahn, 1883.

Capitulare Haristallense. Edited by Alfred Boretius, MGH *Capit.* 1, no. 20. Hanover: Hahn, 1883.

Capitulare missorum item speciale. Edited by Alfred Boretius, MGH *Capit.* 1, no. 35. Hanover: Hahn, 1883.

Cassiodorus. *Cassiodori Senatoris Institutiones*. Edited by R. A. B. Mynors. Oxford: Clarendon Press, 1937.

Cassiodorus. *Institutions of Divine and Secular Learning*. In *Cassiodorus,* Institutions of Divine *and* Secular Learning *and* On the Soul, translated by James W. Halporn. Liverpool: Liverpool University Press, 2004.

Cassius Felix. *Cassii Felicis libri de medicina Concordantiae: Accedunt numeri, voces Graecae Graecis Latinisque litteris scriptae, index nominum notabiliorum, index frequentiae decrescentis formarum*. Edited by Brigitte Maire and Anne Fraisse. Hildesheim: Olms-Weidmann, 2003.

Celsus. *A. Cornelii Celsii quae supersunt*. Edited by Friedrich Marx. CML 1. Leipzig: Teubner, 1915.

Chronique des Abbés de Fontenelle (Saint-Wandrille). Edited and translated by Pascal Pradié. Paris: Belles Lettres, 1999.

Collectio Sangallensis. Edited by Karl Zeumer. MGH *Formulae*. Hanover: Hahn, 1886.

Columbanus, *Saint Columban: His Life, Rule, and Legacy*. Translated by Terrence G. Kardong. Collegeville, MN: Liturgical Press, 2017.

Curae quae ex hominibus atque animalibus fiunt: I. Estudio y edición crítica. Edited by Arsenio Ferraces Rodríguez. Santiago de Compostela: Andavira Editora, 2015.

Dioscorides. *De materia medica*. Translated by Lily Y. Beck. 4th ed. Hildesheim: Olms-Weidmann, 2005.

Dioscorides. *Pedanii Dioscuridis Anazarbei De materia medica libri quinque*. Edited by Max Wellmann. 3 vols. Berlin: Weidmann, 1906–14.

Eigil of Fulda. *Die Vita Sturmi des Eigil von Fulda: Literarkritisch-historische Untersuchung und Edition*. Edited by Pius Engelbert. Marburg: N. G. Elwert, 1968.

Einhard. *The Life of Charlemagne*. In *Two Lives of Charlemagne*, translated by David Ganz. London: Penguin Books, 2008.

Einhard. *Vita Karoli Magni*. Edited by O. Holder-Egger. MGH SS *Rer. Germ.* 25. Hanover: Hahn, 1911.

Ekkehard I of St. Gall. *Waltharius*. Edited and translated by Abram Ring. Leuven: Peeters, 2016.

Ferraces Rodríguez, Arsenio. 'El recetario *Ut pili evulsi non recrescant* (Paris, BNF, Lat. 13955, ff. 146r–147v)'. *Galenos* 5 (2011): 71–90.

Ferraces Rodríguez, Arsenio. 'Un recetario médico altomedieval (Città del Vaticano, BAV, Pal. lat. 1088, ff. 50r–66r): ensayo de edición crítica'. In 'Cui tali cura vel remedio subvenitur'*: De animales y enfermedades en la Edad Media europea*, edited by Gerardo Pérez Barcala, 41–80. Avellino: Edizioni Sinestesie, 2019.

'Die frühmittelalterlichen lateinischen Monatskalendarien. Text, Übersetzung, Kommentar'. Edited and translated by Frank-Dieter Groenke. Diss., Freie Universität Berlin, 1986.

Frühmittelalterliche Rezeptarien. Edited by Julius Jörimann. Zurich: Orell Füssli, 1925.

Fulbert of Chartres. *The Letters and Poems of Fulbert of Chartres*. Edited and translated by Frederick Behrends. Oxford: Clarendon Press, 1976.

Galen. *In Hippocratis Aphorismos*. In *Claudii Galeni Opera Omnia*, edited by Karl Gottlob Kühn, 20 vols. Leipzig: Carl Cnobloch, 1821–33.

Galen. *De simplicium medicamentorum temperamentis ac facultatibus*. In *Claudii Galeni Opera Omnia*, edited by Karl Gottlob Kühn, 20 vols. Leipzig: Carl Cnobloch, 1821–33.

Gregory the Great. *The Book of Pastoral Rule*. Translated by James Barmby. Buffalo: Christian Literature Publishing Co., 1895.

Heiric of Auxerre. *Miracula S. Germani*. PL 124, cols. 1207–72.

Hrabanus Maurus. *De universo*. PL 111, cols. 500–4.

Huneberc. *Hodoeporicon*. In *The Anglo-Saxon Missionaries in Germany*. Translated by Charles Hugh Talbot. London: Sheed and Ward, 1954.

Huneberc. *Vitae Willibaldi et Wynnebaldi*. Edited by O. Holder-Egger. MGH SS 14.1. Hanover: Hahn, 1887.

Isidore of Seville. *Etymologiarum sive originum, libri XX*. Edited by W. M. Lindsay. 2 vols. Oxford: Oxford University Press, 1911.

Isidore of Seville. *The Etymologies of Isidore of Seville*. Translated by Stephen A. Barney, W. J. Lewis, J. A. Beach, and Oliver Berghof. Cambridge: Cambridge University Press, 2006.

Leges Langobardorum. Edited by Friedrich Bluhme. *MGH LL* 4. Hanover: Hahn, 1868.

Das 'Lorscher Arzneibuch': Ein medizinisches Kompendium des 8. Jahrhunderts (Codex Bambergensis medicinalis 1): Text, Übersetzung und Fachglossar. Edited and translated by Ulrich Stoll. Stuttgart: Franz Steiner, 1992.

Loyn, H. R., and John Percival. *The Reign of Charlemagne. Documents on Carolingian Government and Administration*. London: Edward Arnold, 1975.

Marcellus of Bordeaux. *De medicamentis liber*. Edited by Eduard Liechtenhan and Maximilian Niedermann. Translated by Jutta Kollesch and Diethard Nickel. *CML* 5, 2 vols. Berlin: Akademie-Verlag, 1968.

The Medicina Plinii: *Latin Text, Translation, and Commentary*. Translated Yvette Hunt. Abingdon: Routledge, 2020.

Medieval Herbal Remedies: The Old English Herbarium *and Anglo-Saxon Medicine*. Translated by Anne Van Arsdall. New York: Routledge, 2002.

Notker. *Gesta Karoli Magni Imperatoris*. Edited by Hans F. Haefele. *MGH SS Rer. Germ. N. S.* 12. Berlin: Weidmann, 1959.

Notker. *The Deeds of Charlemagne*. In *Two lives of Charlemagne*, translated by David Ganz. London: Penguin Books, 2008.

The Old English Herbarium and Medicina de Quadrupedibus. Edited by Hubert Jan de Vriend. Oxford: Oxford University Press, 1984.

Physica Plinii Bambergensis (Cod. Bamb. med. 2, fol. 93v–232r). Edited by Alf Önnerfors. Hildesheim: Olms, 1975.

Plinii Secundi Iunioris qui feruntur De medicina libri tres. Edited by Alf Önnerfors. *CML* 3. Berlin: Akademie-Verlag, 1964.

Pliny the Elder. *Natural History*. Translated by Harris Rackham, William Henry Samuel Jones, and D. E. Eichholz. 10 vols. Cambridge, MA: Harvard University Press, 1938–63.

Polyptyque de l'abbé Irminon ou dénombrement des manses, des serfs et des revenus de l'abbaye de Saint-Germain-des-Prés sous le règne de Charlemagne. Edited by Benjamin Edme Charles Guérard. 2 vols. Paris: Imprimerie royale, 1844.

Pseudo-Antonius Musa. *De herba vettonica liber*. In *Antonii Musae De herba vettonica liber. Pseudoapulei Herbarius. Anonymi De taxone liber. Sexti Placiti Liber medicinae ex animalibus etc.*, edited by Ernst Howald and Henry E. Sigerist. *CML* 4, 3–11. Leipzig: Teubner, 1927.

Pseudo-Apuleius. *Herbarius*. In *Antonii Musae De herba vettonica liber. Pseudoapulei Herbarius. Anonymi De taxone liber. Sexti Placiti Liber medicinae ex animalibus etc.*, edited by Ernst Howald and Henry E. Sigerist. *CML* 4, 15–225. Leipzig: Teubner, 1927.

Quintus Serenus. *Liber medicinalis (Le livre de médecine)*. Edited and translated by R. Pépin. Paris: Presses universitaires de France, 1950.

Quintus Serenus. *Liber medicinalis*. Edited by F. Vollmer. CML 2.3. Leipzig: Teubner, 1916.

RB *1980: The Rule of St. Benedict in Latin and English with Notes*. Edited and translated by Timothy Fry. Collegeville, MN: Liturgical Press, 1981.

Richer of Reims. *Histoire de France*. Edited and translated by Robert Latouche. 2 vols. Paris: H. Champion, 1930.

Rothair's Edict. In *The Lombard Laws*, translated by Katherine Fischer Drew, 39–130. Philadelphia: University of Pennsylvania Press, 1973.

Soranus. *Sorani quae feruntur* Quaestiones medicinales. *Lateinischer Text beider Versionen mit deutscher Übersetzung und Anmerkungen*. Edited and translated by Klaus-Dietrich Fischer. Cuenca: Ediciones de la Universidad de Castilla-La Mancha, 2017.

Der St. Galler Botanicus*: Ein frühmittelalterliches Herbar: Kritische Edition, Übersetzung und Kommentar*. Edited and translated by Monica Niederer. Bern: Peter Lang, 2005.

Studien und Texte zur frühmittelalterlichen Rezeptliteratur. Edited by Henry E. Sigerist. Leipzig: Johann Ambrosius Barth, 1923.

Tacitus. *Germania*. In *Agricola. Germania. Dialogue on Oratory*, translated by M. Hutton and W. Peterson. Cambridge, MA: Harvard University Press, 1914.

The Trotula*: A Medieval Compendium of Women's Medicine*. Edited and translated by Monica H. Green. Philadelphia: University of Pennsylvania Press, 2001.

Vademecum eines frühmittelalterlichen Arztes: Die gefaltete lateinische Handschrift medizinischen Inhalts im Codex 217 und der Fragmentensammlung 1396 der Stiftsbibliothek in St. Gallen. Edited and translated by Peter Köpp. Aarau: Sauerländer, 1980.

Walahfrid Strabo. *De cultura hortorum*. Edited by Ernst Dümmler. MGH *Poet.* 2. Berlin: Weidmann, 1884.

Walahfrid Strabo. *Hortulus*. Translated by Raef Payne. Pittsburgh: Hunt Botanical Library, 1966.

Wallis, Faith, ed. *Medieval Medicine: A Reader*. Toronto: University of Toronto Press, 2010.

Secondary Scholarship

Abrahams, Harold J. 'Onycha, Ingredient of the Ancient Jewish Incense: An Attempt at Identification'. *Economic Botany* 33, no. 2 (1979): 233–6.

A'lam, Hūšang. 'Camphor'. In *Encyclopædia Iranica*, edited by Ahmad Ashraf, Nicholas Sims-Williams, Mahnaz Moazami, Mohsen Ashtiany, Christopher J. Brunner, Manouchehr Kasheff, and Habib Borjian. Vol. 4/7 (1990): 743–7, https://iranicaonline.org/articles/camphor-npers.

Albritton, Benjamin, Georgia Henley, and Elaine Treharne, eds. *Medieval Manuscripts in the Digital Age*. London: Routledge, 2021.

Amar, Zohar, and Efraim Lev. *Arabian Drugs in Early Medieval Mediterranean Medicine*. Edinburgh: Edinburgh University Press, 2017.

Amoretti, Valeria. 'Analisi paleobiologiche dei resti scheletrici'. In *Lo scavo di San Martino di Ovaro (sec.* V–XII*). Archeologia della cristianizzazione nel territorio di Aquileia*, edited by Aurora Cagnana, 481–536. Mantua: SAP, 2011.

Amoretti, Valeria, Aurora Cagnana, Paola Greppi, and Andrea Saccocci. 'Lo scavo della chiesa di San Vito di Illegio (Tolmezzo, UD). Una "Eigenkirche" carolingia nelle Alpi Carniche'. In *V Congresso Nazionale di Archeologia Medievale. Palazzo della Dogana, Salone del Tribunale (Foggia); Palazzo dei Celestini, Auditorium (Manfredonia); 30 settembre-3 ottobre 2009*, edited by Giuliano Volpe and Pasquale Favia, 487–91. Florence: All'Insegna del Giglio, 2009.

Arnott, Robert, Stanley Finger, and C. U. M. Smith, eds. *Trepanation: History, Discovery, Theory*. Lisse: Swets & Zeitlinger Publishers, 2003.

Arthur, Paul, and Marco Leo Imperiale, eds. *VII Congresso Nazionale di Archeologia Medievale. Palazzo Turrisi. Lecce, 9–12 settembre 2015*. 2 vols. Florence: All'Insegna del Giglio, 2015.

Aufderheide, Arthur C., and Conrado Rodríguez-Martín. *The Cambridge Encyclopedia of Human Paleopathology*. Cambridge: Cambridge University Press, 1998.

Baader, Gerhard. 'Die Anfänge der medizinischen Ausbildung im Abendland bis 1100'. In *La scuola nell'Occidente latino dell'alto medioevo, 15–21 aprile 1971*, Settimane 19, vol. 2, 669–772. Spoleto: Fondazione Centro italiano di studi sull'alto medioevo, 1972.

Baader, Gerhard. 'Early Medieval Latin Adaptations of Byzantine Medicine in Western Europe'. *Dumbarton Oaks Papers* 38 (1984): 251–9. https://doi.org/10.2307/1291509.

Baggieri, Gaspare, and Francesco Mallegni. 'A Probable Case of Gout'. *Medicina Historica* 1, no. 1 (2017): 23–8.

Bakels, Corrie C. 'Crops produced in the southern Netherlands and northern France during the early medieval period: a comparison'. *Vegetation History and Archaeobotany* 14, no. 4 (2005): 394–99. https://doi.org/10.1007/s00334-005-0067-x.

Banham, Debby, and Christine Voth. 'The Diagnosis and Treatment of Wounds in the Old English Medical Collections: Anglo-Saxon Surgery?'. In *Wounds and Wound Repair in Medieval Culture*, edited by Larissa Tracy and Kelly DeVries, 153–74. Leiden: Brill, 2015.

Banniard, Michel. 'Language and Communication in Carolingian Europe'. In *The New Cambridge Medieval History* II, *c. 700-c. 900*, edited by Rosamond McKitterick, 695–708. Cambridge, Cambridge University Press, 1995.

Barnhouse, Lucy, and Winston Black, eds. *Beyond Cadfael: Medieval Medicine and Medical Medievalism*. Budapest: Trivent Publishing, 2023.

Bates, Don G., ed. *Knowledge and the Scholarly Medical Traditions.* Cambridge: Cambridge University Press, 1995.

Battisti, Carlo. 'Ripercussioni lessicali del commercio orientale nel periodo giustinianeo'. In *Moneta e scambi nell'alto medioevo, 21–27 aprile 1960*, Settimane 8, 627–82. Spoleto: Fondazione Centro italiano di studi sull'alto medioevo, 1961.

Beach, Alison I., and Isabelle Cochelin, eds. *The Cambridge History of Medieval Monasticism in the Latin West.* 2 vols. Cambridge: Cambridge University Press, 2020.

Beccaria, Augusto. *I codici di medicina del periodo presalernitano (secoli IX, X e XI).* Rome: Edizioni di Storia e Letteratura, 1956.

Becker, Hilary. 'Pigment nomenclature in the ancient Near East, Greece, and Rome'. *Archaeological and Anthropological Sciences* 14 (2022). https://doi.org/10.1007/s12520-021-01394-1.

Belcastro, Giovanna, Elisa Rastelli, Valentina Mariotti, Chiara Consiglio, Fiorenzo Facchini, and Benedetta Bonfiglioli. 'Continuity or Discontinuity of the Life-Style in Central Italy During the Roman Imperial Age-Early Middle Ages Transition: Diet, Health, and Behaviour'. *American Journal of Physical Anthropology* 132, no. 3 (2007): 381–394. https://doi.org/10.1002/ajpa.20530.

Biggam, C. P., ed. *From Earth to Art: The Many Aspects of the Plant-World in Anglo-Saxon England. Proceedings of the First ASPNS Symposium, University of Glasgow, 5–7 April 2000.* Amsterdam: Rodopi: 2003.

Binder, M., J. Eitler, J. Deutschmann, S. Ladstätter, F. Glaser, and D. Fiedler. 'Prosthetics in Antiquity—An Early Medieval Wearer of a Foot Prosthesis (6th Century AD) from Hemmaberg/Austria'. *International Journal of Paleopathology* 12 (2016): 29–40. https://doi.org/10.1016/j.ijpp.2015.11.003.

Bischoff, Bernhard. 'Wer ist die Nonne von Heidenheim?' *Studien und Mitteilungen zur Geschichte des Benediktinerordens und seiner Zweige* 49 (1931): 387–8.

Bischoff, Bernhard. 'Über gefaltete Handschriften, vornehmlich hagiographischen Inhalts'. In *Mittelalterliche Studien. Ausgewählte Aufsätze zur Schriftkunde und Literaturgeschichte*, edited by Bernhard Bischoff, vol. 1, 93–100. Stuttgart: Hiersemann, 1966.

Bischoff, Bernhard. *Mittelalterliche Studien. Ausgewählte Aufsätze zur Schriftkunde und Literaturgeschichte.* 3 vols. Stuttgart: Hiersemann, 1966–81.

Bischoff, Bernhard. 'Caritas-Leider'. In *Mittelalterliche Studien. Ausgewählte Aufsätze zur Schriftkunde und Literaturgeschichte*, edited by Bernhard Bischoff, vol. 2, 56–76. Stuttgart: Hiersemann, 1967.

Bischoff, Bernhard. 'Das griechische Element in der abendländischen Bildung des Mittelalters'. In *Mittelalterliche Studien. Ausgewählte Aufsätze zur Schriftkunde und Literaturgeschichte*, edited by Bernhard Bischoff, vol. 2, 246–74. Stuttgart: Hiersemann, 1967.

Bischoff, Bernhard. 'Eine Sammelhandschrift Walahfrid Strabos (Cod. Sangall. 878)'. In *Mittelalterliche Studien. Ausgewählte Aufsätze zur Schriftkunde und*

Literaturgeschichte, edited by Bernhard Bischoff, vol. 2, 34–51. Stuttgart: Hiersemann, 1967.

Bischoff, Bernhard. 'Bücher am Hofe Ludwigs des Deutschen und die Privatbibliothek des Kanzlers Grimalt'. In *Mittelalterliche Studien. Ausgewählte Aufsätze zur Schriftkunde und Literaturgeschichte*, edited by Bernhard Bischoff, vol. 3, 187–212. Stuttgart: Hiersemann, 1981.

Bischoff, Bernhard. 'Übersicht über die nichtdiplomatischen Geheimschriften des Mittelalters'. In *Mittelalterliche Studien. Ausgewählte Aufsätze zur Schriftkunde und Literaturgeschichte*, edited by Bernhard Bischoff, vol. 3, 120–48. Stuttgart: Hiersemann, 1981.

Bischoff, Bernhard. 'Italienische Handschriften des neunten bis elften Jahrhunderts in frühmittelalterlichen Bibliotheken ausserhalb Italiens'. In *Il libro e il testo: Atti del Convegno Internazionale, Urbino, 20–23 Settembre 1982*, edited by Cesare Questa and Renato Raffaelli, 169–94. Urbino: Università degli Studi di Urbino, 1984.

Bischoff, Bernhard. 'Maße und Gewichte zur Zeit Papst Hadrians I. (772–795)'. In *Anecdota novissima. Texte des vierten bis sechzehnten Jahrhunderts*. Edited by Bernhard Bischoff, 169–70. Stuttgart: Hiersemann, 1984.

Bischoff, Bernhard. *Die Abtei Lorsch im Spiegel ihrer Handschriften*. 2nd ed. Lorsch: Laurissa, 1989.

Bischoff, Bernhard. *Katalog der festländischen Handschriften des neunten Jahrhunderts* (*mit Ausnahme der wisigotischen*). 3 vols. Wiesbaden: Harrassowitz, 1998–2014.

Bischoff, Bernhard. *Manuscripts and Libraries in the Age of Charlemagne*. Translated by Michael M. Gorman. Cambridge: Cambridge University Press, 2007.

Bliquez, Lawrence J. 'Two Lists of Greek Surgical Instruments and the State of Surgery in Byzantine Times'. *Dumbarton Oaks Papers* 38 (1984): 187–204. https://doi.org/10.2307/1291505.

Bloch, R. Howard. *God's Plagiarist: Being an Account of the Fabulous Industry and Irregular Commerce of the Abbé Migne*. Chicago, University of Chicago Press, 1994.

Blockley, Paul, Roberto Caimi, Donatella Caporusso, Cristina Cattaneo, Paola Marina De Marchi, Lucia Miazzo, Davide Porta, and Cristina Ravedoni. 'Campione d'Italia. Scavi archeologici nella ex chiesa di San Zeno'. In *Carte di famiglia. Strategie, rappresentazione e memoria del gruppo familiare di Totone di Campione (721–877)*, edited by Stefano Gasparri and Cristina La Rocca, 29–80. Rome: Viella, 2005.

Blondiaux, Joël, Anne Cotten, Christian Fontaine, Catherine Hänni, Anne Bera, René-Marc Flipo. 'Two Roman and Medieval Cases of Symmetrical Erosive Polyarthropathy from Normandy: Anatomico-pathological and Radiological Evidence for Rheumatoid Arthritis'. *International Journal of Osteoarchaeology* 7, no. 5 (1997): 451–66. https://doi.org/10.1002/(SICI)1099-1212(199709/10)7:5%3C451::AID-OA334%3E3.0.CO;2-4.

Bowers, Barbara S., ed. *The Medieval Hospital and Medical Practice*. Aldershot: Ashgate, 2007.

Bowersock, G. W., Peter Brown, and Oleg Grabar, eds. *Late Antiquity: A Guide to the Postclassical World*. Cambridge, MA: Belknap Press, 1999.

Brackmann, Rebecca. '"It Will Help Him Wonderfully": Placebo and Meaning Responses in Early Medieval English Medicine'. *Speculum* 97, no. 4 (2022): 1012–39. https://doi.org/10.1086/721680.

Brall, Artur, ed. *Von der Klosterbibliothek zur Landesbibliothek. Beiträge zum zweihundertjährigen Bestehen der Hessischen Landesbibliothek Fulda*. Stuttgart: Hiersemann, 1978.

Brennessel, Barbara, Michael D. C. Drout, and Robyn Gravel. 'A Reassessment of the Efficacy of Anglo-Saxon Medicine'. *Anglo-Saxon England* 34 (2005): 183–95.

Bricout, Sébastien. 'Note sur deux laïcs carolingiens et la médecine au ixᵉ siècle'. *Latomus* 65, no. 2 (2006): 458–61.

Brown, Giles. 'Introduction: The Carolingian Renaissance'. In *Carolingian Culture: Emulation and Innovation*, edited by Rosamond McKitterick, 1–51. Cambridge: Cambridge University Press, 1994.

Brown, Peter. *The Making of Late Antiquity*. Cambridge, MA: Harvard University Press, 1978.

Brown, T. S. *Gentlemen and Officers: Imperial Administration and Aristocratic Power in Byzantine Italy, AD 554–800*. London: British School at Rome, 1984.

Brown, T. S. 'Byzantine Italy, *c.* 680-*c.* 876'. In *The New Cambridge Medieval History* II, *c. 700-c. 900*, edited by Rosamond McKitterick, 320–48. Cambridge: Cambridge University Press, 1995.

Brown, Thomas S. 'Ravenna and Other Early Rivals of Venice: Comparative Urban and Economic Development in the Upper Adriatic c.751–1050'. In *Byzantium, Venice and the Medieval Adriatic: Spheres of Maritime Power and Influence, c. 700–1453*, edited by Magdalena Skoblar, 173–87. Cambridge: Cambridge University Press, 2021.

Brown, Warren C. *Violence in Medieval Europe*. Harlow: Pearson Education Limited, 2011.

Brubaker, Leslie. 'The Vienna Dioskorides and Anicia Juliana'. In *Byzantine Garden Culture*, edited by Antony Robert Littlewood, Henry Maguire, and Joachim Wolschke-Bulmahn, 189–214. Washington, D.C.: Dumbarton Oaks, 2002.

Buora, Maurizio, and Licia Usai. 'La tomba del cavaliere longobardo Moechis a Lovaria (Comune di Pradamano, Provincia di Udine): Un caso di acculturazione dopo la metà del VII sec'. In *I Congresso Nazionale di Archeologia Medievale. Auditorium del Centro Studi della Cassa di Risparmio di Pisa (ex Benedettine), Pisa, 29–31 maggio 1997*, edited by Sauro Gelichi, 261–4. Florence: All'Insegna del Giglio, 1997.

Burridge, Claire. 'Incense in Medicine: An Early Medieval Perspective'. *Early Medieval Europe* 28, no. 2 (2020): 219–55. https://doi.org/10.1111/emed.12394.

Burridge, Claire. 'Healing Body and Soul in Early Medieval Europe: Medical Remedies with Christian Elements'. *Studies in Church History* 58 (2022): 46–67. https://doi.org/10.1017/stc.2022.3.

Caffaro, Adriano. *Scrivere in oro: Ricettari medievali d'arte e artigianato (secoli IX–XI). Codici di Lucca e Ivrea*. Naples: Liguori, 2003.

Cagnana, Aurora, ed. *Lo scavo di San Martino di Ovaro (UD) (sec. V–XII). Archeologia della cristianizzazione rurale nel territorio di Aquileia*. Mantua: SAP, 2011.

Cambornac, Michel. *Plantes et jardins du Moyen Âge*. Paris: Hartmann, 2001.

Cameron, Averil. *The Mediterranean World of Late Antiquity, 395–700 AD*. 2nd ed. Abingdon: Routledge, 2012.

Cameron, M. L., 'Anglo-Saxon Medicine and Magic'. *Anglo-Saxon England* 17 (1988): 191–215.

Cameron, M. L. *Anglo-Saxon Medicine*. Cambridge: Cambridge University Press, 1993.

Campbell, Sheila, Bert Hall, and David Klausner, eds. *Health, Disease and Healing in Medieval Culture*. Houndmills: Macmillan, 1992.

Canci, Alessandro, Alexandra Chavarría Arnau, and Maurizio Marinato. 'Il cimitero della chiesa altomedievale di San Lorenzo di Desenzano (BS): note di bioarcheologia'. In *VI Congresso Nazionale di Archeologia Medievale. Sala Conferenze "E. Sericchi", Centro Direzionale CARISPAQ "Strinella 88". L'Aquila, 12–15 settembre 2012*, edited by Fabio Redi and Alfonso Forgione, 452–5. Florence: All'Insegna del Giglio, 2012.

Cappelli, Adriano. *Dizionario di abbreviature latine ed italiane*. 6th ed. Milan: Hoepli, 1990.

Cardon, Dominique. *Natural Dyes: Sources, Tradition, Technology and Science*. London: Archetype, 2007.

Caseau, Béatrice. 'La parfum de Dieu'. In *Parfums et odeurs au Moyen Âge. Science, usage, symboles*, edited by Agostino Paravicini Bagliani, 3–22. Florence: SISMEL Edizioni del Galluzzo, 2015.

Cattaneo, Cristina, and Andrea Mazzucchi. 'Popolazioni tardo antiche e dell'alto medioevo narrate dai resti ossei: il progetto di una banca dati lombarda'. In *La via Carolingia: uomini e idee sulle strade d'Europa. Dal sistema viario al sistema informativo*, edited by Paola Marina De Marchi and Stefano Pilato, 87–98. Mantua: SAP, 2013.

Chavarría, Alexandra, and Maurizio Marinato. 'Frammentazione e complessità nelle pratiche funerarie altomedievali in Italia settentrionale'. In *VII Congresso Nazionale di Archeologia Medievale. Palazzo Turrisi. Lecce, 9–12 settembre 2015*, edited by Paul Arthur and Marco Leo Imperiale, vol. 2, 61–8. Florence: All'Insegna del Giglio, 2015.

Chen, Pei, Jianghao Sun, and Paul Ford. 'Differentiation of the Four Major Species of Cinnamons (*C. burmannii, C. verum, C. cassia*, and *C. loureiroi*) Using a Flow Injection Mass Spectrometric (FIMS) Fingerprinting Method'. *Journal of Agricultural and Food Chemistry* 62, no. 12 (2014): 2516–21. https://doi.org/10.1021/jf405580c.

Clarke, Robert C., and Mark D. Merlin. *Cannabis: Evolution and Ethnobotany*. Berkeley: University of California Press, 2013.

Cohen, Mark Nathan, James W. Wood, and George R. Milner. 'The Osteological Paradox Reconsidered'. *Current Anthropology* 35, no. 5 (1994): 629–37.

Collins, Minta. *Medieval Herbals: The Illustrative Traditions*. London: British Library, 2000.

Conrad, Lawrence I., Michael Neve, Vivian Nutton, Roy Porter, and Andrew Wear. *The Western Medical Tradition: 800 BC to AD 1800*. Cambridge: Cambridge University Press, 1995.

Contreni, John J. 'Masters and Medicine in Northern France in the Reign of Charles the Bald'. In *Charles the Bald: Court and Kingdom. Papers Based on a Colloquium Held in London in April 1979*, edited by Margaret T. Gibson and Janet Nelson, 2nd ed., 267–82. Aldershot: Variorum, 1990.

Contreni, John J. *Carolingian Learning, Masters and Manuscripts*. Aldershot: Variorum, 1992.

Contreni, John J. 'The Carolingian Renaissance: Education and Literary Culture'. In *The New Cambridge Medieval History* II, *c. 700-c. 900*, edited by Rosamond McKitterick, 709–57. Cambridge: Cambridge University Press, 1995.

Corbineau, Rémi, and Patrice Georges-Zimmermann. 'Le parfum de la mort. Plantes et aromates pour la préparation des corps (Moyen Âge et période moderne)'. In *Parfums et odeurs au Moyen Âge. Science, usage, symboles*, edited by Agostino Paravicini Bagliani, 161–80. Florence: SISMEL Edizioni del Galluzzo, 2015.

Córdoba, Ricardo, ed. *Craft Treatises and Handbooks: The Dissemination of Technical Knowledge in the Middle Ages*. Turnhout: Brepols, 2013.

Corradini, Richard. 'Pieces of a Puzzle: Time and History in Walahfrid's *Vademecum*'. *Early Medieval Europe* 22, no. 4 (2014): 476–91. https://doi.org/10.1111/emed.12083.

Corradini, Richard. 'Wissenschaft und Zeitdiagnose. Zur Transformation antiken Wissens in Walahfrid Strabos Vademecum'. In *Neue Wege der Frühmittelalterforschung: Bilanz und Perspektiven*, edited by Walter Pohl, Maximilian Diesenberger, and Bernhard Zeller, 287–308. Vienna: Österreichischen Akademie der Wissenschaften, 2018.

Corradini, Richard, Max Diesenberger, and Helmut Reimitz, eds. *The Construction of Communities in the Early Middle Ages. Texts, Resources and Artefacts*. Leiden: Brill, 2003.

Costambeys, Marios, Matthew Innes, and Simon MacLean, *The Carolingian World*. Cambridge: Cambridge University Press, 2011.

Coupland, Simon, 'Carolingian Arms and Armor in the Ninth Century', *Viator* 21 (1990): 29–50.

Courcelle, Pierre, *Late Latin Writers and Their Greek Sources*. Translated by Harry E. Wedeck. Cambridge, MA: Harvard University Press, 1969.

Crislip, Andrew T. *From Monastery to Hospital: Christian Monasticism & the Transformation of Health Care in Late Antiquity*. Ann Arbor: University of Michigan Press, 2005.

Crislip, Andrew, *Thorns in the Flesh: Illness and Sanctity in Late Ancient Christianity*. Philadelphia: University of Pennsylvania Press, 2013.

Cunningham, Andrew. 'Identifying Disease in the Past: Cutting the Gordian Knot'. *Asclepio* 54, no. 1 (2002): 13–34. https://doi.org/10.3989/asclepio.2002.v54.i1.133.

Curtis, Robert I. *Garum and Salsamenta: Production and Commerce in Materia Medica*. Leiden: Brill, 1991.

Dalbeth, Nicola, Tony R. Merriman, and Lisa K. Stamp. 'Gout'. *The Lancet* 388 (2016): 2039–52. https://doi.org/10.1016/S0140-6736(16)00346-9.

Dal Poz, Marco, Francesca Ricci, Bruno Reale, Maddalena Malvone, Loretana Salvadei, and Giorgio Manzi. 'Paleobiologia della popolazione altomedievale di San Lorenzo di Quingentole, Mantova'. In *San Lorenzo di Quingentole: archeologia, storia ed antropologia*, edited by Alberto Manicardi, 151–98. Mantua: SAP, 2001.

D'Aronco, Maria Amalia. 'Anglo-Saxon Plant Pharmacy and the Latin Medical Tradition'. In *From Earth to Art: The Many Aspects of the Plant-World in Anglo-Saxon England. Proceedings of the First ASPNS Symposium, University of Glasgow, 5–7 April 2000*, edited by C. P. Biggam, 133–51. Amsterdam: Rodopi: 2003.

D'Aronco, Maria Amalia. 'The Transmission of Medical Knowledge in Anglo-Saxon England: The Voices of Manuscripts'. In *Form and Content of Instruction in Anglo-Saxon England in the Light of Contemporary Manuscript Evidence: Papers Presented at the International Conference, Udine, 6–8 April 2006*, edited by Patrizia Lendinara, Loredana Lazzari, and Maria Amalia D'Aronco, 35–58. Turnhout: Brepols, 2007.

D'Aronco, Maria Amalia, and Malcolm L. Cameron. *The Old English Illustrated Pharmacopoeia*. Copenhagen: Rosenkilde and Bagger, 1998.

Davis, Jennifer R., and Michael McCormick, 'The Early Middle Ages: Europe's Long Morning'. In *The Long Morning of Medieval Europe: New Directions in Early Medieval Studies*, edited by Jennifer R. Davis and Michael McCormick, 1–10. Aldershot: Ashgate, 2008.

Davis, Jennifer R., and Michael McCormick, eds. *The Long Morning of Medieval Europe: New Directions in Early Medieval Studies*. Aldershot: Ashgate, 2008.

Delogu, Paolo. 'Lombard and Carolingian Italy'. In *The New Cambridge Medieval History* II, *c. 700-c. 900*, edited by Rosamond McKitterick, 290–319. Cambridge: Cambridge University Press, 1995.

Demaitre, Luke, '"Is It Lupus?"—The Wolf in a Disease, from Metaphor to Medicine'. In *Beyond Cadfael: Medieval Medicine and Medical Medievalism*, edited by Lucy Barnhouse and Winston Black, 31–56. Budapest: Trivent Publishing, 2023.

De Marchi, Paola Marina, and Stefano Pilato, eds. *La via Carolingia: uomini e idee sulle strade d'Europa. Dal sistema viario al sistema informativo*. Mantua: SAP, 2013.

Dendle, Peter, and Alain Touwaide, eds. *Health and Healing from the Medieval Garden*. Woodbridge: Boydell & Brewer, 2008.

DeWitte, Sharon N., and Christopher M. Stojanowski. 'The Osteological Paradox 20 Years Later: Past Perspectives, Future Directions'. *Journal of Archaeological Research* 23 (2015): 397–450. https://doi.org/10.1007/s10814-015-9084-1.

Diem, Albrecht. 'Inventing the Holy Rule: Some Observations on the History of Monastic Normative Observance in the Early Medieval West'. In *Western Monasticism* ante litteram*: The Spaces of Monastic Observance in Late Antiquity and the Early Middle Ages*, edited by Hendrik Dey and Elizabeth Fentress, 53–84. Turnhout: Brepols, 2011.

Diem, Albrecht, and Claudia Rapp. 'The Monastic Laboratory: Perspectives of Research in Late Antique and Early Medieval Monasticism'. In *The Cambridge History of Medieval Monasticism in the Latin West*, edited by Alison I. Beach and Isabelle Cochelin, vol. 1, 19–39. Cambridge: Cambridge University Press, 2020.

Diem, Albrecht, and Philip Rousseau. 'Monastic Rules (Fourth to Ninth Century)'. In *The Cambridge History of Medieval Monasticism in the Latin West*, edited by Alison I. Beach and Isabelle Cochelin, vol. 1, 162–94. Cambridge: Cambridge University Press, 2020.

Dittmar, Jenna M., Piers D. Mitchell, Peter M. Jones, Bram Mulder, Sarah A. Inskip, Craig Cessford, and John E. Robb. 'Gout and 'Podagra' in medieval Cambridge, England'. *International Journal of Paleopathology* 33 (2021): 170–81. https://doi.org/10.1016/j.ijpp.2021.04.007.

Doody, Aude. 'Authority and Authorship in the *Medicina Plinii*'. In *Authorial Voices in Greco-Roman Technical Writing*, edited by Liba Taub and Aude Doody, 93–105. Trier: Wissenschaftlicher Verlag, 2009.

Doody, Aude. *Pliny's Encyclopedia: The Reception of the* Natural History. Cambridge: Cambridge University Press, 2010.

Dörnemann, Michael. 'Einer ist Arzt, Christus: Medizinales Verständnis von Erlösung in der Theologie der griechischen Kirchenväter des zweiten bis vierten Jahrhunderts'. *Zeitschrift für antikes Christentum/Journal of Ancient Christianity* 17 (2013): 102–24. https://doi.org/10.1515/zac-2013-0006.

Dorofeeva, Anna. 'Miscellanies, Christian Reform and Early Medieval Encyclopaedism: A Reconsideration of the Pre-Bestiary *Physiologus* Manuscripts'. *Historical Research* 90 (2017): 665–82. https://doi.org/10.1111/1468-2281.12198.

Dorofeeva, Anna. 'Strategies of Knowledge Organisation in Early Medieval Latin Glossary Miscellanies: The Example of Munich, Bayerische Staatsbibliothek, Clm 14388'. In *Writing the Early Medieval West*, edited by Elina Screen and Charles West, 146–68. Cambridge: Cambridge University Press, 2018.

Doyle, Conan T., *The Reception of Latin Medicine in Anglo-Saxon England: Evidence from Old English Medical Texts*. York: York Medieval Press, forthcoming.

Drabkin, Miriam. 'Select Pages from Mediaeval Medical Manuscripts'. *Bulletin of the History of Medicine* 11, no. 4 (1942): 409–36.

Dronke, Peter. *Women Writers of the Middle Ages: A Critical Study of Texts from Perpetua (†203) to Marguerite Porete (†1310)*. Cambridge: Cambridge University Press, 1984.

Engs, Ruth C. 'Do Traditional Western European Drinking Practices Have Origins in Antiquity?' *Addiction Research* 2, no. 3 (1995): 227–39. https://doi.org/10.3109/16066359509005208.

Everett, Nicholas. *Literacy in Lombard Italy, c. 568–774*. Cambridge: Cambridge University Press, 2003.

Everett, Nicholas. 'The Manuscript Evidence for Pharmacy in the Early Middle Ages'. In *Writing the Early Medieval West*, edited by Elina Screen and Charles West, 115–30. Cambridge: Cambridge University Press, 2018.

Evers, Kasper Grønland. *Worlds Apart Trading Together: The Organisation of Long-Distance Trade Between Rome and India in Antiquity*. Oxford: Archaeopress, 2017.

Fear, Andrew, and Jamie Wood, eds. *Isidore of Seville and His Reception in the Early Middle Ages: Transmitting and Transforming Knowledge*. Amsterdam: Amsterdam University Press, 2016.

Ferngren, Gary B. *Medicine and Health Care in Early Christianity*. Baltimore: Johns Hopkins University Press, 2009.

Ferraces Rodríguez, Arsenio. 'El Pseudo-Dioscórides *De herbis femininis*, los *Dynamidia* e Isidoro de Sevilla, *Etym.* XVII, 7–11'. In *Tradición e Innovación de la Medicina Latina de la Antigüedad y de la Alta Edad Media: Actas del IV Coloquio Internacional sobre los "textos médicos latinos antiguos"*, edited by Manuel Enrique Vázquez Buján, 183–203. Santiago de Compostela: Servicio de Publicacións e Intercambio Científico da Universidade de Santiago de Compostela, 1994.

Ferraces Rodríguez, Arsenio. 'Isidoro de Sevilla y los textos de medicina'. In *"Isidorus medicus": Isidoro de Sevilla y los textos de medicina*, edited by Arsenio Ferraces Rodríguez, 11–37. A Coruña: Servizio de Publicacións, Universidade da Coruña, 2005.

Ferraces Rodríguez, Arsenio, ed. *"Isidorus medicus": Isidoro de Sevilla y los textos de medicina*. A Coruña: Servizio de Publicacións, Universidade da Coruña, 2005.

Ferraces Rodríguez, Arsenio, ed. *Tradición griega y textos médicos latinos en el período presalernitano: actas del VIII Coloquio Internacional "Textos Médicos Latinos Antiguos" (A Coruña, 2–4 septiembre 2004)*. A Coruña: Servizio de Publicacións, Universidade da Coruña, 2007.

Ferraces Rodríguez, Arsenio. 'Accidentes de transmisión y fuentes de una compilación alfabética altomedieval (Florencia, Biblioteca Medicea Laurenziana, 73. 41, ff. 1v–8v)'. In *Tradición griega y textos médicos latinos en el período presalernitano: actas del VIII Coloquio Internacional "Textos Médicos Latinos Antiguos" (A Coruña, 2–4 septiembre 2004)*, edited by Arsenio Ferraces Rodríguez, 85–104. A Coruña: Servizio de Publicacións, Universidade da Coruña, 2007.

Ferraces Rodríguez, Arsenio. 'Tradición indirecta del *De materia medica* de Dioscórides y del *De plantis* atribuido a Tésalo de Tralles: la reutilización de dos fragmentos en traducción latina'. In *Body, Disease and Treatment in a Changing World: Latin Texts and Contexts in Ancient and Medieval Medicine. Proceedings of the Ninth*

International Conference "Ancient Latin Medical Texts", Hulme Hall, University of Manchester, 5–8 September 2007, edited by David Langslow and Brigitte Maire, 201–12. Lausanne: Éditions BHMS, 2010.

Ferraces Rodríguez, Arsenio. 'Reutilización de fuentes en recetarios médicos de la antigüedad tardía: Teodoro Prisciano-*Teraupetica-Tereoperica*'. *Acta Classica: Proceedings of the Classical Association of South Africa* 64, no. 1 (2021): 212–36.

Fiddyment, Sarah, Matthew D. Teasdale, Jirí Vnouček, Élodie Lévêque, Annelise Binois, and Matthew J. Collins. 'So you want to do biocodicology? A field guide to the biological analysis of parchment'. *Heritage Science* 7 (2019). https://doi.org/10.1186/s40494-019-0278-6.

Fiddyment, Sarah, Natalie J. Goodison, Elma Brenner, Stefania Signorello, Kierri Price, and Matthew J. Collins. 'Girding the loins? Direct evidence of the use of a medieval English parchment birthing girdle from biomolecular analysis'. *Royal Society Open Science* 8, no. 3 (2021). https://doi.org/10.1098/rsos.202055.

Fischer, Klaus-Dietrich. '*Universorum ferramentorum nomina*. Frühmittelalterliche Listen chirurgischer Instrumente und ihr griechisches Vorbild'. *Mittellateinisches Jahrbuch* 22 (1987): 28–44.

Fischer, Klaus-Dietrich. 'Der *Liber medicinalis* des Pseudo-Democritus'. *Tradición e Innovación de la Medicina Latina de la Antigüedad y de la Alta Edad Media: Actas del IV Coloquio Internacional sobre los "textos médicos latinos antiguos"*, edited by Manuel Enrique Vázquez Buján, 45–56. Santiago de Compostela: Servicio de Publicacións e Intercambio Científico da Universidade de Santiago de Compostela, 1994.

Fischer, Klaus-Dietrich. *Bibliographie des textes médicaux latins. Antiquité et haut Moyen Âge: premier supplément*. Saint-Étienne: Publications de l'Université de St. Étienne, 2000.

Fischer, Klaus-Dietrich. *Bibliographie des textes médicaux latins. Antiquité et haut Moyen Âge: second supplément*. Saint-Étienne: Bibliothèque Interuniversitaire de Médecine, 2000. https://www.biusante.parisdescartes.fr/histoire/medicina/documents/fischer.php.

Fischer, Klaus-Dietrich. 'Dr Monk's Medical Digest'. *Social History of Medicine* 13, no. 2 (2000): 239–51. https://doi.org/10.1093/shm/13.2.239.

Fischer, Klaus-Dietrich. *Bibliographie des textes médicaux latins. Antiquité et haut Moyen Âge: addendum 2002*. Saint-Étienne: Bibliothèque Interuniversitaire de Médecine, 2002. https://www.biusante.parisdescartes.fr/histoire/medicina/documents/fischer2002.php.

Fischer, Klaus-Dietrich. 'Die Quellen des *Liber passionalis*'. In *Tradición griega y textos médicos latinos en el período presalernitano: actas del VIII Coloquio Internacional "Textos Médicos Latinos Antiguos" (A Coruña, 2–4 septiembre 2004)*, edited by Arsenio Ferraces Rodríguez, 105–25. A Coruña: Servizio de Publicacións, Universidade da Coruña, 2007.

Fischer, Klaus-Dietrich. 'Galen, Pardalas, and Sundry Delights for the Student of Ancient Greek Medicine'. *Galenos* 3 (2009): 161–76.

Fischer, Klaus-Dietrich. 'Die Antidotos des Zopyros und andere Fundstücke zu Scribonius Largus'. In *Body, Disease and Treatment in a Changing World: Latin Texts and Contexts in Ancient and Medieval Medicine. Proceedings of the Ninth International Conference "Ancient Latin Medical Texts", Hulme Hall, University of Manchester, 5–8 September 2007*, edited by David Langslow and Brigitte Maire, 147–60. Lausanne: Éditions BHMS, 2010.

Fischer, Klaus-Dietrich. 'Das Lorscher Arzneibuch im Widerstreit der Meinungen'. *Medizinhistorisches Journal* 45, no. 2 (2010): 165–88.

Fischer, Klaus-Dietrich. '*Antidotum cui nomen est acharistum*'. In *Between Text and Patient: The Medical Enterprise in Medieval and Early Modern Europe*, edited by Florence Eliza Glaze and Brian K. Nance, 173–99. Florence: SISMEL Edizioni del Galluzzo, 2011.

Fischer, Klaus-Dietrich. 'Wenn kein Arzt erreichbar ist—Medizinische Literatur für Laien in der Spätantike'. *Medicina nei Secoli* 24, no. 2 (2012): 379–401.

Fischer, Klaus-Dietrich. 'Unbekannter und seltener Wortschatz in den Pseudosoranischen *Quaestiones medicinales*'. *Voces* 23–24 (2012–13): 29–74.

Fischer, Klaus-Dietrich. 'Two Latin Pre-Salernitan medical manuals, the *Liber passionalis* and the *Tereoperica* (Ps. Petroncellus)'. In *Medical Books in the Byzantine World*, edited by Barbara Zipser, 35–56. Bologna: Università di Bologna, 2013.

Fischer, Klaus-Dietrich. 'Die vorsalernitanischen lateinischen Galenübersetzungen'. *Medicina nei secoli* 25, no. 3 (2013): 673–714.

Fischer, Klaus-Dietrich. 'Drugs to Declare. Two Pharmaceutical Works Attributed to Galen'. *Cuadernos de Filología Clásica. Estudios griegos e indoeuropeos* 28 (2018): 225–41. https://doi.org/10.5209/CFCG.59395.

Fischer, Klaus-Dietrich. 'In Augusto Beccarias Fuszstapfen'. In *La conoscenza scientifica nell'alto medioevo: Spoleto, 25 aprile-1 maggio 2019*, Settimane 67, vol. 1, 439–73. Spoleto: Fondazione Centro italiano di studi sull'alto medioevo, 2020.

Fischer, Klaus-Dietrich. 'A Most Sovereign Herb: Pseudo-Antonius Musa on Betony'. *Cuadernos de Filología Clásica. Estudios griegos e indoeuropeos* 30 (2020): 131–48. https://doi.org/10.5209/cfcg.68480.

Fischer Drew, Katherine. *Law and Society in Early Medieval Europe: Studies in Legal History*. London: Variorum, 1988.

Fleming, Robin. 'Bones for Historians: Putting the Body Back into Biography'. In *Writing Medieval Biography, 750–1250: Essays in Honour of Frank Barlow*, edited by David Bates, Julia Crick, and Sarah Hamilton, 29–48. Woodbridge: Boydell & Brewer, 2006.

Fleming, Robin. 'Writing Biography at the Edge of History'. *The American Historical Review* 114, no. 3 (2009): 606–14.

Flint, Valerie J. 'The Early Medieval 'Medicus', the Saint—and the Enchanter'. *Social History of Medicine* 2, no. 2 (1989): 127–45. https://doi.org/10.1093/shm/2.2.127.

Fontaine, Jacques. 'Isidore de Séville et la mutation de l'encyclopédisme antique'. *Cahiers d'Histoire Mondiale* 9, no. 1 (1966): 519–38.

Fornaciari, Gino, and Valentina Giuffra, 'The "Gout of the Medici": Making the Modern Diagnosis Using Paleopathology'. *Gene* 528, no. 1 (2013): 46–50. https://doi.org/10.1016/j.gene.2013.04.056.

Foscati, Alessandra. *Ignis sacer. Una storia culturale del 'fuoco sacro' dall'antichità al Settecento*. Florence: SISMEL Edizioni del Galluzzo, 2013.

Foscati, Alessandra. *Saint Anthony's Fire from Antiquity to the Eighteenth Century*. Translated by Francis Gordon. Amsterdam: Amsterdam University Press, 2020.

Freedman, Paul. 'Spices and Late-Medieval European Ideas of Scarcity and Value'. *Speculum* 80, no. 4 (2005): 1209–27. https://doi.org/10.1017/S0038713400001391.

Fried, Johannes. 'The Frankish Kingdoms, 817–911: The East and Middle Kingdoms'. In *The New Cambridge Medieval History* II, *c. 700-c. 900*, edited by Rosamond McKitterick, 142–68. Cambridge: Cambridge University Press, 1995.

Furdell, Elizabeth Lane, ed. *Textual Healing: Essays on Medieval and Early Modern Medicine*. Leiden: Brill, 2005.

Gamillscheg, Ernst. 'Das Geschenk für Juliana Anicia: Überlegungen zur Struktur und Entstehung des Wiener Dioskurides'. In *Byzantina Mediterranea. Festschrift für Johannes Koder zum 65. Geburtstag*, edited by Klaus Belke, Ewald Kislinger, Andreas Külzer, and Maria A. Stassinopoulou, 187–95. Vienna: Böhlau, 2007.

Ganz, David. 'Book Production in the Carolingian Empire and the Spread of Caroline Minuscule'. In *The New Cambridge Medieval History* II, *c. 700-c. 900*, edited by Rosamond McKitterick, 786–808. Cambridge: Cambridge University Press, 1995.

Garcin, V., P. Velemínsky, P. Trefny, A. Alduc-Le Bagousse, A. Lefebvre, and J. Bruzek. 'Dental Health and Lifestyle in Four Early Mediaeval Juvenile Populations: Comparisons between Urban and Rural Individuals, and between Coastal and Inland Settlements'. *HOMO—Journal of Comparative Human Biology* 61, no. 6 (2010): 421–39. https://doi.org/10.1016/j.jchb.2010.06.004.

Garofalo, Ivan, and Amneris Roselli, eds. *Galenismo e medicina tardoantica. Fonti greche, latine e arabe. Atti del Seminario internazionale di Siena, Certosa di Pontignano, 9 e 10 settembre 2002*. Naples: Istituto Universitario Orientale, 2003.

Gasparri, Stefano, and Cristina La Rocca, eds. *Carte di famiglia. Strategie, rappresentazione e memoria del gruppo familiare di Totone di Campione (721–877)*. Rome: Viella, 2005.

Geber, J. 'Comparative Study of Perimortem Weapon Trauma in Two Early Medieval Skeletal Populations (AD 400–1200) from Ireland'. *International Journal of Osteoarchaeology* 25, no. 3 (2015): 253–64. https://doi.org/10.1002/oa.2281.

Geldof, M. R. '"And to describe the shapes of the dead": Making Sense of the Archaeology of Armed Violence'. In *Wounds and Wound Repair in Medieval Culture*, edited by Larissa Tracy and Kelly DeVries, 57–80. Leiden: Brill, 2015.

Gelichi, Sauro, ed. I *Congresso Nazionale di Archeologia Medievale. Auditorium del Centro Studi della Cassa di Risparmio di Pisa (ex Benedettine), Pisa, 29–31 maggio 1997*. Florence: All'Insegna del Giglio, 1997.

Gelichi, Sauro, Diego Calaon, Elena Grandi, and Claudio Negrelli. 'The History of a Forgotten Town: Comacchio and its Archaeology'. In *From One Sea to Another. Trading Places in the European and Mediterranean Early Middle Ages: Proceedings of the International Conference, Comacchio 27th-29th March 2009*, edited by Sauro Gelichi and Richard Hodges, 169–205. Turnhout: Brepols, 2012.

Gelichi, Sauro, and Richard Hodges, eds. *From One Sea to Another. Trading Places in the European and Mediterranean Early Middle Ages: Proceedings of the International Conference, Comacchio 27th-29th March 2009*. Turnhout: Brepols, 2012.

George, Alain. 'Direct Sea Trade Between Early Islamic Iraq and Tang China: From the Exchange of Goods to the Transmission of Ideas'. *Journal of the Royal Asiatic Society* 25, no. 4 (2015): 579–624. https://doi.org/10.1017/S1356186315000231.

Gibson, Margaret T., and Janet Nelson, eds. *Charles the Bald: Court and Kingdom. Papers Based on a Colloquium Held in London in April 1979*. 2nd ed. Aldershot: Variorum, 1990.

Gilchrist, Roberta. *Medieval Life: Archaeology and the Life Course*. Woodbridge: Boydell & Brewer, 2012.

Gilman, Sharon Larimer, and Florence Eliza Glaze, '"How Science Survived"—Medieval Manuscripts as Fossils', *Science* 307 (2005): 1208–9. https://doi.org/10.1126/science.1109679.

Giuffra, V., L. Pejrani Baricco, M. Subbrizio, and G. Fornaciari. 'Weapon-related Cranial Lesions from Medieval and Renaissance Turin, Italy'. *International Journal of Osteoarchaeology* 25, no. 5 (2015): 690–700. https://doi.org/10.1002/oa.2334.

Glaze, Florence Eliza. 'The Perforated Wall: The Ownership and Circulation of Medical Books in Medieval Europe, ca. 800–1200'. PhD diss., Duke University, 1999.

Glaze, Florence Eliza. 'Master-Student Medical Dialogues: The Evidence of London, British Library, Sloane 2839'. In *Form and Content of Instruction in Anglo-Saxon England in the Light of Contemporary Manuscript Evidence: Papers Presented at the International Conference, Udine, 6–8 April 2006*, edited by Patrizia Lendinara, Loredana Lazzari, and Maria Amalia D'Aronco, 467–94. Turnhout: Brepols, 2007.

Glaze, Florence Eliza. 'Gariopontus and the Salernitans: Textual Traditions in the Eleventh and Twelfth Centuries'. In *La* Collectio Salernitana *di Salvatore De Renzi. Convegno internazionale, Università degli Studi di Salerno, 18–19 giugno 2007*, edited by Danielle Jacquart and Agostino Paravicini Bagliani, 149–90. Florence: SISMEL Edizioni del Galluzzo, 2008.

Glaze, Florence Eliza. 'Salerno's Lombard Prince: Johannes 'Abbas de Curte' as Medical Practitioner'. *Early Science and Medicine* 23, no. 3 (2018): 177–216. https://doi.org/10.1163/15733823-00233P01.

Glaze, Florence Eliza, and Brian K. Nance, eds. *Between Text and Patient: The Medical Enterprise in Medieval and Early Modern Europe*. Florence: SISMEL Edizioni del Galluzzo, 2011.

Glick, Thomas, Steven J. Livesey, and Faith Wallis, eds. *Medieval Science, Technology and Medicine: An Encyclopedia*. London: Routledge, 2005.

Goodman, Jordan, Paul E. Lovejoy, and Andrew Sherratt, eds. *Consuming Habits: Global and Historical Perspectives on How Cultures Define Drugs*. 2nd ed. London: Routledge, 2007.

Goodrich, James Tait. 'Cervical Spine Surgery in the Ancient and Medieval Worlds'. *Neurosurgical Focus* 23, no. 1 (2007): 1–22. https://doi.org/10.3171/FOC-07/07/E7.

Goodson, Caroline. *Cultivating the City in Early Medieval Italy*. Cambridge: Cambridge University Press, 2021.

Goullet, Monique, Martin Heinzelmann, and Christiane Veyrard-Cosme, eds. *L'hagiographie mérovingienne à travers ses réécritures*. Ostfildern: Thorbecke, 2010.

Grattan, J. H. G. and Charles Singer, *Anglo-Saxon Magic and Medicine: Illustrated Specially from the Semi-Pagan Text* Lacnunga. Oxford: Oxford University Press, 1952.

Grauer, Anne L., ed. *A Companion to Paleopathology*. Chichester: Wiley-Blackwell, 2012.

Green, Monica H. *Women's Healthcare in the Medieval West*. Aldershot: Ashgate, 2000.

Green, Monica H. 'Bodies, Gender, Health, Disease: Recent Work on Medieval Women's Medicine'. *Studies in Medieval and Renaissance History* 3 (2005): 1–46.

Green, Monica H. 'Gendering the History of Women's Healthcare'. *Gender & History* 20, no. 3 (2008): 487–518. https://doi.org/10.1111/j.1468-0424.2008.00534.x.

Green, Monica H. 'Integrative Medicine: Incorporating Medicine and Health into the Canon of Medieval European History'. *History Compass* 7, no. 4 (2009): 1218–45. https://doi.org/10.1111/j.1478-0542.2009.00618.x.

Green, Monica H. ''History of Medicine' or 'History of Health'?'. *Past and Future: The Magazine of the Institute of Historical Research* 9 (2011): 7–9.

Green, Monica H. 'Moving from Philology to Social History: The Circulation and Uses of Albucasis's Latin *Surgery* in the Middle Ages'. In *Between Text and Patient: The Medical Enterprise in Medieval and Early Modern Europe*, edited by Florence Eliza Glaze and Brian K. Nance, 331–72. Florence: SISMEL Edizioni del Galluzzo, 2011.

Green, Monica H., 'Genetics as a Historicist Discipline: A New Player in Disease History', *Perspectives on History* 52, no. 9 (1 December 2014), https://www.historians.org/research-and-publications/perspectives-on-history/december-2014/genetics-as-a-historicist-discipline.

Green, Monica H., ed. *Pandemic Disease in the Medieval World: Rethinking the Black Death*. Kalamazoo, MI: Arc Humanities Press, 2015.

Green, Monica H. 'The Four Black Deaths'. *American Historical Review* 125, no. 5 (2020): 1601–31. https://doi.org/10.1093/ahr/rhaa511.

Green, Monica H. 'A New Definition of the Black Death: Genetic Findings and Historical Interpretations'. *De Medio Aevo* 11, no. 2 (2022): 139–55. https://doi.org/10.5209/dmae.83788.

Grimm, Jacob, and Wilhelm Grimm, eds. *Deutsches Wörterbuch*. 32 vols. Leipzig: S. Hirzel, 1854–1961.

Grotans, Anna, Julian Hendrix, and Bernice Kaczynski. 'Understanding Medieval Manuscripts: St. Gall's Virtual Library'. *History Compass* 7, no. 3 (2009): 955–80. https://doi.org/10.1111/j.1478-0542.2009.00603.x.

Hakenbeck, Susanne. 'Potentials and Limitations of Isotope Analysis in Early Medieval Archaeology'. *European Journal of Post-Classical Archaeologies* 3 (2013): 95–111.

Haldon, John, Lee Mordechai, Timothy P. Newfield, Arlen F. Chase, Adam Izdebski, Piotr Guzowski, Inga Labuhn, and Neil Roberts. 'History meets palaeoscience: Consilience and collaboration in studying past societal responses to environmental change'. *PNAS* 115, no. 13 (2018): 3210–18. https://doi.org/10.1073/pnas.1716912115.

Halsall, Guy. *Settlement and Social Organization: The Merovingian Region of Metz*. Cambridge: Cambridge University Press, 1995.

Halsall, Guy. *Cemeteries and Society in Merovingian Gaul: Selected Studies in History and Archaeology, 1992–2009*. Leiden: Brill, 2010.

Hamilton, Bernard, ed. *The Leper King and His Heirs: Baldwin IV and the Crusader Kingdom of Jerusalem*. Cambridge: Cambridge University Press, 2000.

Hansen, Inge Lyse, and Chris Wickham, eds. *The Long Eighth Century. Production, Distribution and Demand*. Leiden: Brill, 2000.

Hansen, J. L., and K. W. Alt. 'An Exceptional Case of Dental Calculus in a Merovingian Skeleton from Mannheim-Seckenheim'. *Bulletin of the International Association for Paleodontology* 6, no. 2 (2012): 70–6.

Hardy, Gavin, and Laurence Totelin. *Ancient Botany*. London: Routledge, 2016.

Harris, William V., ed. *Popular Medicine in Graeco-Roman Antiquity: Explorations*. Leiden: Brill, 2016.

Harrison, Freya, Aled E. L. Roberts, Rebecca Gabrilska, Kendra P. Rumbaugh, Christina Lee, and Stephen P. Diggle. 'A 1,000-Year-Old Antimicrobial Remedy with Antistaphylococcal Activity'. *mBio* 6, no. 4 (2015). https://doi.org/10.1128/mBio.01129-15.

Häse, Angelika. *Mittelalterliche Bücherverzeichnisse aus Kloster Lorsch. Einleitung, Edition und Kommentar*. Wiesbaden: Harrassowitz, 2002.

Henderson, John. *The Medieval World of Isidore of Seville: Truth from Words*. Cambridge: Cambridge University Press, 2007.

Herrin, Judith. *Ravenna: Capital of Empire, Crucible of Europe*. London: Allen Lane, 2020.

Higgins, Valerie. 'The People of San Vincenzo in Late Antiquity and the Early Middle Ages'. In *San Vincenzo al Volturno 3: The Finds from the 1980–86 Excavations*, edited by John Mitchell and Inge Lyse Hansen, vol. 1, 425–37. Spoleto: Centro italiano di studi sull'alto medioevo, 2001.

Hillson, Simon. 'Recording Dental Caries in Archaeological Human Remains'. *International Journal of Osteoarchaeology* 11, no. 4 (2001): 249–89. https://doi.org/10.1002/oa.538.

Hillson, Simon. *Dental Anthropology*. Cambridge: Cambridge University Press, 1996.

Hodges, Richard. 'Adriatic Sea Trade in an European Perspective'. In *From One Sea to Another. Trading Places in the European and Mediterranean Early Middle Ages: Proceedings of the International Conference, Comacchio 27th-29th March 2009*, edited by Sauro Gelichi and Richard Hodges, 207–34. Turnhout: Brepols, 2012.

Hodges, Richard, John Mitchell, and Lucy Watson. 'The discovery of Abbot Talaricus' (817–3 October 823) tomb at San Vincenzo al Volturno'. *Antiquity* 71 (1997): 453–6. https://doi.org/10.1017/S0003598X00085082.

Horden, Peregrine. 'The Millennium Bug: Health and Medicine Around the Year 1000'. *Social History of Medicine* 13, no. 2 (2000): 201–19. https://doi.org/10.1093/shm/13.2.201.

Horden, Peregrine. 'Alms and the Man: Hospital Founders in Byzantium'. In *The Impact of Hospitals, 300–2000*, edited by John Henderson, Peregrine Horden, and Alessandro Pastore, 59–76. Oxford: Peter Lang, 2007.

Horden, Peregrine. 'Sickness and Healing'. In *The Cambridge History of Christianity 3: Early Medieval Christianities, c. 600–1100*, edited by Thomas F. X. Noble and Julia M. H. Smith, 416–32. Cambridge: Cambridge University Press, 2008.

Horden, Peregrine. *Hospitals and Healing from Antiquity to the Later Middle Ages*. Aldershot: Ashgate, 2008.

Horden, Peregrine. 'What's Wrong with Early Medieval Medicine?' *Social History of Medicine* 24, no. 1 (2011): 5–25. https://doi.org/10.1093/shm/hkp052.

Horden, Peregrine. 'Poverty, Charity, and the Invention of the Hospital'. In *The Oxford Handbook of Late Antiquity*, edited by Scott Fitzgerald Johnson, 715–43. Oxford: Oxford University Press, 2012.

Horden, Peregrine. 'Prefatory Note: The Uses of Medical Manuscripts'. In *Medical Books in the Byzantine World*, edited by Barbara Zipser, 1–6. Bologna: Università di Bologna, 2013.

Horden, Peregrine. 'Cities Within Cities: Early Hospital Foundations and Urban Space'. In *Stiftungen zwischen Politik und Wirtshaft. Ein Dialog zwischen Geschichte und Gegenwart*, edited by Sitta von Reden, 157–75. Berlin: De Gruyter, 2015.

Horden, Peregrine. *Cultures of Healing: Medieval and After*. Abingdon: Routledge, 2019.

Horn, Walter, and Ernest Born. *The Plan of St. Gall: A Study of the Architecture and Economy of, and Life in a Paradigmatic Carolingian Monastery*. 3 vols. Berkeley, CA: University of California Press, 1979.

Hymes, Robert, and Monica H. Green. *New Evidence for the Dating and Impact of the Black Death in Asia*, edited by Carol Symes. Leeds: Arc Humanities Press, 2022.

Internullo, Dario. 'Du papyrus au parchemin. Les origines médiévales de la mémoire archivistique en Europe occidentale'. *Annales. Histoire, Sciences Sociales* 74, nos. 3–4 (2019): 523–57. https://doi.org/10.1017/ahss.2020.52.

Israelowich, Ido. 'Medical Care in the Roman Army during the High Empire'. In *Popular Medicine in Graeco-Roman Antiquity: Explorations*, edited by William V. Harris, 215–30. Leiden: Brill, 2016.

Janick, Jules, and Kim E. Hummer. 'The 1500th Anniversary (512–2012) of the *Juliana Anicia Codex*: An Illustrated Dioscoridean Recension'. *Chronica Horticulturae* 52, no. 3 (2012): 9–15.

Joosten, Leo A. B., Mihai G. Netea, Eleni Mylona, Marije I. Koenders, R. K. Subbarao Malireddi, Marije Oosting, Rinke Stienstra, et al. 'Engagement of Fatty Acids with Toll-like Receptor 2 Drives Interleukin-1β Production via the ASC/Caspase 1 Pathway in Monosodium Urate Monohydrate Crystal-Induced Gouty Arthritis'. *Arthritis & Rheumatism* 62, no. 11 (2010): 3237–48. https://doi.org/10.1002/art.27667.

Judd, Margaret A., and Rebecca Redfern. 'Trauma'. In *A Companion to Paleopathology*, edited by Anne L. Grauer, 359–79. Chichester: Wiley-Blackwell, 2012.

Jurmain, Robert D., and Lynn Kilgore. 'Skeletal Evidence of Osteoarthritis: A Palaeopathological Perspective'. *Annals of the Rheumatic Diseases* 54 (1995): 443–50. https://doi.org/10.1136/ard.54.6.443.

Karenberg, Axel. 'Retrospective Diagnosis: Use and Abuse in Medical Historiography'. *Prague Medical Report* 110, no. 2 (2009): 140–5.

Keil, Gundolf. 'Möglichkeiten und Grenzen frühmittelalterlicher Medizin'. In *Das Lorscher Arzneibuch und die frühmittelalterliche Medizin: Verhandlungen des medizinhistorischen Symposiums im September 1989 in Lorsch*, edited by Gundolf Keil and Paul Schnitzer, 219–52. Lorsch: Laurissa, 1991.

Keil, Gundolf, and Paul Schnitzer, eds. *Das Lorscher Arzneibuch und die frühmittelalterliche Medizin: Verhandlungen des medizinhistorischen Symposiums im September 1989 in Lorsch*. Lorsch: Laurissa, 1991.

Kieckhefer, Richard. *Magic in the Middle Ages*. Cambridge: Cambridge University Press, 1990.

King, Anya H. *Scent from the Garden of Paradise: Musk and the Medieval Islamic World*. Leiden: Brill, 2017.

Knapp, C. W., G. E. Christidis, D. Venieri, I. Gounaki, J. Gibney-Vamvakari, M. Stillings, and E. Photos-Jones. 'The ecology and bioactivity of some Greco-Roman medicinal minerals: The case of Melos earth pigments'. *Archaeological and Anthropological Sciences* 13 (2021). https://doi.org/10.1007/s12520-021-01396-z.

Knibbs, Eric. 'How to Use Modern Critical Editions of Medieval Latin Texts'. *History Compass* 5, no. 5 (2007): 1521–49. https://doi.org/10.1111/j.1478-0542.2007.00452.x.

Knipp, David. 'The Chapel of Physicians at Santa Maria Antiqua'. *Dumbarton Oaks Papers* 56 (2002): 1–23. https://doi.org/10.2307/1291851.

Knowles, David. *Great Historical Enterprises. Problems in Monastic History*. London: Nelson, 1963.

Knowles, M. D. 'Presidential Address: Great Historical Enterprises IV. The Rolls Series'. *Transactions of the Royal Historical Society* 11 (1961): 137–159.

Kramer, Rutger. *Rethinking Authority in the Carolingian Empire: Ideals and Expectations during the Reign of Louis the Pious (813–828)*. Amsterdam: Amsterdam University Press, 2019.

Kramer, Rutger. 'Monasticism, Reform, and Authority in the Carolingian Era'. In *The Cambridge History of Medieval Monasticism in the Latin West*, edited by Alison I. Beach and Isabelle Cochelin, vol. 1, 432–49. Cambridge: Cambridge University Press, 2020.

Kreiner, Jamie. *Legions of Pigs in the Early Medieval West*. New Haven: Yale University Press, 2020.

Kristjánsdóttir, Steinunn. 'The Tip of the Iceberg: The Material of Skriðuklaustur Monastery and Hospital'. *Norwegian Archaeological Review* 43, no. 1 (2010): 44–62. https://doi.org/10.1080/00293651003798796.

Kropp, Claus, Anne-Karin Kirsch, Wilfried Rosendahl, Jörg Orschiedt, and Lukas Fischer. *Begraben und Vergessen? Knochen erzählen Geschichte: Anthropologische Ausstellung im Schaudepot Zehntscheune des UNESCO Welterbe Kloster Lorsch*. Bad Homburg v. d. Höhe: Verwaltung der Staatlichen Schlösser und Gärten, 2017.

Kwakkel, Erik, Rosamond McKitterick, and Rodney Thomson. *Turning Over a New Leaf: Change and Development in the Medieval Book*. Leiden: Leiden University Press, 2012.

Lake, Justin. 'Current Approaches to Medieval Historiography'. *History Compass* 13, no. 3 (2015): 89–109. https://doi.org/10.1111/hic3.12222.

Landgraf, Erhard. 'Ein frühmittelalterlicher Botanicus'. *Kyklos* 1 (1928): 114–46.

Langsjoen, Odin M. 'Diseases of the Dentition'. In *The Cambridge Encyclopedia of Human Paleopathology*, edited by Arthur C. Aufderheide and Conrado Rodríguez-Martín, 393–412. Cambridge: Cambridge University Press, 1998.

Langslow, David R., 'Some historical developments in the terminology and style of Latin medical writings'. In *Tradición e Innovación de la Medicina Latina de la Antigüedad y de la Alta Edad Media: Actas del IV Coloquio Internacional sobre los "textos médicos latinos antiguos"*, edited by Manuel Enrique Vázquez Buján, 225–40. Santiago de

Compostela: Servicio de Publicacións e Intercambio Científico da Universidade de Santiago de Compostela, 1994.

Langslow, D. R. 'The Language of Poetry and the Language of Science: The Latin Poets and 'Medical Latin''. *Proceedings of the British Academy* 93 (1999): 183–225.

Langslow, D. R. *Medical Latin in the Roman Empire*. Oxford: Oxford University Press, 2000.

Langslow, David, and Brigitte Maire, eds. *Body, Disease and Treatment in a Changing World: Latin Texts and Contexts in Ancient and Medieval Medicine. Proceedings of the Ninth International Conference "Ancient Latin Medical Texts", Hulme Hall, University of Manchester, 5–8 September 2007*. Lausanne: Éditions BHMS, 2010.

Laurioux, Bruno. 'Parfums d'Orient. La science des épices au Moyen Âge'. In *Parfums et odeurs au Moyen Âge. Science, usage, symboles*, edited by Agostino Paravicini Bagliani, 61–87. Florence: SISMEL Edizioni del Galluzzo, 2015.

Lavan, Luke, and Michael Mulryan, eds. *Field Methods and Post-Excavation Techniques in Late Antique Archaeology*. Leiden: Brill, 2015.

Leggett, Sam. 'A Hierarchical Meta-Analytical Approach to Western European Dietary Transitions in the First Millennium AD'. *European Journal of Archaeology* 25, no. 4 (2022): 523–43. https://doi.org/10.1017/eaa.2022.23.

Leggett, Sam, and Tom Lambert. 'Food and Power in Early Medieval England: A Lack of (Isotopic) Enrichment'. *Anglo-Saxon England* 49 (2020): 155–96. https://doi.org/10.1017/S0263675122000072.

Leja, Meg. 'The Sacred Art: Medicine in the Carolingian Renaissance'. *Viator* 47, no. 2 (2016): 1–34. https://doi.org/10.1484/J.VIATOR.5.111224.

Leja, Meg. *Embodying the Soul: Medicine and Religion in Carolingian Europe*. Philadelphia: University of Pennsylvania Press, 2022.

Lendinara, Patrizia, Loredana Lazzari, and Maria Amalia D'Aronco, eds. *Form and Content of Instruction in Anglo-Saxon England in the Light of Contemporary Manuscript Evidence: Papers Presented at the International Conference, Udine, 6–8 April 2006*. Turnhout: Brepols, 2007.

Lestocquoy, Jean. 'Épices, médecine et abbayes', In *Études mérovingiennes. Actes des journées de Poitiers, 1er-3 mai 1952*, 179–86. Paris: A. et J. Picard, 1953.

Lev, Efraim. 'Botanical View of the Use of Plants in Medieval Medicine in the Eastern Mediterranean According to the Cairo Genizah'. *Israel Journal of Plant Sciences* 62, nos. 1–2 (2015): 122–40. https://doi.org/10.1080/07929978.2014.887380.

Lev, Efraim, and Zohar Amar. *Practical* Materia Medica *of the Medieval Eastern Mediterranean According to the Cairo Genizah*. Leiden: Brill, 2008.

Lev, Efraim, and Leigh Chipman. *Medical Prescriptions in the Cambridge Genizah Collections: Practical Medicine and Pharmacology in Medieval Egypt*. Leiden: Brill, 2012.

Lewis, Charlton T., and Charles Short. *A Latin Dictionary*. Oxford: The Clarendon Press, 1879.

Licata, Marta, Melania Borgo, Giuseppe Armocida, Luca Nicosia, and Elena Ferioli. 'New Paleoradiological Investigations of Ancient Human Remains from North West Lombardy Archaeological Excavations'. *Skeletal Radiology* 45 (2016): 323–31. https://doi.org/10.1007/s00256-015-2266-6.

Licata, Marta, Mario Ronga, Paolo Cherubino, and Giuseppe Armocida. 'Different Types of Traumatic Lesions on Mediaeval Skeletons from Archaeological Sites in Varese (North Italy): Diagnosis on *ante mortal* Fractures Using Macroscopic, Radiological and CT Analysis'. *Injury* 45, no. 2 (2014): 457–9. https://doi.org/10.1016/j.injury.2013.10.013.

Lifshitz, Felice. 'The Historiography of Central Medieval Western Monasticism'. In *The Cambridge History of Medieval Monasticism in the Latin West*, edited by Alison I. Beach and Isabelle Cochelin, vol. 1, 365–81. Cambridge: Cambridge University Press, 2020.

Lindberg, David C., and Michael H. Shank, eds. *The Cambridge History of Science 2: Medieval Science*. Cambridge: Cambridge University Press, 2013.

Liuzza, Roy Michael. 'The Sphere of Life and Death: Time, Medicine, and the Visual Imagination'. In *Latin Learning and English Lore: Studies in Anglo-Saxon Literature for Michael Lapidge*, edited by Katherine O'Brien O'Keeffe and Andy Orchard, vol. 2, 28–52. Toronto: University of Toronto Press, 2005.

López Figueroa, Laura. 'From Cassius Felix to *Tereoperica*: New Considerations on Indirect Tradition'. In *'Greek' and 'Roman' in Latin Medical Texts: Studies in Cultural Change and Exchange in Ancient Medicine*, edited by Brigitte Maire, 383–401. Leiden: Brill, 2014.

López Martínez, Belén, Antonio Fernández Pardiñas, Eva García Vázquez, and Eduardo Dopico Rodríguez. 'Socio-Cultural Factors in Dental Diseases in the Medieval and Early Modern Age of Northern Spain'. *HOMO—Journal of Comparative Human Biology* 63, no. 1 (2012): 21–42. https://doi.org/10.1016/j.jchb.2011.12.001.

López-Sampson, Arlene, and Tony Page. 'History of Use and Trade of Agarwood'. *Economic Botany* 72 (2018): 107–129. https://doi.org/10.1007/s12231-018-9408-4.

Lowe, E. A. *Codices Latini antiquiores: A Palaeographical Guide to Latin Manuscripts Prior to the Ninth Century*, 11 vols. Oxford: Clarendon Press, 1934–66.

Lukacs, John R. 'Oral Health in Past Populations: Context, Concepts and Controversies'. In *A Companion to Paleopathology*, edited by Anne L. Grauer, 553–81. Chichester: Wiley-Blackwell, 2012.

MacKinney, Loren C. 'Tenth-Century Medicine as Seen in the *Historia* of Richer of Rheims', *Bulletin of the Institute of the History of Medicine* 2, no. 6 (1934): 347–75.

MacKinney, Loren C. '"Dynamidia" in Medieval Medical Literature', *Isis* 24, no. 2 (1936): 400–14.

MacKinney, Loren C. *Early Medieval Medicine, With Special Reference to France and Chartres*. Baltimore: Johns Hopkins Press, 1937.

MacKinney, Loren C. 'An Unpublished Treatise on Medicine and Magic from the Age of Charlemagne'. *Speculum* 18, no. 4 (1943): 494–6. https://doi.org/10.2307/2853665.

MacKinney, Loren C. 'Medical Education in the Middle Ages'. *Cahiers d'histoire mondiale* 2, no. 4 (1955): 835–61.

Maire, Brigitte. 'Proposition d'un nouveau *stemma codicum* de la tradition manuscrite du *De medicina* d'Aulus Cornelius Celsus'. In *Tradición e Innovación de la Medicina Latina de la Antigüedad y de la Alta Edad Media: Actas del IV Coloquio Internacional sobre los "textos médicos latinos antiguos"*, edited by Manuel Enrique Vázquez Buján, 87–99. Santiago de Compostela: Servicio de Publicacións e Intercambio Científico da Universidade de Santiago de Compostela, 1994.

Maire, Brigitte. 'Apport de Mustio à la représentation de la femme antique'. In *Body, Disease and Treatment in a Changing World: Latin Texts and Contexts in Ancient and Medieval Medicine. Proceedings of the Ninth International Conference "Ancient Latin Medical Texts", Hulme Hall, University of Manchester, 5–8 September 2007*, edited by David Langslow and Brigitte Maire, 49–60. Lausanne: Éditions BHMS, 2010.

Maire, Brigitte, ed. *'Greek' and 'Roman' in Latin Medical Texts: Studies in Cultural Change and Exchange in Ancient Medicine*. Leiden: Brill, 2014.

Mallegni, Francesco, Elena Bedini, Angelica Vitiello, Laura Paglialunga, and Fulvio Bartoli. 'Su alcuni gruppi umani del territorio piemontese dal IV al XVIII secolo: aspetti di paleobiologia'. In *Archeologia in Piemonte*, edited by Liliana Mercando, Marica Venturino Gambari, and Egle Micheletto, vol. 3, 233–61. Turin: Allemandi, 1998.

Manicardi, Alberto, ed. *San Lorenzo di Quingentole: archeologia, storia ed antropologia*. Mantua: SAP, 2001.

Mariotti, Valeria, ed. *Un monastero nei secoli. Santa Maria Assunta di Cairate: scavi e ricerche*. Mantua: SAP, 2014.

Martin, Elizabeth A., ed. *Oxford Concise Medical Dictionary*. 9th ed. Oxford: Oxford University Press, 2015. https://doi.org/10.1093/acref/9780199687817.001.0001.

Martínez, Javier, and Patricia González. 'Knowledge and Specialised Trade in the Late Antique West: Medicine vs Engineering'. *Journal for Late Antique Religion and Culture* 11 (2017): 38–58. https://doi.org/10.18573/j.2017.10451.

Martínez Prieto, Rocío. 'A Short Approach to the Analysis of the Textual Tradition of an Extract about Phytotherapy from the Codex Sangallensis 751'. In *II Jornadas Predoctorales en Estudios de la Antigüedad y de la Edad Media. Κτῆμα ἐς αἰεὶ: el texto como herramienta común para estudiar el pasado: Proceedings of the Second Postgraduate Conference in Studies of Antiquity and Middle Ages, Universitat Autònoma de Barcelona, 19–21st November 2014*, edited by Núria Olaya Montero, Manuel Montoza Coca, Alba Aguilera Felipe and Roser Gómez Guiu, 115–19. Oxford: BAR, 2015.

Mattucci, Anny, Cristina Ravedoni, and Elena Rettore. 'Analisi antropologica e paleopatologica della popolazione rinvenuta nel monastero dell'Assunta di Cairate'. In

Un monastero nei secoli. Santa Maria Assunta di Cairate: scavi e ricerche, edited by Valeria Mariotti, 519–32. Mantua: SAP, 2014.

Mayali, Laurent, and Stephanie A. J. Tibbetts, eds. *The Two Laws: Studies in Medieval Legal History Dedicated to Stephan Kuttner*. Washington, DC: Catholic University of America Press, 1990.

Mays, S. A. 'A Possible Case of Surgical Treatment of Cranial Blunt Force Injury from Medieval England'. *International Journal of Osteoarchaeology* 16, no. 2 (2006): 95–103. https://doi.org/10.1002/oa.806.

Mays, Simon. 'A Biomechanical Study of Activity Patterns in a Medieval Human Skeletal Assemblage'. *International Journal of Osteoarchaeology* 9, no. 1 (1999): 68–73. https://doi.org/10.1002/(SICI)1099-1212(199901/02)9:1%3C68::AID-OA468%3E3.0.CO;2-M.

Mazzini, Innocenzo. 'Les traductions latines d'Oribase et d'Hippocrate'. In *Les écoles médicales à Rome: Actes du 2ème Colloque international sur les textes médicaux latins antiques, Lausanne, septembre 1986*, edited by Philippe Mudry and Jackie Pigeaud, 286–93. Geneva: Droz, 1991.

Mazzini, Innocenzo. 'Il sapone di Costantino'. In *Costantino il grande: dall'Antichità all'umanesimo: colloquio sul Cristianesimo nel mondo antico, Macerata, 18-20 Dicembre 1990*, edited by Giorgio Bonamente and Franca Fusco, vol. 2, 693–9. Macerata: Università degli studi di Macerata, 1992–3.

Mazzini, Innocenzo. 'References to Medical Authors in Non-Medical Latin Literature'. In *'Greek' and 'Roman' in Latin Medical Texts: Studies in Cultural Change and Exchange in Ancient Medicine*, edited by Brigitte Maire, 77–91. Leiden: Brill, 2014.

McCormick, Michael. 'Byzantium and the West, 700–900'. In *The New Cambridge Medieval History* II, *c. 700-c. 900*, edited by Rosamond McKitterick, 349–80. Cambridge: Cambridge University Press, 1995.

McCormick, Michael. *Origins of the European Economy: Communications and Commerce, AD 300–900*. Cambridge: Cambridge University Press, 2001.

McCormick, Michael. 'Molecular Middle Ages: Early Medieval Economic History in the Twenty-First Century'. In *The Long Morning of Medieval Europe: New Directions in Early Medieval Studies*, edited by Jennifer R. Davis and Michael McCormick, 83–97. Aldershot: Ashgate, 2008.

McCormick, Michael. 'Comparing and Connecting: Comacchio and the Early Medieval Trading Towns'. In *From One Sea to Another. Trading Places in the European and Mediterranean Early Middle Ages: Proceedings of the International Conference, Comacchio 27th-29th March 2009*, edited by Sauro Gelichi and Richard Hodges, 477–502. Turnhout: Brepols, 2012.

McKinley, Jacqueline I. 'A Probable Trepanation from an Early Anglo-Saxon Cemetery at Oxborough, Norfolk'. *International Journal of Osteoarchaeology* 2, no. 4 (1992): 333–35. https://doi.org/10.1002/oa.1390020409.

McKitterick, Rosamond. *The Frankish Kingdoms under the Carolingians, 751–987*. London: Longman, 1983.

McKitterick, Rosamond. *The Carolingians and the Written Word*. Cambridge: Cambridge University Press, 1989.

McKitterick, Rosamond, ed. *Carolingian Culture: Emulation and Innovation*. Cambridge: Cambridge University Press, 1994.

McKitterick, Rosamond, ed. *The New Cambridge Medieval History* II, *c. 700-c. 900*. Cambridge: Cambridge University Press, 1995.

McKitterick, Rosamond. 'Eighth-Century Foundations'. In *The New Cambridge Medieval History* II, *c. 700-c. 900*, edited by Rosamond McKitterick, 681–94. Cambridge: Cambridge University Press, 1995.

McKitterick, Rosamond. 'Introduction: Sources and Interpretation'. In *The New Cambridge Medieval History* II, *c. 700-c. 900*, edited by Rosamond McKitterick, 3–17. Cambridge: Cambridge University Press, 1995.

McKitterick, Rosamond. *History and Memory in the Carolingian World*. Cambridge: Cambridge University Press, 2004.

McKitterick, Rosamond. 'The Carolingian Renaissance of Culture and Learning'. In *Charlemagne: Empire and Society*, edited by Joanna Story, 151–66. Manchester: Manchester University Press, 2005.

McKitterick, Rosamond. *Charlemagne: The Formation of a European Identity*. Cambridge: Cambridge University Press, 2008.

McVaugh, Michael R. *Medicine before the Plague: Practitioners and their Patients in the Crown of Aragon, 1285–1345*. Cambridge: Cambridge University Press, 1993.

McVaugh, Michael. *The Rational Surgery of the Middle Ages*. Florence: SISMEL Edizioni del Galluzzo, 2006.

Meaney, Audrey L. 'The Anglo-Saxon View of the Causes of Illness'. In *Health, Disease and Healing in Medieval Culture*, edited by Sheila Campbell, Bert Hall, and David Klausner, 12–33. Houndmills: Macmillan, 1992.

Meaney, Audrey. 'The Practice of Medicine in England about the Year 1000'. *Social History of Medicine* 13, no. 2 (2000): 221–37. https://doi.org/10.1093/shm/13.2.221.

Meaney, Audrey L. 'Extra-Medical Elements in Anglo-Saxon Medicine'. *Social History of Medicine* 24, no. 1 (2011): 41–56. https://doi.org/10.1093/shm/hkq105.

Meens, Rob, Dorine van Espelo, Bram van den Hoven van Genderen, Janneke Raaijmakers, Irene van Renswoude, and Carine van Rhijn, eds. *Religious Franks. Religion and Power in the Frankish Kingdoms: Studies in Honour of Mayke de Jong*. Manchester: Manchester University Press, 2016.

Meinl, A., G. M. Rottensteiner, C. D. Huber, S. Tangl, G. Watzak, and G. Watzek. 'Caries frequency and distribution in an early medieval Avar population from Austria'. *Oral Diseases* 16, no. 1 (2010): 108–16. https://doi.org/10.1111/j.1601-0825.2009.01624.x.

Mercando, Liliana, Marica Venturino Gambari, and Egle Micheletto, eds. *Archeologia in Piemonte*. 3 vols. Turin: Allemandi, 1998.

Mistry, Zubin. *Abortion in the Early Middle Ages, c. 500–900*. Woodbridge: Boydell & Brewer, 2015.

Mitchell, John, Lucy Watson, Flavia De Rubeis, Richard Hodges, and Ian Wood. 'Cult, Relics and Privileged Burial at San Vincenzo al Volturno in the Age of Charlemagne: The Discovery of the Tomb of Abbot Talaricus (817–3 October 823)'. In *I Congresso Nazionale di Archeologia Medievale. Auditorium del Centro Studi della Cassa di Risparmio di Pisa (ex Benedettine), Pisa, 29–31 maggio 1997*, edited by Sauro Gelichi, 315–21. Florence: All'Insegna del Giglio, 1997.

Mitchell, Piers D. 'An Evaluation of the Leprosy of King Baldwin IV of Jerusalem in the Context of the Medieval World'. In *The Leper King and His Heirs: Baldwin IV and the Crusader Kingdom of Jerusalem*, edited by Bernard Hamilton, 245–58. Cambridge: Cambridge University Press, 2000.

Mitchell, Piers D. *Medicine in the Crusades: Warfare, Wounds and the Medieval Surgeon*. Cambridge: Cambridge University Press, 2004.

Mitchell, Piers D. 'Retrospective Diagnosis and the Use of Historical Texts for Investigating Disease in the Past'. *International Journal of Paleopathology* 1, no. 2 (2011): 81–8. https://doi.org/10.1016/j.ijpp.2011.04.002.

Mitchell, Piers D. 'Palaeopathology of the Crusades'. In *Crusader Landscapes in the Medieval Levant: The Archaeology and History of the Latin East*, edited by Micaela Sinibaldi, Kevin J. Lewis, Balázs Major, and Jennifer A. Thompson, 349–59. Cardiff: University of Wales Press, 2016.

Mitchell, Piers D. 'Improving the Use of Historical Written Sources in Paleopathology'. *International Journal of Paleopathology* 19 (2017): 88–95. https://doi.org/10.1016/j.ijpp.2016.02.005.

Montanari, Armando, ed. *Food and Environment: Geographies of Taste*. Rome: Società Geografica Italiana, 2002.

Mostert, Marco. *The Library of Fleury. A Provisional List of Manuscripts*. Hilversum: Verloren, 1989.

Motto, Monica. 'Sepolture nel monastero di Cairate: tipologia e organizzazione delle aree cimiteriali, uno sguardo di sintesi'. In *Un monastero nei secoli. Santa Maria Assunta di Cairate: scavi e ricerche*, edited by Valeria Mariotti, 501–18. Mantua: SAP, 2014.

Müller, Antonia, and Kais Hussein. 'Meta-Analysis of Teeth from European Populations Before and After the 18th Century Reveals a Shift Towards Increased Prevalence of Caries and Tooth Loss'. *Archives of Oral Biology* 73 (2017): 7–15. https://doi.org/10.1016/j.archoralbio.2016.08.018.

Muramoto, Osamu. 'Retrospective Diagnosis of a Famous Historical Figure: Ontological, Epistemic, and Ethical Considerations'. *Philosophy, Ethics, and Humanities in Medicine* 9 (2014). https://doi.org/10.1186/1747-5341-9-10.

Navitainuck, Denise, Christian Meyer, and Kurt W. Alt. 'Degenerative Alterations of the Spine in an Early Mediaeval Population from Mannheim-Seckenheim, Germany'. *HOMO—Journal of Comparative Human Biology* 64, no. 3 (2013): 179–89. https://doi.org/10.1016/j.jchb.2013.03.007.

Nelson, Janet L. 'The Frankish Kingdoms, 814–898: The West'. In *The New Cambridge Medieval History* II, *c. 700-c. 900*, edited by Rosamond McKitterick, 110–41. Cambridge: Cambridge University Press, 1995.

Nelson, Janet L., 'Revisiting the Carolingian Renaissance'. In *Motions of Late Antiquity: Essays on Religion, Politics, and Society in Honour of Peter Brown*, edited by Jamie Kreiner and Helmut Reimitz, 331–46. Turnhout: Brepols, 2016.

Nelson, Max. *The Barbarian's Beverage: A History of Beer in Ancient Europe*. London: Routledge, 2005.

Nelson, Max. 'The Geography of Beer in Europe from 1000 BC to AD 1000'. In *The Geography of Beer: Regions, Environments, and Societies*, edited by Mark Patterson and Nancy Hoalst-Pullen, 9–21. Dordrecht: Springer, 2014.

Newfield, Timothy P. 'Domesticates, Disease and Climate in Early Post-Classical Europe: The Cattle Plague of c.940 and its Environmental Context'. *Postclassical Archaeologies* 5 (2015): 95–126.

Newfield, Timothy P. 'Malaria and Malaria-like Disease in the Early Middle Ages'. *Early Medieval Europe* 25, no. 3 (2017): 251–300. https://doi.org/10.1111/emed.12212.

Newfield, Timothy P. 'Mysterious and Mortiferous Clouds: The Climate Cooling and Disease Burden of Late Antiquity'. In *Environment and Society in the Long Late Antiquity*, edited by Adam Izdebski and Michael Mulryan, 271–97. Leiden: Brill, 2019.

Niermeyer, Jan Frederik. *Mediae Latinitatis Lexicon Minus*. 2nd ed. Leiden: Brill, 2002.

Nievergelt, Andreas, Rudolf Gamper, Marina Bernasconi Reusser, Birgit Ebersperger, and Ernst Tremp, eds. *Scriptorium: Wesen, Funktion, Eigenheiten. Comité international de paléographie latine. XVIII. Kolloquium, St. Gallen, 11.-14. September 2013*. Munich: Beck, 2015.

Noble, Thomas F. X., and Julia M. H. Smith, eds. *The Cambridge History of Christianity 3: Early Medieval Christianities, c. 600–1100*. Cambridge: Cambridge University Press, 2008.

Norri, Juhani. 'Translation from Latin and French as a Source of New Medical Terms in Late Medieval England'. *Romance Philology* 71, no. 2 (2017): 563–622. https://doi.org/10.1484/J.RPH.5.114789.

Nuki, George, and Peter A. Simkin. 'A concise history of gout and hyperuricemia and their treatment'. *Arthritis Research and Therapy* 8 (2006). https://doi.org/10.1186/ar1906.

Nutton, Vivian. 'From Galen to Alexander, Aspects of Medicine and Medical Practice in Late Antiquity'. *Dumbarton Oaks Papers* 38 (1984): 1–14. https://doi.org/10.2307/1291489.

Nutton, Vivian. 'Medicine in Late Antiquity and the Early Middle Ages'. In *The Western Medical Tradition: 800 BC to AD 1800*, edited by Lawrence I. Conrad, Michael Neve, Vivian Nutton, Roy Porter, and Andrew Wear, 71–88. Cambridge: Cambridge University Press, 1995.

Nutton, Vivian. 'Medicine in the Greek World, 800–50 BC'. In *The Western Medical Tradition: 800 BC to AD 1800*, edited by Lawrence I. Conrad, Michael Neve, Vivian Nutton, Roy Porter, and Andrew Wear, 11–38. Cambridge: Cambridge University Press, 1995.

Nutton, Vivian. 'Roman Medicine, 250 BC to AD 200'. In *The Western Medical Tradition: 800 BC to AD 1800*, edited by Lawrence I. Conrad, Michael Neve, Vivian Nutton, Roy Porter, and Andrew Wear, 39–70. Cambridge: Cambridge University Press, 1995.

Nutton, Vivian. *Ancient Medicine*. 2nd ed. Abingdon: Routledge, 2013.

Nutton, Vivian. 'Early Medieval Medicine and Natural Science'. In *The Cambridge History of Science 2: Medieval Science*, edited by David C. Lindberg and Michael H. Shank, 323–40. Cambridge: Cambridge University Press, 2013.

Nutton, Vivian. *Galen: A Thinking Doctor in Imperial Rome*. Abingdon: Routledge, 2020.

O'Brien O'Keeffe, Katherine, and Andy Orchard, eds. *Latin Learning and English Lore: Studies in Anglo-Saxon Literature for Michael Lapidge*. 2 vols. Toronto: University of Toronto Press, 2005.

OED Online. Oxford: Oxford University Press, 2023. https://www.oed.com.

Oliver, Lisi. *The Body Legal in Barbarian Law*. Toronto: University of Toronto Press, 2011.

Olsen, Karin E., Antonina Harbus, and Tette Hofstra, eds. *Germanic Texts and Latin Models: Medieval Reconstructions*. Leuven: Peeters, 2001.

Opsomer, Carmélia. *Index de la pharmacopée du Ier au Xe siècle*. 2 vols. Hildesheim: Olms-Weidmann, 1989.

Ortner, Donald J. 'What Skeletons Tell Us: The Story of Human Paleopathology'. *Virchows Archiv* 459 (2011): 247–54. https://doi.org/10.1007/s00428-011-1122-x.

Ostorero, Martine. 'L'odeur fétide des démons: une preuve de leur présence corporelle au sabbat'. In *Parfums et odeurs au Moyen Âge. Science, usage, symboles*, edited by Agostino Paravicini Bagliani, 259–88. Florence: SISMEL Edizioni del Galluzzo, 2015.

Palmer, James T. 'Merovingian Medicine between Practical Art and Philosophy', *Traditio* (forthcoming).

Palmieri, Nicoletta. 'Les commentaires de Galien'. In *Les écoles médicales à Rome: Actes du 2ème Colloque international sur les textes médicaux latins antiques, Lausanne, septembre 1986*, edited by Philippe Mudry and Jackie Pigeaud, 294–310. Geneva: Droz, 1991.

Palmieri, Nicoletta. 'Il commento latino-ravennate all'*Ars medica* di Galeno e la tradizione alessandrina'. In *Tradición e Innovación de la Medicina Latina de la Antigüedad y de la Alta Edad Media: Actas del IV Coloquio Internacional sobre los "textos médicos latinos antiguos"*, edited by Manuel Enrique Vázquez Buján, 57–75. Santiago de Compostela: Servicio de Publicacións e Intercambio Científico da Universidade de Santiago de Compostela, 1994.

Palmieri, Nicoletta. 'Nouvelles remarques sur les commentaires à Galien de l'école médicale de Ravenne'. In *«Docente natura». Mélanges de médecine ancienne et médiévale offerts à Guy Sabbah*, edited by Armelle Debru and Nicoletta Palmieri, 209–46. Saint-Étienne: Publications de l'Université de Saint-Étienne, 2001.

Palmieri, Nicoletta. 'Il galenismo alessandrino in Italia tra antichità tarda e alto medioevo'. In *La conoscenza scientifica nell'alto medioevo: Spoleto, 25 aprile-1 maggio 2019*, Settimane 67, vol. 1, 237–70. Spoleto: Fondazione Centro italiano di studi sull'alto medioevo, 2020.

Panhuysen, Raphaël G. A. M. 'Het scherp van de snede: Sporen van geweld in vroegmiddeleeuws Maastricht'. *Archeologie in Limburg* 92 (2002): 2–7.

Panhuysen, Raphaël G. A. M. 'Demography and Health in Early Medieval Maastricht: Prosopographical Observations on Two Cemeteries'. Diss., Universiteit Maastricht, 2005.

Paravicini Bagliani, Agostino, ed. *Parfums et odeurs au Moyen Âge. Science, usage, symboles*. Florence: SISMEL Edizioni del Galluzzo, 2015.

Parejko, Ken. 'Pliny the Elder's Silphium: First Recorded Species Extinction'. *Conservation Biology* 17, no. 3 (2003): 925–7.

Park, Katharine. 'Medicine and Society in Medieval Europe, 500–1500'. In *Medicine in Society: Historical Essays*, edited by Andrew Wear, 59–90. Cambridge: Cambridge University Press, 1992.

Patterson, Mark, and Nancy Hoalst-Pullen, eds. *The Geography of Beer: Regions, Environments, and Societies*. Dordrecht: Springer, 2014.

Paxton, Frederick S. '*Bonus Liber*: A Late Carolingian Clerical Manual from Lorsch (Biblioteca Vaticana MS Pal. lat. 485)'. In *The Two Laws: Studies in Medieval Legal History Dedicated to Stephan Kuttner*, edited by Laurent Mayali and Stephanie A. J. Tibbetts, 1–30. Washington, DC: Catholic University of America Press, 1990.

Paxton, Frederick S. 'Curing Bodies—Curing Souls: Hrabanus Maurus, Medical Education, and the Clergy in Ninth-Century Francia'. *Journal of the History of Medicine and Allied Sciences* 50, no. 2 (1995): 230–252.

Pearce, John. 'Beyond the Grave: Excavating the Dead in the Late Roman Provinces'. In *Field Methods and Post-Excavation Techniques in Late Antique Archaeology*, edited by Luke Lavan and Michael Mulryan, 441–82. Leiden: Brill, 2015.

Pezo Lanfranco, Luis, and Sabine Eggers, 'Caries Through Time: An Anthropological Overview'. In *Contemporary Approach to Dental Caries*, edited by Ming-Yu Li, 3–34. Rijeka: IntechOpen, 2012. https://doi.org/10.5772/38059.

Pilsworth, Clare. 'Could you just sign this for me John? Doctors, charters and occupational identity in early medieval northern and central Italy'. *Early Medieval Europe* 17, no. 4 (2009): 363–88. https://doi.org/10.1111/j.1468-0254.2009.00282.x.

Pilsworth, Clare. 'Beyond the Medical Text: Health and Illness in Early Medieval Italian Sources'. *Social History of Medicine* 24, no. 1 (2011): 26–40. https://doi.org/10.1093/shm/hkq115.

Pilsworth, Clare. *Healthcare in Early Medieval Northern Italy: More to Life than Leeches?* Turnhout: Brepols, 2014.

Platte, Adelheid, and Karlheinz Platte, eds. *Das Lorscher Arzneibuch: Klostermedizin in der Karolingerzeit*. Lorsch: Laurissa, 1990.

Questa, Cesare, and Renato Raffaelli, eds. *Il libro e il testo: atti del Convegno Internazionale, Urbino, 20–23 Settembre 1982*. Urbino: Università degli Studi di Urbino, 1984.

Radini, A., M. Tromp, A. Beach, E. Tong, C. Speller, M. McCormick, J. V. Dudgeon, et al. 'Medieval women's early involvement in manuscript production suggested by lapis lazuli identification in dental calculus'. *Science Advances* 5, no. 1 (2019). https://doi.org/10.1126/sciadv.aau7126.

Ragab, Gaafar, Mohsen Elshahaly, and Thomas Bardin. 'Gout: An old disease in new perspective—A review'. *Journal of Advanced Research* 8, no. 5 (2017): 495–511. https://doi.org/10.1016/j.jare.2017.04.008.

Rajamma, Rajasree K., Audhesh K. Paswan, and Lou E. Pelton. 'Flipping the script: Consumers' propensity for self-medication'. *Journal of Marketing Theory and Practice* 29, no. 4 (2021): 448–62. https://doi.org/10.1080/10696679.2020.1870240.

Redi, Fabio, and Alfonso Forgione, eds. *VI Congresso Nazionale di Archeologia Medievale. Sala Conferenze "E. Sericchi", Centro Direzionale CARISPAQ "Strinella 88". L'Aquila, 12–15 settembre 2012*. Florence: All'Insegna del Giglio, 2012.

Riddle, John M. 'The Introduction and Use of Eastern Drugs in the Early Middle Ages'. *Sudhoffs Archiv für Geschichte der Medizin und der Naturwissenschaften* 49, no. 2 (1965): 185–98.

Riddle, John M. 'Theory and Practice in Medieval Medicine'. *Viator* 5 (1974): 157–84. https://doi.org/10.1484/J.VIATOR.2.301620.

Riddle, John M. 'Pseudo-Dioscorides' *Ex herbis femininis* and Early Medieval Medical Botany'. *Journal of the History of Biology* 14, no. 1 (1981): 43–81.

Riddle, John M. *Dioscorides on Pharmacy and Medicine*. Austin: University of Texas Press, 1985.

Riddle, John M. 'The Pseudo-Hippocratic *Dynamidia*'. *Sudhoffs Archiv für Geschichte der Medizin und der Naturwissenschaften* 27 (1989): 283–311.

Riddle, John M. *Contraception and Abortion from the Ancient World to the Renaissance.* Cambridge, MA: Harvard University Press, 1992.

Riddle, John M. *Quid pro quo: Studies in the History of Drugs*. Aldershot: Variorum, 1992.

Riddle, John M. 'Research Procedures in Evaluating Medieval Medicine'. In *The Medieval Hospital and Medical Practice,* edited by Barbara S. Bowers, 3–17. Aldershot: Ashgate, 2007.

Rio, Alice. *Legal Practice and the Written Word in the Early Middle Ages: Frankish Formulae, c. 500–1000*. Cambridge: Cambridge University Press, 2009.

Roberts, Charlotte A. *Human Remains in Archaeology: A Handbook.* Rev. ed. York: Council for British Archaeology, 2012.

Roberts, Charlotte A., and Jacqueline McKinley. 'A Review of Trepanations in British Antiquity Focusing on Funerary Context to Explain Their Occurrence'. In *Trepanation: History, Discovery, Theory*, edited by Robert Arnott, Stanley Finger, and C. U. M. Smith, 55–78. Lisse: Swets & Zeitlinger Publishers, 2003.

Rogers, Juliet, and Tony Waldron. 'DISH and the Monastic Way of Life'. *International Journal of Osteoarchaeology* 11, no. 5 (2001): 357–65. https://doi.org/10.1002/oa.574.

Rogers, Juliet, Iain Watt, and Paul Dieppe. 'Arthritis in Saxon and Mediaeval Skeletons'. *British Medical Journal* 283 (1981): 1668–70. https://doi.org/10.1136/bmj.283.6307.1668.

Roosen, Joris, and Monica H. Green, 'The Mother of All Pandemics: The State of Black Death Research in the Era of COVID-19—Bibliography'. Last modified 26 February 2024. https://drive.google.com/file/d/1xoD_dwyAwp9xi9sMCW5UvpGfEVH5J2ZA/view?usp=sharing.

Roulet, Jean-François, and Susi Ulrich-Bochsler. 'Zahnärztliche Untersuchung frühmittelalterlicher Schädel aus Biel-Mett'. *Schweizerische Monatsschrift für Zahnheilkunde* 89, no. 6 (1979): 526–40.

Ruas, Marie-Pierre. 'Productions agricoles en Auvergne carolingienne d'après un dépotoir découvert à Saint-Germain-des-Fossés (Allier)'. *Revue archéologique du centre de la France* 39 (2000): 137–60. https://doi.org/10.3406/racf.2000.2849.

Sabbah, Guy, Pierre-Paul Corsetti, and Klaus-Dietrich Fischer. *Bibliographie des textes médicaux latins: Antiquité et haut Moyen Âge*. Saint-Étienne: Publications de l'Université de St. Étienne, 1987.

Santamaría Hernández, María Teresa. 'La denominación verbal de las cualidades humorales'. In *Tradición e Innovación de la Medicina Latina de la Antigüedad y de la Alta Edad Media: Actas del IV Coloquio Internacional sobre los "textos médicos latinos antiguos"*, edited by Manuel Enrique Vázquez Buján, 297–315. Santiago de Compostela: Servicio de Publicacións e Intercambio Científico da Universidade de Santiago de Compostela, 1994.

Santamaría Hernández, María Teresa. 'La toxicología en los textos médicos latinos de la Antigüedad'. In *Tradición griega y textos médicos latinos en el período presalernitano: actas del VIII Coloquio Internacional "Textos Médicos Latinos Antiguos" (A Coruña, 2–4 septiembre 2004)*, edited by Arsenio Ferraces Rodríguez, 289–316. A Coruña: Servizio de Publicacións, Universidade da Coruña, 2007.

Santamaría Hernández, María Teresa. *Estudios sobre Galeno Latino y sus fuentes*. Cuenca: Ediciones de la Universidad de Castilla-La Mancha, 2021.

Schedl, Barbara. *Der Plan von St. Gallen: Ein Modell europäischer Klosterkultur*. Vienna: Böhlau, 2014.

Schipperges, Heinrich. *Die Benediktiner in der Medizin des frühen Mittelalters*. Leipzig: St. Benno, 1964.

Schleissner, Margaret R., ed. *Manuscript Sources of Medieval Medicine: A Book of Essays*. London: Garland, 1995.

Schmuki, Karl, Ernst Tremp, and Nina Otto. *Heilkräuter und Gartenanlagen im Kloster St. Gallen: Katalog zur Jahresausstellung in der Stiftsbibliothek St. Gallen (30. November 2009–7. November 2010)*. St. Gallen: Verlag am Klosterhof St. Gallen, 2010.

Schnell, Bernhard. 'Prolegomena to a History of Medieval German Medical Literature: The Twelfth Century'. In *Manuscript Sources of Medieval Medicine: A Book of Essays*, edited by Margaret R. Schleissner, 3–15. London: Garland, 1995.

Screen, Elina, and Charles West, eds. *Writing the Early Medieval West*. Cambridge: Cambridge University Press, 2018.

Sherratt, Andrew. 'Alcohol and its Alternatives: Symbol and Substance in Pre-Industrial Cultures'. In *Consuming Habits: Global and Historical Perspectives on How Cultures Define Drugs*, edited by Jordan Goodman, Paul E. Lovejoy, and Andrew Sherratt, 2nd ed., 11–45. London: Routledge, 2007.

Sigerist, Henry E. 'Maße und Gewichte in den medizinischen Texten des frühen Mittelalters'. *Kyklos* 3 (1930): 439–44.

Sigerist, Henry E. 'A Summer of Research in European Libraries'. *Bulletin of the Institute of the History of Medicine* 2, no. 10 (1934): 559–610.

Sigerist, Henry E. 'Materia Medica in the Middle Ages: A Review'. *Bulletin of the History of Medicine* 7, no. 4 (1939): 417–23.

Sigerist, Henry E. '"The Sphere of Life and Death" in Early Medieval Manuscripts'. *Bulletin of the History of Medicine* 11, no. 3 (1942): 292–303.

Sigerist, Henry E. 'The Latin Medical Literature of the Early Middle Ages'. *Journal of the History of Medicine and Allied Sciences* 13, no. 2 (1958): 127–45.

Singer, Charles. 'A Review of the Medical Literature of the Dark Ages, with a New Text of about 1110'. *Proceedings of the Royal Society of Medicine* 10 (1917): 107–60.

Siraisi, Nancy G. *Medieval and Early Renaissance Medicine: An Introduction to Knowledge and Practice*. Chicago, University of Chicago Press, 1990.

Skemer, Don C. '*Armis Gunfe*: Remembering Egyptian Days'. *Traditio* 65 (2010): 75–106.

Skinner, Patricia. *Health and Medicine in Early Medieval Southern Italy*. Leiden: Brill, 1997.

Skinner, Patricia. 'Visible Prowess?: Reading Men's Head and Face Wounds in Early Medieval Europe to 1000 CE'. In *Wounds and Wound Repair in Medieval Culture*, edited by Larissa Tracy and Kelly DeVries, 81–101. Leiden: Brill, 2015.

Sofaer Derevenski, Joanna R. 'Sex Differences in Activity-related Osseous Change in the Spine and the Gendered Division of Labor at Ensay and Wharram Percy, UK'. *American Journal of Biological Anthropology* 111, no. 3 (2000): 333–54. https://doi.org/10.1002/(sici)1096-8644(200003)111:3%3C333::aid-ajpa4%3E3.0.co;2-k.

Somers, J., C. Cooper, A. Alterauge, and S. Lösch. 'A Medieval/Early Modern Alpine Population from Zweisimmen, Switzerland: A Comparative Study of Anthropology and Palaeopathology'. *International Journal of Osteoarchaeology* 27, no. 6 (2017): 958–72. https://doi.org/10.1002/oa.2607.

Spilling, Herrad. 'Angelsächsische Schrift in Fulda'. In *Von der Klosterbibliothek zur Landesbibliothek. Beiträge zum zweihundertjährigen Bestehen der Hessischen Landesbibliothek Fulda*, edited by Artur Brall, 47–98. Stuttgart: Hiersemann, 1978.

Spyrou, Maria A., Kirsten I. Bos, Alexander Herbig, and Johannes Krause, 'Ancient pathogen genomics as an emerging tool for infectious disease research', *Nature Reviews Genetics* 20 (2019): 323–40. https://doi.org/10.1038/s41576-019-0119-1.

Squatriti, Paolo. *Landscape and Change in Early Medieval Italy: Chestnuts, Economy, and Culture*. Cambridge: Cambridge University Press, 2013.

Squatriti, Paolo. *Weeds and the Carolingians: Empire, Culture, and Nature in Frankish Europe, AD 750–900*. Cambridge: Cambridge University Press, 2022.

Stannard, Jerry. 'The Plant Called Moly'. *Osiris* 14 (1962): 254–307.

Stannard, Jerry. 'The Herbal as a Medical Document'. *Bulletin of the History of Medicine'* 43, no. 3 (1969): 212–20.

Stannard, Jerry. 'Marcellus of Bordeaux and the Beginnings of Medieval *Materia Medica*'. *Pharmacy in History* 15, no. 2 (1973): 47–53.

Stannard, Jerry. 'Aspects of Byzantine *Materia Medica*'. *Dumbarton Oaks Papers* 38 (1984): 205–11. https://doi.org/10.2307/1291506.

Stannard, Jerry. *Herbs and Herbalism in the Middle Ages and Renaissance*. Aldershot: Ashgate, 1999.

Stannard, Jerry. *Pristina Medicamenta: Ancient and Medieval Medical Botany*. Aldershot: Ashgate, 1999.

Steinová, Evina. 'The Oldest Manuscript Tradition of the *Etymologiae* (Eighty Years after A. E. Anspach)'. *Visigothic Symposium* 4 (2020–21): 100–43. https://doi.org/10.17613/ehr8-5c39.

Stevenson, Angus, ed. *Oxford Dictionary of English*. 3rd ed. Oxford: Oxford University Press, 2010.

Stoll, Clemens. 'Arznei und Arzneiversorgung in frühmittelalterlichen Klöstern'. In *Das Lorscher Arzneibuch und die frühmittelalterliche Medizin: Verhandlungen des medizinhistorischen Symposiums im September 1989 in Lorsch*, edited by Gundolf Keil and Paul Schnitzer, 149–218. Lorsch: Laurissa, 1991.

Stoll, Ulrich. 'Das 'Lorscher Arzneibuch'. Ein Überblick über Herkunft, Inhalt und Anspruch des ältesten Arzneibuchs deutscher Provenienz'. In *Das Lorscher Arzneibuch und die frühmittelalterliche Medizin: Verhandlungen des medizinhistorischen Symposiums im September 1989 in Lorsch*, edited by Gundolf Keil and Paul Schnitzer, 61–80. Lorsch: Laurissa, 1991.

Story, Joanna, ed. *Charlemagne: Empire and Society*. Manchester: Manchester University Press, 2005.

Stuart, Malcolm, ed. *The Encyclopedia of Herbs and Herbalism*. London: Orbis Books, 1979.

Teasdale, M. D., N. L. van Doorn, S. Fiddyment, C. C. Webb, T. O'Connor, M. Hofreiter, M. J. Collins, and D. G. Bradley. 'Paging through history: parchment as a reservoir of ancient DNA for next generation sequencing'. *Philosophical Transactions of the Royal Society B* 370 (2015), https://doi.org/10.1098/rstb.2013.0379.

Teasdale, Matthew D., Sarah Fiddyment, Jirí Vnouček, Valeria Mattiangeli, Camilla Speller, Annelise Binois, Martin Carver, et al. 'The York Gospels: A 1000-year biological palimpsest'. *Royal Society Open Science* 4, no. 10 (2017), https://doi.org/10.1098/rsos.170988.

Temkin, Owsei. *The Double Face of Janus and Other Essays in the History of Medicine*. Baltimore: Johns Hopkins University Press, 1977.

Temkin, Owsei. *Hippocrates in a World of Pagans and Christians*. Baltimore: Johns Hopkins University Press, 1995.

Theuws, Frans, and Janet L. Nelson, eds. *Rituals of Power: From Late Antiquity to the Early Middle Ages*. Leiden: Brill, 2000.

Theuws, Frans, and Mirjam Kars, eds. *The Saint-Servatius complex in Maastricht: The Vrijthof excavations (1969–1970): Roman Infrastructure—Merovingian Cemetery—Carolingian Cemetery—Early Town Development*. Bonn: Habelt, 2017.

Theuws, Frans, and Mirjam Kars. 'The Carolingian Cemetery 5'. In *The Saint-Servatius complex in Maastricht: The Vrijthof excavations (1969–1970): Roman Infrastructure—Merovingian Cemetery—Carolingian Cemetery—Early Town Development*, edited by Frans Theuws and Mirjam Kars, 354–63. Bonn: Habelt, 2017.

Thompson, Pauline. 'The Disease We Call Cancer'. In *Health, Disease and Healing in Medieval Culture*, edited by Sheila Campbell, Bert Hall, and David Klausner, 1–11. Houndmills: Macmillan, 1992.

Timpanaro, Sebastiano. *The Genesis of Lachmann's Method*. Translated by Glenn W. Most. Chicago: University of Chicago Press, 2005.

Tosi, Adelaide, Paola Badino, Barbara Pezzoni. 'Medical Conditions Observed in Osteoarchaeological Remains: Arthropathies, Traumatic Lesions, Tumours, Metabolic Diseases and Dental Pathologies'. *Medicina Historica* 1, no. 1 (2017): 29–34.

Totelin, Laurence M. V. 'Mithridates' Antidote—A Pharmacological Ghost'. *Early Science and Medicine* 9, no. 1 (2004): 1–19.

Touati, François-Olivier, 'Raban Maur et la médecine carolingienne'. In *Raban Maur et son temps*, edited by Philippe Depreux, Stéphane Lebecq, Michel J.-L. Perrin, and Olivier Szerwiniack, 173–202. Turnhout: Brepols, 2010.

Touwaide, Alain. 'Dioscorides'. In *Medieval Science, Technology and Medicine: An Encyclopedia*, edited by Thomas Glick, Steven J. Livesey, and Faith Wallis, 152–4. London: Routledge, 2005.

Touwaide, Alain. 'Pharmaceutic Handbooks'. In *Medieval Science, Technology and Medicine: An Encyclopedia*, edited by Thomas Glick, Steven J. Livesey, and Faith Wallis, 393–4. London: Routledge, 2005.

Touwaide, Alain. 'Pharmacy and *Materia medica*'. In *Medieval Science, Technology and Medicine: An Encyclopedia*, edited by Thomas Glick, Steven J. Livesey, and Faith Wallis, 397–9. London: Routledge, 2005.

Touwaide, Alain. 'Pharmaceutical Literature'. In *Handbook of Medieval Studies. Terms—Methods—Trends*, edited by Albrecht Classen, vol. 3, 1979–2000. Berlin: De Gruyter, 2010.

Touwaide, Alain. 'Quid pro Quo: Revisiting the Practice of Substitution in Ancient Pharmacy'. In *Herbs and Healers from the Ancient Mediterranean through the Medieval West: Essays in Honor of John M. Riddle*, edited by Anne Van Arsdall and Timothy Graham, 19–61. Farnham: Ashgate, 2012.

Tracy, Larissa, and Kelly DeVries, eds. *Wounds and Wound Repair in Medieval Culture*. Leiden: Brill, 2015.

Tsutaya, Takumi, and Minoru Yoneda. 'Reconstruction of breastfeeding and weaning practices using stable isotope and trace element analyses: A review'. *American Journal of Biological Anthropology* 156, supplement 59 (2015): 2–21. https://doi.org/10.1002/ajpa.22657.

Van Arsdall, Anne. 'Reading Medieval Medical Texts with an Open Mind'. In *Textual Healing: Essays on Medieval and Early Modern Medicine*, edited by Elizabeth Lane Furdell, 9–29. Leiden: Brill, 2005.

Van Arsdall, Anne. 'Challenging the "Eye of Newt" Image of Medieval Medicine'. In *The Medieval Hospital and Medical Practice*, edited by Barbara S. Bowers, 195–205. Aldershot: Ashgate, 2007.

Van Arsdall, Anne. 'Medical Training in Anglo-Saxon England: An Evaluation of the Evidence'. In *Form and Content of Instruction in Anglo-Saxon England in the Light of Contemporary Manuscript Evidence: Papers Presented at the International Conference, Udine, 6–8 April 2006*, edited by Patrizia Lendinara, Loredana Lazzari, and Maria Amalia D'Aronco, 415–34. Turnhout: Brepols, 2007.

Van Arsdall, Anne. 'The Transmission of Knowledge in Early Medieval Medical Texts: An Exploration'. In *Between Text and Patient: The Medical Enterprise in Medieval and

Early Modern Europe, edited by Florence Eliza Glaze and Brian K. Nance, 201–15. Florence: SISMEL Edizioni del Galluzzo, 2011.

Van Arsdall, Anne. 'Evaluating the Content of Medieval Herbals'. In *Critical Approaches to the History of Western Herbal Medicine: From Classical Antiquity to the Early Modern Period*, edited by Susan Francia and Anne Stobart, 47–66. London: Bloomsbury Academic, 2014.

Van Arsdall, Anne, and Timothy Graham, eds. *Herbs and Healers from the Ancient Mediterranean through the Medieval West: Essays in Honor of John M. Riddle*. Farnham: Ashgate, 2012.

van Es, Willem A., and Willem J. H. Verwers. *Excavations at Dorestad 4: The Settlement on the River Bank Area*. Amersfoort: Cultural Heritage Agency of the Netherlands, 2015.

van Minnen, Peter. 'Medical care in late antiquity'. In *Ancient Medicine in Its Socio-Cultural Context, Volume 1: Papers Read at the Congress Held at Leiden University, 13–15 April 1992*, edited by H. F. J. Horstmanshoff, Philip J. van der Eijk, and P. H. Schrijvers, 153–169. Amsterdam: Rodopi, 1995.

Vannier, Marie-Anne. 'L'image du Christ médecin chez les pères'. In *Les Pères de l'Église face à la science médicale de leur temps*, edited by Véronique Boudon-Millot and Bernard Pouderon, 525–34. Paris: Beauchesne, 2005.

van Rhijn, Carine. 'Manuscripts for local priests and the Carolingian Reforms'. In *Men in the Middle: Local Priests in Early Medieval Europe*, edited by Steffen Patzold and Carine van Rhijn, 177–98. Berlin: De Gruyter, 2016.

van Rhijn, Carine. 'Pastoral Care and Prognostics in the Carolingian Period. The Case of El Escorial, Real Biblioteca di San Lorenzo, ms L III 8'. *Revue Bénédictine* 127, no. 2 (2017): 272–97. https://doi.org/10.1484/J.RB.5.114639.

van Rhijn, Carine. 'Charlemagne's *correctio*: A Local Perspective'. In *Charlemagne: les temps, les espaces, les hommes. Construction et déconstruction d'un règne*, edited by Rolf Grosse and Michel Sot, 43–59. Turnhout: Brepols, 2018.

van Rhijn, Carine. *Leading the Way to Heaven: Pastoral Care and Salvation in the Carolingian Period*. London: Routledge, 2022.

Vázquez Buján, Manuel Enrique, ed. *Tradición e Innovación de la Medicina Latina de la Antigüedad y de la Alta Edad Media: Actas del IV Coloquio Internacional sobre los "textos médicos latinos antiguos"*. Santiago de Compostela: Servicio de Publicacións e Intercambio Científico da Universidade de Santiago de Compostela, 1994.

Vázquez Buján, Manuel Enrique. 'De nuevo sobre los textos del Oribasio latino'. In *Tradición griega y textos médicos latinos en el período presalernitano: actas del VIII Coloquio Internacional "Textos Médicos Latinos Antiguos" (A Coruña, 2–4 septiembre 2004)*, edited by Arsenio Ferraces Rodríguez, 373–90. A Coruña: Servizio de Publicacións, Universidade da Coruña, 2007.

Vázquez Buján, Manuel Enrique. 'Éléments complémentaires en vue de l'édition critique de l'ancienne version latine des *Aphorismes* hippocratiques'. In *Body, Disease and Treatment in a Changing World: Latin Texts and Contexts in Ancient and Medieval Medicine. Proceedings of the Ninth International Conference "Ancient Latin Medical Texts", Hulme Hall, University of Manchester, 5–8 September 2007*, edited by David Langslow and Brigitte Maire, 119–30. Lausanne: Éditions BHMS, 2010.

Ventura, Iolanda. '"Sume tibi aromata prima": Profumi ed aromi nell'esegesi ad *Ex.* 30'. In *Parfums et odeurs au Moyen Âge. Science, usage, symboles*, edited by Agostino Paravicini Bagliani, 349–428. Florence: SISMEL Edizioni del Galluzzo, 2015.

Vezin, Jean. 'Le point d'interrogation, un élément de datation et de localisation des manuscrits. L'exemple de Saint-Denis au IXᵉ siècle'. *Scriptorium* 34, no. 2 (1980): 181–96.

Vezin, Jean. 'Les manuscrits copiés à Saint-Denis en France pendant l'époque carolingienne'. *Paris et Île-de-France. Mémoires* 32 (1981): 273–87.

Voigts, Linda E. 'Anglo-Saxon Plant Remedies and the Anglo-Saxons'. *Isis* 70, no. 2 (1979): 250–68.

Voigts, Linda Ehrsam. 'The Significance of the Name Apuleius to the *Herbarium Apulei*'. *Bulletin of the History of Medicine* 52, no. 2 (1978): 214–27.

Volpe, Giuliano, and Pasquale, Favia, eds. *V Congresso Nazionale di Archeologia Medievale. Palazzo della Dogana, Salone del Tribunale (Foggia); Palazzo dei Celestini, Auditorium (Manfredonia); 30 settembre-3 ottobre 2009*. Florence: All'Insegna del Giglio, 2009.

von Steinmeyer, Emil Elias, and Eduard Sievers. *Die althochdeutschen Glossen*. 5 vols. Berlin: Weidmann, 1879–1922.

Waldron, Tony. *Palaeopathology*. Cambridge: Cambridge University Press, 2009.

Waldron, Tony. 'Joint Disease'. In *A Companion to Paleopathology*, edited by Anne L. Grauer, 513–30. Chichester: Wiley-Blackwell, 2012.

Wallis, Faith. 'The Experience of the Book: Manuscripts, Texts, and the Role of Epistemology in Early Medieval Medicine'. In *Knowledge and the Scholarly Medical Traditions*, edited by Don G. Bates, 101–26. Cambridge: Cambridge University Press, 1995.

Wallis, Faith. 'Medicine in Medieval Calendar Manuscripts'. In *Manuscript Sources of Medieval Medicine*, edited by Margaret R. Schleissner, 105–43. London: Garland, 1995.

Wallis, Faith. 'Signs and Senses: Diagnosis and Prognosis in Early Medieval Pulse and Urine Texts'. *Social History of Medicine* 13, no. 2 (2000): 265–78. https://doi.org/10.1093/shm/13.2.265.

Wallis, Faith. 'Counting All the Bones: Measure, Number and Weight in Early Medieval Texts About the Body'. In *Was zählt. Ordnungsangebote, Gebrauchsformen und Erfahrungsmodalitäten des "numerus" im Mittelalter*, edited by Moritz Wedell, 185–208. Cologne: Böhlau, 2012.

Wang, Tianyi, Craig Cessford, Jenna M. Dittmar, Sarah Inskip, Peter M. Jones, and Piers D. Mitchell. 'Intestinal parasite infection in the Augustinian friars and general population of medieval Cambridge, UK'. *International Journal of Paleopathology* 39 (2022): 115–21. https://doi.org/10.1016/j.ijpp.2022.06.001.

Wang, Weiwei, Khanh Trung Kien Nguyen, Chunguang Zhao, and Hsiao-Chun Hung, 'Earliest curry in Southeast Asia and the global spice trade 2000 years ago'. *Science Advances* 9, no. 29 (2023): https://doi.org/10.1126/sciadv.adh5517.

Watkins, Frances, Barbara Pendry, Alberto Sanchez-Medina, and Olivia Corcoran. 'Antimicrobial Assays of Three Native British Plants Used in Anglo-Saxon Medicine for Wound Healing Formulations in 10th-Century England'. *Journal of Ethnopharmacology* 144, no. 2 (2012): 408–15. https://doi.org/10.1016/j.jep.2012.09.031.

Wayens, Benjamin, Isabelle van den Steen, and Marie-Eve Ronveaux. 'A Short Historical Geography of Beer'. In *Food and Environment: Geographies of Taste*, edited by Armando Montanari, 93–114. Rome: Società Geografica Italiana, 2002.

Wear, Andrew, ed. *Medicine in Society: Historical Essays*. Cambridge: Cambridge University Press, 1992.

Weber, Jochen, and Alfred Czarnetzki. 'Brief Communication: Neurotraumatological Aspects of Head Injuries Resulting from Sharp and Blunt Force in the Early Medieval Period of Southwestern Germany'. *American Journal of Biological Anthropology* 114, no. 4 (2001): 352–6. https://doi.org/10.1002/ajpa.1047.

Wexler, Philip, ed. *Toxicology in Antiquity*. 2nd ed. London: Academic Press, 2019.

Wickersheimer, Ernest. *Les manuscrits latins de médecine du haut Moyen Âge dans les bibliothèques de France*. Paris: Éditions du Centre national de la Recherche scientifique, 1966.

Wickham, Chris. *Framing the Early Middle Ages: Europe and the Mediterranean, 400–800*. Oxford: Oxford University Press, 2005.

Wickham, Chris. 'Comacchio and the Central Mediterranean'. In *From One Sea to Another. Trading Places in the European and Mediterranean Early Middle Ages: Proceedings of the International Conference, Comacchio 27th-29th March 2009*, edited by Sauro Gelichi and Richard Hodges, 503–10. Turnhout: Brepols, 2012.

Wieland, Gernot R., Carin Ruff, and Ross G. Arthur, eds. *Insignis Sophiae Arcator: Medieval Latin Studies in Honour of Michael Herren on his 65th Birthday*. Turnhout: Brepols, 2006.

Wood, James W., George R. Milner, Henry C. Harpending, and Kenneth M. Weiss. 'The Osteological Paradox: Problems of Inferring Prehistoric Health from Skeletal Samples'. *Current Anthropology* 33, no. 4 (1992): 343–70.

Woosnam-Savage, Robert C., and Kelly DeVries, 'Battle Trauma in Medieval Warfare: Wounds, Weapons and Armor'. In *Wounds and Wound Repair in Medieval Culture*, edited by Larissa Tracy and Kelly De Vries, 27–56. Leiden: Brill, 2015.

Yearl, Mary K. K. 'Bloodletting as Recreation in the Monasteries of Medieval Europe'. In *Between Text and Patient: The Medical Enterprise in Medieval and Early Modern*

Europe, edited by Florence Eliza Glaze and Brian K. Nance, 217–43. Florence: SISMEL Edizioni del Galluzzo, 2011.

Zecher, Jonathan L. *Spiritual Direction as a Medical Art in Early Christian Monasticism*. Oxford: Oxford University Press, 2022.

Zeller, Bernhard, Charles West, Francesca Tinti, Marco Stoffella, Nicolas Schroeder, Carine van Rhijn, Steffen Patzold, Thomas Kohl, Wendy Davies, and Miriam Czock. *Neighbours and Strangers: Local Societies in Early Medieval Europe*. Manchester: Manchester University Press, 2020.

Zimmerman, Michael R. 'The Analysis and Interpretation of Mummified Remains'. In *A Companion to Paleopathology*, edited by Anne L. Grauer, 152–69. Chichester: Wiley-Blackwell, 2012.

Ziolkowski, Jan M. 'Fighting Words: Wordplay and Swordplay in the *Waltharius*'. In *Germanic Texts and Latin Models: Medieval Reconstructions*, edited by Karin E. Olsen, Antonina Harbus, and Tette Hofstra, 29–51. Leuven: Peeters, 2001.

Ziolkowski, Jan M. 'Blood, Sweat and Tears in the *Waltharius*'. In *Insignis Sophiae Arcator: Medieval Latin Studies in Honour of Michael Herren on his 65th Birthday*, edited by Gernot R. Wieland, Carin Ruff, and Ross G. Arthur, 149–64. Turnhout: Brepols, 2006.

Zipser, Barbara, ed. *Medical Books in the Byzantine World*. Bologna: Università di Bologna, 2013.

Zörnig, Heinrich. *Arzneidrogen als Nachschlagebuch für den Gebrauch der Apotheker, Ärzte, Veterinärärzte, Drogisten und Studierenden der Pharmazie*. 2 vols. Leipzig: Klinkhardt, 1909.

Index

Printed in the United States
by Baker & Taylor Publisher Services